Young People's Lives and Sexual Relationships in Rural Africa

Young People's Lives and Sexual Relationships in Rural Africa

Findings from a Large Qualitative Study in Tanzania

Mary Louisa Plummer and Daniel Wight

LEXINGTON BOOKS
Lanham • Boulder • New York • Toronto • Plymouth, UK

Published by Lexington Books
A wholly owned subsidiary of The Rowman & Littlefield Publishing Group, Inc.
4501 Forbes Boulevard, Suite 200, Lanham, Maryland 20706
www.lexingtonbooks.com

Estover Road, Plymouth PL6 7PY, United Kingdom

British Library Cataloguing in Publication Information Available

Library of Congress Cataloging-in-Publication Data

Plummer, Mary Louisa.
  Young people's lives and sexual relationships in rural Africa : findings from a large
qualitative study in Tanzania / Mary Louisa Plummer & Daniel Wight.
    p. cm.
  Includes bibliographical references and index.
  ISBN 978-0-7391-3578-5 (cloth : alk. paper) — ISBN 978-0-7391-3580-8 (ebook)
  1. Teenagers—Sexual behavior—Tanzania. 2. Rural youth—Sexual behavior—
Tanzania. 3. Sex customs—Tanzania. 4. HIV infections—Tanzania. 5. Intergenerational
relations—Tanzania I. Wight, Daniel. II. Title.
  HQ27.P586 2011
  306.70835096—dc22

                                                                                2011013036

∞™ The paper used in this publication meets the minimum requirements of American
National Standard for Information Sciences—Permanence of Paper for Printed Library
Materials, ANSI/NISO Z39.48-1992.

Printed in the United States of America

This book is dedicated to the memory of Henry Nyalali,
one of countless vibrant, gifted, humorous,
and loving individuals who have been lost to AIDS.

Contents

Case Study Series 2
"He Told Me, 'Just Come and Live at My House'":

Case Study Series 3
"The Fever Went Away but Always Returned":

Tables

Figures

Case Studies

Case Study Series 3
"The Fever Went Away but Always Returned":
HIV-Positive Young People's Lives and Sexual Relationships   367

Boxes

Acknowledgments

Kidole kimoja hakivunji chawa
One finger will not kill a louse.
[More than one person is needed to achieve a goal.]

—Swahili proverb

This book and its companion volume would not have been possible without the dedicated efforts of many people. First and foremost, we thank the villagers in Mwanza, Tanzania who participated in this study. We are especially grateful to the families that hosted participant observation researchers, to the young people who researchers accompanied in their daily activities, and to those who participated in formal and informal interviews.

We are also indebted to the extraordinary qualitative researchers in the Health and Lifestyles Research (HALIRA) Project, who collected almost all of the data presented in these two books: Halima Abdallah, Neema Busali, Gerry Mshana, Kija Nyalali, Zachayo Salamba Shigongo, and Joyce Wamoyi. Each of these individuals demonstrated remarkable fortitude and adaptability in collecting sensitive data in often trying field conditions. All of them also contributed to data coding, data summarizing, and report writing post-fieldwork. We are grateful to each of them for their many unique contributions, in particular Joyce's prolific, discerning documentation; Zachayo's invaluable critical reflections; Kija's enthusiastic and astute questioning; Gerry's articulate analytical skills; Neema's thoughtful diligence; and Halima's cheerful adaptability. It was a pleasure and an honor to work with such good-natured, hardworking, and insightful individuals.

Our colleagues within the broader *MEMA kwa Vijana* adolescent sexual health intervention trial were also crucial in the creation of this book and its companion volume. David Ross, the *MEMA kwa Vijana* director, provided essential input and support at every stage of the HALIRA study, from its inception and design, to fieldwork and management, to data analysis and chapter review. Angela Obasi, the *MEMA kwa Vijana* intervention coordinator, developed and implemented a high quality, culturally appropriate, and sustainable intervention, enabling close examination of the real-world potential and challenges of adolescent sexual health promotion. Richard Hayes, a principal investigator for both *MEMA kwa Vijana* and HALIRA, was generous in his time and critical input throughout the research process. We also thank Alessandra Anemona, John Changalucha, Kenneth Chima, Bernadette Cleophas-Mazige, Heiner Grosskurth, Maende Makokha, Pieter Remes, Jim Todd, Deborah Watson-Jones, and Helen Weiss, all of whom provided us with important logistical assistance and discerning advice during data collection and beyond.

Throughout the study we benefited from the support of many other administrative, intervention, and trial staff at the Tanzanian National Institute for Medical Research, the African Medical and Research Foundation, and the London School of Hygiene and Tropical Medicine. Of particular note are the trilingual translators, Stanslaus Shitindi, Samuel Gogomoka, Eustadius Kabika, William Kasubi, Deogratius Mazula, Daudi Ngosha, and Henry Nyalali, who brought great skill and patience to their work, as did the bilingual transcribers, Mbango Mhamba, Happiness Ng'habi, Mwanahawa Maporo, and Fatma Bakshi. Nicola Desmond, Caroline Ingall, and Tom Ingall provided very valuable assistance in data coding and/or summarizing.

We are also grateful to the dozens of people who read and commented on the individual paper drafts that were later adapted within book chapters. We are particularly indebted to Karen Coen Flynn and Janet Seeley for their painstaking and insightful reviews of many book chapters. At Lexington Books we thank our acquisition editors, Justin Race and Michael Sisskin, our production editor Gwen E. Kirby, and our typesetter Rhonda Baker, for their patience, advice, and assistance in bringing this book to press.

Many of the people mentioned above are our friends as well as colleagues and gave us invaluable personal support during the decade of work that culminated in this book and its companion volume. Each of us has other individuals who we would also like to thank below.

Mary: I am very grateful for the humor, caring and assistance of many dear friends throughout this time, including Alexandra Terninko, Anna Sassi, Ben Steinberg, Graham Anderson, Jennifer Schoenstadt, Kathy White, Kulindwa Kasubi, Lida Junghans, Ma-nee Chacaby, and Susan Cook. Members of my family—Amina, Munir and Yasmin Kudrati-Plummer, Bascom and Nancy M. Plummer, Bob and Nancy D. Plummer, Kaye Carmichael Plummer,

Gulamabbas Kudrati, and Shirin, Azher, and Mariya Karimjee—were also sources of great love and support during this work. My deepest thanks go to my husband, Mustafa Kudrati, who was patient and enthusiastic during every day, week, month, and year of this project. My final stretch of work on these books included over two years of long hours, no pay, and many sacrifices for our family, but Mustafa's loving support never wavered. Neither book would have happened without it.

Daniel: I very much appreciate the support and encouragement of my immediate family—Erica Wimbush, and Ruby and Megan Wight—and their tolerance of my preoccupation with this book on numerous "family" weekends and holidays. I am also very grateful to Sally Macintyre, director of the Medical Research Council Social and Public Health Sciences Unit, for her support throughout the HALIRA Project and the drafting of this book, and to my immediate colleagues for tolerating my reduced input to collaborative work with them.

The HALIRA Project fieldwork and preliminary data analysis were funded by a UK Medical Research Council grant. Subsequent data analysis and publication writing were partially funded by the Medical Research Council Social and Public Health Sciences Unit and a British Academy Post-Doctoral Fellowship held by Mary Plummer from 2006 to 2008.

Chapter One

Introduction

Ndila is an 18-year-old man who recently finished Year 7 of primary school. Like most pupils he failed his leaving examination, so he did not get a place in secondary school. However, Ndila's mother has arranged for him to repeat a year of primary school and re-sit the examination. In the last two to three years, Ndila has had several sexual relationships with younger girls he first met while on errands. He meets his partners for sex outdoors or in the girl's room at night, each time giving them Tshs[1] 200–500 ($0.24–$0.60). Ndila tested negative for sexually transmitted infections in a large survey. When asked how he would feel if a girl requested that he use a condom, he immediately replies, "I would think that girl has diseases, and reject her."

—Case Study 1.1

Flora is a 16-year-old girl who recently passed her Year 7 leaving examination. Flora's parents will not pay for her to go to secondary school, so she plans to become a tailor instead. Flora has been sexually pursued by boys and men since she was 13 years old, and she finally agreed to have sex when she was 14. Since then Flora has had several sexual partners who were many years older than her. Her partners typically give her Tshs 1,000–2,000 ($1.20–$2.40) for each sexual encounter. Flora participated in a sexual health intervention and successfully negotiated condom use a couple of times. Nonetheless, she has severe symptoms of sexually transmitted infection. She does not seek medical treatment because, she explains, "The doctor . . . will ask me a lot of questions. Really, I just can't do it."

—Case Study 1.4

1

In sub-Saharan Africa, Ndila's and Flora's experiences are not unusual. Many young people become sexually active in their early teens. Boys typically have younger and same-aged partners while girls typically have same-aged and older partners. It is also typical for unmarried girls and women to receive money or gifts in exchange for sexual encounters. Sexually transmitted infections are very prevalent by the late teen years, particularly for girls.

Thirty years have passed since the identification of the Acquired Immunodeficiency Syndrome (AIDS), and the subsequent discovery of its biological cause, the Human Immunodeficiency Virus (HIV). However, new infections with HIV remain an urgent problem, particularly in sub-Saharan Africa. In 2008, 22 million (67 percent) of the 33 million people living with HIV globally were sub-Saharan Africans, although sub-Saharan Africa only holds about 10 percent of the world's population (UNAIDS and WHO 2009). Young people are especially vulnerable, as over half of new infections in high prevalence countries occur amongst 15–24-year-olds (World Bank 2006). An estimated five million 15–24-year-olds are living with HIV globally, and there were 900,000 new infections in this age group in 2008 alone (UNAIDS 2010). In sub-Saharan Africa, the vast majority of HIV infections are acquired through heterosexual sex (UNAIDS and WHO 2009). Nonetheless, most young Africans pursue their sexual relationships with little thought about the epidemic. A central aim of this book is to understand why the risk of HIV infection is *not* a salient concern for most young people in sub-Saharan Africa. Only by better understanding this are we likely to identify more effective ways to reduce HIV transmission.

In this book we will bring together findings from an unusually large and in-depth qualitative study of young people's lives and sexual relationships in rural Tanzania. Relying primarily on participant observation research, we consider young people's sexual behavior within their social context, attempting to understand it in relation to their everyday lives, their family and peer relationships, and the dominant norms within their villages. Personal accounts such as Ndila's and Flora's are the backbone of this book. Their particular stories will be described in detail later, within a series of case studies.

In this introduction, we will first outline general conditions in sub-Saharan Africa at the start of the twenty-first century, and then summarize key aspects of sexual and reproductive health and behavior. We will then describe the study setting, background, purpose, and design, and discuss our findings' relative validity and representativeness within the broader research literature. Next we will introduce one of the book's key themes: the complex, ambivalent, and sometimes inconsistent ways that young rural Tanzanians manage sexual norms and expectations. Finally, this chapter will provide an overview of the chapters to come.

SUB-SAHARAN AFRICA AT THE START
OF THE TWENTY-FIRST CENTURY

Africa south of the Sahara desert is very diverse, with forty-eight countries and over a thousand ethnic groups and languages (National Research Council 2002), so any general overview risks gross simplification. Nevertheless, it is indisputable that most sub-Saharan countries are amongst the poorest in the world at the start of the new millennium. Socioeconomic circumstances vary within and between countries, but most Africans have extremely limited financial and material resources, and very poor access to health, education, water, and sanitation services (World Bank 2006).

An estimated 63 percent of Africans and 72 percent of Tanzanians live in rural areas, which have particularly poor infrastructures and services (IFAD 2001; National Bureau of Statistics and ORC Macro 2005). Rural residents have lower quality health, higher rates of infant mortality, and more stunted growth than urban residents (World Bank 2005). Most rural households cope with poverty by diversifying their sources of income, for example, raising small livestock or fishing while also cultivating cash crops and food staples, such as maize, millet, sorghum, yams, or cassava (IFAD 2001). However, even in relatively productive seasons most rural families' diets are based almost exclusively on a few staples. In less productive seasons, consumption of even those staples can be substantially reduced, causing malnourishment (IFAD 2001).

The majority of people in both urban and rural Africa are young, largely due to high fertility and the impact of HIV/AIDS on older populations (United Nations 2007). In 2005, 41 percent of Africans were 14 years old or younger. By 2030, the global population of youth aged 15–24 years is expected to increase by 17 percent, but in Africa it is expected to increase by 84 percent (United Nations 2004).

SEXUAL AND REPRODUCTIVE HEALTH

To better understand the risk and impact of HIV for young Africans, it is important to first consider broader sexual and reproductive health beliefs and practices. Historically, fertility has been highly valued in Africa (Caldwell and Caldwell 1987; Cohen 1998). Traditionally almost all women married at an early age, and couples prioritized conceiving a pregnancy very soon after marriage. Efficient contraception has been extremely low. This has resulted in women giving birth to an average of six or seven children in their lifetimes. However, in recent decades fertility has declined in rural and especially urban areas of Africa, primarily due to greater use of modern contraception (Kirk and Pillet 1998), and to a lesser extent, older age at first marriage (Cohen 1998; Harwood-Lejeune 2000) and the HIV epidemic (Hinde and Mturi 2000; Terceira et al. 2003). Contraceptive use has generally increased because unmarried women seek to delay childbearing (Gage-Brandon and Meekers 1993), while married women wish to increase intervals between children, to protect their children's health and their own future reproductive capacity (Cohen 1998).

Less is known about the history of sexually transmitted infections in sub-Saharan Africa, as there are few historical studies and they are of highly variable and questionable quality (Setel 1999a). During the colonial period, for example, venereal syphilis was often confused with yaws, a nonsexually transmitted illness caused by a similar bacterium to the one that causes syphilis (Setel 1999a). Similarly, in Africa there have been few historical studies of Herpes Simplex Virus 2 (hereafter simply referred to as "herpes"). Blood samples collected in the early 1980s provide some of the earliest data, revealing that herpes was very prevalent among adults in urban areas such as Brazzaville, Congo (71 percent in 1982) and Kinshasa, Zaire (41 percent in 1985) (O'Farrell 1999). In general, sexually transmitted infections are prone to being underestimated because they may not have obvious symptoms, and even when they do, people may be reluctant to seek treatment because of potential stigma and cost (Gerbase et al. 1998; O'Farrell 1999). Poor health services and inconsistent collection of medical data in most African countries only exacerbates such problems (Caldwell, Caldwell, and Quiggin 1989; Setel 1999a). Based on the available studies, the World Health Organization estimated that in 1999 12 percent of adults in sub-Saharan Africa had a curable sexually transmitted infection (Chlamydia, gonorrhea, syphilis or Trichomonas), which was a far higher rate than found in any other region in the world (WHO 2001). Prevalence of incurable sexually transmitted infections such as HIV, herpes, or human papilloma virus is often higher, because once people become infected they remain infected for life.

HIV AND AIDS

The condition that came to be known as AIDS was first identified in Africa in the United Republic of Tanzania, Uganda, and the Democratic Republic of Congo in the early 1980s, although later tests of stored blood found evidence of HIV in central Africa in the 1950s (Caraël 2006). Three decades since AIDS was first identified an estimated 5 percent of sub-Saharan Africans aged 15–49 are infected with HIV (UNAIDS and WHO 2009). The vast majority of HIV-positive Africans do not know that they are infected with HIV and that they are potentially infectious (UNAIDS and WHO 2009). A proportion of these individuals will eventually develop symptoms, be tested, and obtain therapy, but others may never have an accurate test or diagnosis, and even those who are correctly diagnosed may not succeed in accessing antiretroviral therapy. A study in rural Mwanza, Tanzania recently estimated that, in the absence of antiretroviral therapy, only half of those infected with HIV survived for twelve years or longer (Isingo et al. 2007). Similarly, a study in rural Uganda found that HIV-infected individuals typically lived about nine years before developing AIDS, and another nine months before dying, similar to what has been found in high income countries (Morgan et al. 2002; United Nations 2007).

The advent of antiretroviral therapy has had a tremendous impact on the epidemic, improving quality of life and reducing illness and death for the HIV-positive individuals who are fortunate enough to receive it. In eastern and southern Africa, almost 3 million people with HIV were on antiretroviral therapy in 2008, which represented 48 percent of those estimated to need the treatment at the time (UNAIDS and WHO 2009). Despite this great progress, there remain daunting challenges to comprehensive provision of antiretroviral therapy in sub-Saharan Africa, including the need for accurate diagnoses and proper care and management in areas with very poor health services (Mills, Nachega, Bangsberg, et al. 2006; Heimer 2007; UNAIDS and WHO 2009). Even in the best of circumstances, people receiving antiretroviral therapy face a daily drug regime for the rest of their lives, a range of possible side effects, and the possibility that the virus will become resistant (Oyugi et al. 2007; Fox et al. 2010).

The great benefits of antiretroviral therapy also do not reduce the fact that the HIV epidemic has already had a severe impact on health, education, and economic growth in sub-Saharan Africa (World Bank 2006). The epidemic has contributed to an increase in already high infant mortality rates, and a reduction in already low average life expectancies (UNAIDS and WHO 2009). In Swaziland, for example, a country that has been severely affected by the epidemic, the average life expectancy halved between 1990 and 2007, dropping to only 37 years (UNAIDS and WHO 2009).

The severe impact of HIV/AIDS in sub-Saharan Africa relative to the rest of the world raises the question: Why has sub-Saharan Africa borne the brunt of the global HIV epidemic? This is a compelling and urgent question, particularly given that key patterns in Africa—such as heterosexual transmission, or the original concentration amongst commercial sex workers—are also found in less affected areas of the world, such as southeast Asia (Buvé 2006). Many explanations have been proposed, but their relationship to one another and their relative importance is still debated. Biological factors such as the high prevalence of sexually transmitted infections are clearly important, as sexually transmitted infections and HIV can facilitate each other's transmission (Aral and Over 2006; Smith et al. 2010). Social factors such as very limited services to diagnose and treat sexually transmitted infections also play an important role (Schomogyi, Wald, and Corey 1998; Buvé, Bishikwabo-Nsarhaza, and Mutangadura 2002). Added to these factors are broad socioeconomic, cultural, and historical features such as poverty, labor migration, wars and conflicts, and the subordinate position of women (Setel 1999a; Parker, Easton, and Klein 2000; Buvé et al. 2002; Kim and Watts 2005). The role that sexual behavior has played in the African HIV epidemic has been the subject of much controversy, so it will be discussed in more detail in the next section.

Despite the severity of the HIV epidemic in Africa overall, it varies enormously both between and within countries (Buvé et al. 2002; Boerma et al. 2003). Northern Africa has been fortunate to largely escape the epidemic, as in almost every north African country no more than 0.1 percent of 15–49-year-olds are believed to be HIV-positive (UNAIDS and WHO 2009). Broadly speaking, the epidemic varies between four areas south of the Sahara. In western Africa, most countries have an HIV prevalence of 4 percent or less, including in Nigeria (4 percent), a country of 117 million people that makes up almost half of the population of West Africa. Similarly, most central African countries have an HIV prevalence of 3 percent or less, including in the Democratic Republic of Congo (1 percent), which with 52 million people holds approximately two-thirds of the central African population. In eastern Africa, most countries instead have an HIV prevalence of 6–8 percent, including the three largest countries, Kenya (8 percent), Tanzania (6 percent) and Uganda (6 percent), which together represent 99 million people, or more than 90 percent of the total East African population. HIV prevalence is by far the highest in southern Africa, however, where almost all countries have HIV prevalence of 14–26 percent. This includes the largest southern African country, South Africa (17 percent), which constitutes almost half of the people in southern Africa with a population of 50 million.

To determine which factors are most important in the spread of HIV, Buvé and colleagues (2001) conducted a study comparing two cities with relatively low HIV prevalence in western and central Africa, with two cities with relatively high prevalence in eastern and southern Africa (Buvé et al. 2001). The authors found some significant differences in reported behavior: the higher prevalence cities were characterized by earlier age at first sex, earlier marriage, and larger age differences between spouses (Caraël and Holmes 2001). However, these differences were outweighed by biological factors which alter the likelihood of HIV transmission during intercourse: in high prevalence cities, there were significantly lower rates of male circumcision, and significantly higher rates of infections that cause genital ulcerations, such as herpes and syphilis (Buvé et al. 2001).

Another striking pattern of the HIV epidemic in sub-Saharan Africa is that adolescent girls consistently have had far higher rates of infection than boys of the same age. In Tanzania, for example, 15–24-year-old women face nine times the risk of HIV infection of young men (Hallet et al. 2010). A number of issues are believed to contribute to this phenomenon, including biological factors, such as easier genital transmission and higher rates of non-symptomatic sexually transmitted infections, as well as behavioral factors, such as earlier age at first sex and generally older sexual partners (Laga et al. 2001; Pettifor et al. 2004; Leclerc-Madlala 2008).

Throughout sub-Saharan Africa, the HIV epidemic has been most concentrated and severe in cities, with the exception of certain high risk areas, such as fishing villages and mines (Campbell and Williams 1999; Béné and Merten 2008). Most research and intervention work has thus focused on urban areas, and/or on highly vulnerable subpopulations, such as truck drivers, soldiers, miners, migrant workers, or commercial sex workers (Dyson 2003). However, as already noted the majority of sub-Saharan Africans live in rural areas, where people may have sexual behaviors that are equally or more risky than those of urban populations (Voeten et al. 2004; Coffee et al. 2005; Sambisa, Curtis, and Stokes 2010). Particularly vulnerable are settlements on truck routes or near mines, and those that experience high mobility or migration rates, such as fishing villages (Boerma et al. 2002; Cowan et al. 2005; Desmond et al. 2005; Ferguson and Morris 2007; Béné and Merten 2008). In some countries, for example, large sections of the rural male population are migrant workers who live apart from their families for much of the year, contributing to very high rates of extramarital relationships (Campbell 2003).

The severity of the HIV epidemic in eastern and southern Africa has meant that even very remote villages have seen residents die of AIDS, and awareness of it is widespread. AIDS-related illness and death has been particularly severe at a household level in rural areas, maintaining poverty and reducing development (Seeley, Dercon, and Barnett 2010). The agricultural sector has been affected in many African countries, which can have consequences far beyond rural areas, because agriculture is essential for national employment, food supply, and export. By 2020, it has been estimated that agricultural workforces in the twelve highest prevalence countries will be over 10 percent smaller than they would have been in the absence of AIDS, and in certain countries, 20 percent to 25 percent smaller (UNAIDS and WHO 2006). Nonetheless, recent research suggests that the long-term impact over the larger rural population may be less profound than initially expected (Seeley, Dercon, and Barnett 2010). The authors attribute this to the resilience and coping skills which rural Africans have used to face drought, pests, and other human diseases in the past, drawing on the support of family, friends, and local organizations.

There is also increasing evidence of positive sexual behavior change in some rural settings, particularly where there have been intensive intervention efforts, as in Uganda (Pool, Kamali, and Whitworth 2006; UNAIDS and WHO 2009). For example, HIV prevalence trends in 15–24-year-olds have declined in rural or urban areas in 16 of the 25 countries most affected by AIDS, and this is associated with a reduction in young people's reported sexual risk behaviors (UNAIDS 2010). However, there are many parts of rural Africa where HIV prevalence has not declined, and the epidemic and sexual risk reduction do not appear to be salient concerns in villagers' daily lives (e.g., Eaton, Flisher, and Aarø 2003; Sambisa and Stokes 2006; Nzioka 2004; Adelore, Olujide, and Popoola 2006).

SEXUAL BEHAVIOR

There has been considerable debate about the role that sexual behavior has played in the course of the African HIV epidemic (Hrdy 1987; Caldwell, Caldwell, and Quiggin 1989; Rushton and Bogaert 1989; Le Blanc, Meintel, and Piche 1991; Ahlberg 1994; Heald 1995; Undie and Benaya 2006). Sexual behavior is influenced by three types of factors and how they interact together: those within an individual (such as their sexual preferences, or beliefs about HIV/AIDS), those within interpersonal relationships and physical environment (such as a couple's sexual negotiation, or access to condoms), and those within the specific cultural and structural context (such as whether premarital sex is socially acceptable, or whether poverty creates incentives for higher risk sex) (Eaton, Flisher, and Aarø 2003; Bandura 2004). Given this complexity and the tremendous cultural diversity found within the African continent, any attempt to generalize and describe common aspects of African sexuality is problematic. However, broad patterns are worth considering given the particularly severe course that the HIV epidemic has taken in much of sub-Saharan Africa.

In sub-Saharan Africa, as elsewhere in the world, behavioral factors believed to increase risk of HIV exposure or transmission include having particular sexual mixing patterns, concurrent or overlapping sexual relationships, high rates of partner change, a high number of lifetime sexual partners, and/or not using condoms (Caldwell, Caldwell, and Quiggin 1989; Halperin and Epstein 2004; Buvé 2006; Harrison and O'Sullivan 2010). Sexual mixing patterns refer to how people with similar or distinct characteristics tend to be linked to each other sexually (Aral and Foxman 2003). Specific populations can be "bridged" by individuals who have partners in different groups, affecting viral transmission and the course of an epidemic. Most research on young people's sexual activity in sub-Saharan Africa, for example, has found that young men tend to have sexual partners who are the same age or younger, while young women commonly have relationships with men 5–10 years older than themselves (Gregson et al. 2002; Buvé 2006). Older men are more likely to have had the greatest number of lifetime sexual partners and also to be HIV infected than either younger men or women. This sexual mixing pattern is believed to be an important reason why young African women have higher rates of HIV infection than young men (Gregson et al. 2002; Doherty et al. 2006). In Tanzania, for example, the age groups at most risk of HIV infection are 15–19-year-old women and 25–39-year-old men (Hallet et al. 2010).

Another common aspect of sexual behavior in sub-Saharan Africa is the exchange of money or gifts for sex. Unmarried women often rely on one, or sometimes more, sexual partners to provide them with gifts or financial support (Caldwell, Caldwell, and Quiggin 1989). These relationships are rarely perceived as commercial sex or prostitution, which many Africans associate with risk of HIV or other sexually transmitted infections (Helle-Valle 2004; Halperin and Epstein 2004). Material exchange for sex is generally depicted in the research literature as a result of women's poverty and economic dependence on men (e.g., Schoepf 1991; Schoepf 1992a; Seeley et al. 1994; Balmer et al. 1997; Hunter 2002; Dunkle et al. 2004). However, African women may sometimes engage in transactional sex for reasons other than immediate material need, such as a desire for attractive consumer goods, or traditional understandings of service, self-esteem, and reciprocity (e.g., Caldwell, Caldwell, and Quiggin 1989; Nyanzi, Kinsman, and Pool 2001; Silberschmidt and Rasch 2001; Tawfik and Watkins 2007; Wamoyi, Fenwick et al. 2010).

In this book we will explore the extent to which material exchange motivates rural young people's sexual relationships, and we will demonstrate that transactional sex, combined with concealment of young people's sexual relationships, contributes to greater vulnerability to HIV through short relationship duration, high partner change, and concurrent or overlapping relationships.

STUDY SETTING AND POPULATION

The qualitative study that is the basis of this book focused on young people's lives, sexual relationships, and vulnerability to sexually transmitted infections and HIV in rural Mwanza Region, northern Tanzania (figures 1.1 and 1.2).

As a study setting, Tanzania is similar to many other sub-Saharan African countries in numerous ways, including that it gained national independence from colonial powers in the mid-twentieth century, it underwent tremendous political and economic change since then, and at the start of the twenty-first century it has a largely rural population, limited financial and material resources, and very poor health, education, water, and sanitation services (World Bank 2006). From 1990–2003, for example, 60 percent of Tanzanians lived on less than $2 per day and 29 percent of children under 5 years were underweight (Palmer et al. 2007).

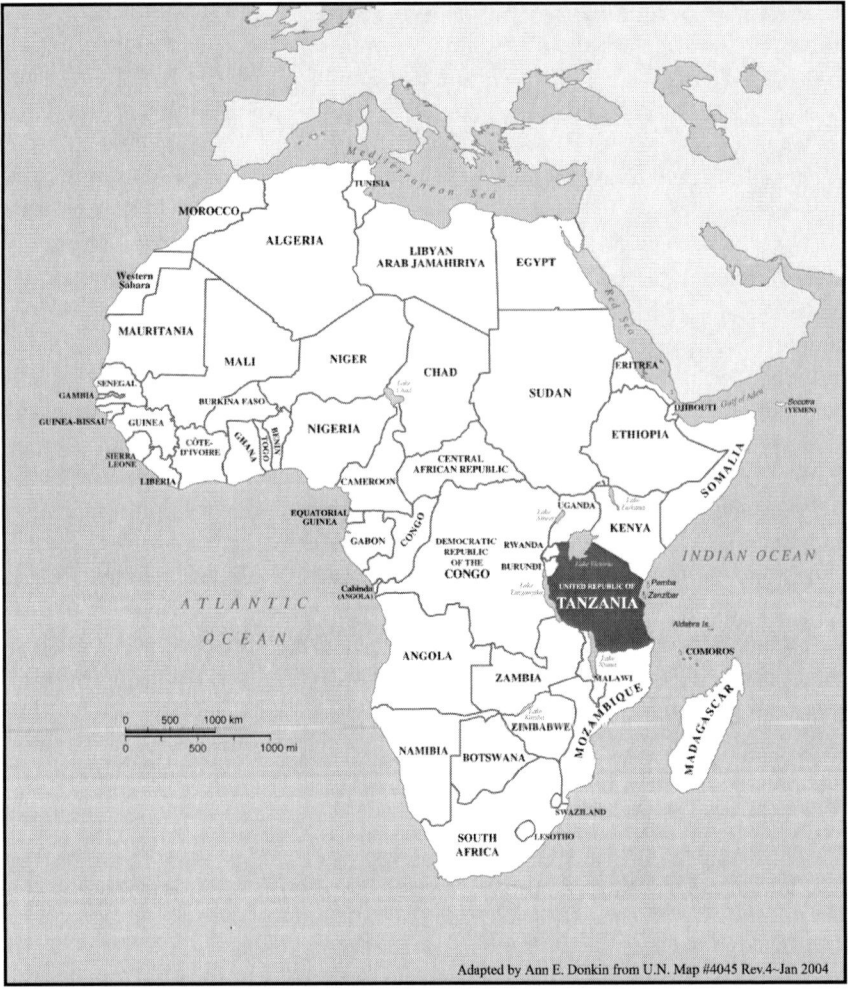

Adapted by Ann E. Donkin from U.N. Map #4045 Rev.4–Jan 2004

Figure 1.1.   The continent of Africa, with Tanzania highlighted. Used with permission of Karen Coen Flynn. 2005. *Food, culture, and survival in an African city*. Palgrave: NY.

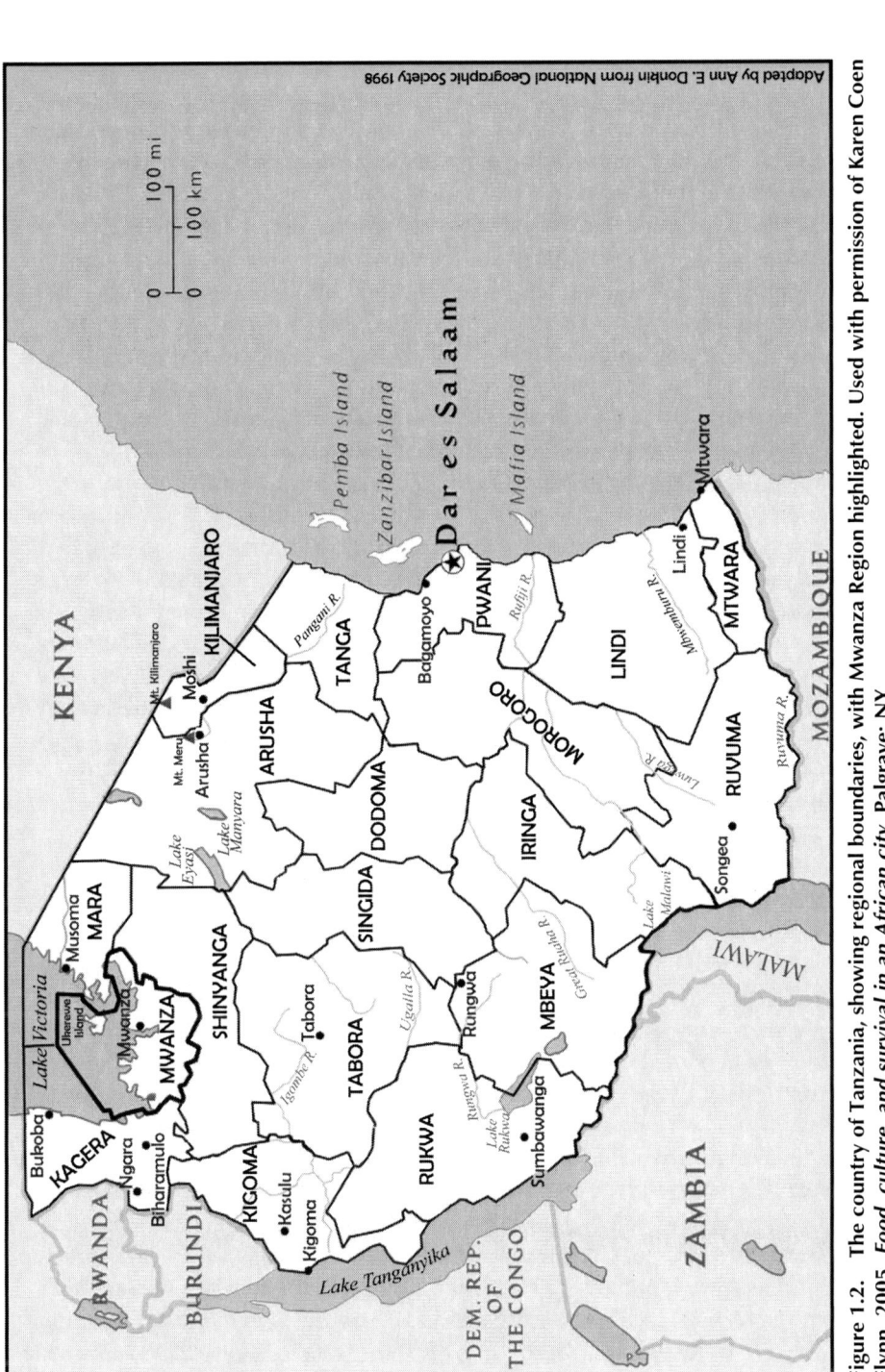

Figure 1.2.   The country of Tanzania, showing regional boundaries, with Mwanza Region highlighted. Used with permission of Karen Coen Flynn. 2005. *Food, culture, and survival in an African city.* Palgrave: NY.

Important ways that Tanzania differs from other sub-Saharan African countries include that: its primary national language (Swahili) is indigenous to Africa; it has been extraordinarily stable politically since independence; and it has one of the smallest secondary and higher education systems in the world (Cooksey and Riedmiller 1997; Topan 2008). In 2002–2003, for example, the average number of students enrolled in secondary education as a percentage of the population of official school age was 28 percent for sub-Saharan Africa overall, but only 7 percent for Tanzania (Palmer et al. 2007).

Mwanza Region is a 19,592 km^2 area just south of the equator on the southern shore of Lake Victoria (figure 1.2). At the start of the twenty-first century, this region was home to almost 3 million people, 90 percent of whom were of Sukuma ethnicity and 80 percent of whom lived in rural areas (United Republic of Tanzania 1997; National Bureau of Statistics and ORC Macro 2004). Other ethnic groups common to the area are the Zinza, Haya, Sumbwa, Nyamwezi, Luo, Kurya, Jita and Kerewe (United Republic of Tanzania 1997).

The people described in this book are fairly typical of rural populations throughout sub-Saharan Africa. They lived in settlements of varying remoteness, some on international thoroughfares or near economically vibrant towns, and others relatively isolated. They were mainly small farmers reliant on a combination of subsistence and cash crops and cattle. The vast majority lived in mud-built houses without electricity and used traditional pit toilets. Women in most households had to walk for approximately half an hour every day to obtain water for domestic use, and most of the population were poorly served by education and health services (National Bureau of Statistics and ORC Macro 2005).

Sukumas make up the largest ethnic group in Tanzania and numbered approximately 5–6 million people at the time of the study. In chapter 3 we will describe some of the unique beliefs and traditions of Sukuma culture, so here we will only note some broad similarities between the Sukuma and many other African ethnic groups. Caldwell, Caldwell, and Quiggin (1989) argue that most Africa societies share characteristics which the authors define as part of an "African system." Historically, Sukuma culture has shared most of those characteristics, including: placing great importance in ancestry, descent, and fertility; believing in ancestral spirit intervention in the affairs of the living; respecting the old (particularly men) and typically valuing intergenerational links over marital bonds; payment of bridewealth to the bride's family upon marriage; marked spousal separation of economic activities and responsibilities; husbands usually being much older than wives; polygyny (i.e., a man having multiple wives) being more common than in the Eurasian system; and divorce also being fairly common (Caldwell, Caldwell, and Quiggin 1989).

Almost half of Mwanza Region's population was under 15 years of age at the time of the study (National Bureau of Statistics and ORC Macro 2004). A 2007–2008 survey found that 1 percent of males and 6 percent females aged 15–24 years in Mwanza Region were HIV-positive; no statistics were available for those under 15 years of age (TACAIDS et al. 2008).

STUDY BACKGROUND AND PURPOSE

This book is primarily based upon the findings of the Health and Lifestyles Research (HALIRA) Project, a large qualitative study that involved data collection in four rural districts of Mwanza Region from 1999–2002. HALIRA initially was developed as a complement to the *MEMA kwa Vijana* adolescent sexual and reproductive health trial. The HALIRA Project had four main objectives: to investigate the lives and sexual behavior of adolescents; to determine behaviors which put young people at risk of infection with HIV or other sexually transmitted infections; to develop and evaluate quantitative and qualitative research methodologies for use with rural African adolescents; and to contribute to the evaluation of the *MEMA kwa Vijana* adolescent sexual health intervention. The first three of these objectives will be examined in-depth in this book. The fourth will be the focus of a companion volume (Plummer, forthcoming).

The *MEMA kwa Vijana* intervention consisted of four components: a teacher-led, peer-assisted primary school program; training of health facility workers to encourage youth friendliness; the promotion and distribution of condoms by out-of-school youth; and community mobilization (Obasi et al. 2006). The impact of the *MEMA kwa Vijana* intervention was evaluated through a community randomized trial, in which 20 communities were assigned to either the intervention or a control group on the basis of chance (Hayes et al. 2005). Each community was roughly equivalent to a local administrative ward and consisted of 5–6 villages, 5–6 primary schools, 1–2 government health units and an average total population of 17,000 people. To assess intervention impact, three surveys were conducted with 9,645 adolescents and young adults between 1998 and 2002. Ninety-four percent of trial participants were 14–17 years old in the first year of the intervention. The trial surveys collected data on participants' knowledge, their self-reported attitudes and behavior, and their biomedical outcomes such as HIV, sexually transmitted infection, and pregnancy (Ross et al. 2007).

The *MEMA kwa Vijana* trial found that intervention participants had significantly improved sexual health knowledge, more desirable reported attitudes, and fewer reported risk behaviors at a group level than young people who had not received the intervention (Ross et al. 2007). However, intervention status was not significantly associated with the two primary biological outcomes, HIV and herpes. It was also not associated with any other sexually transmitted infections or pregnancy, except that gonorrhea was slightly higher amongst female intervention participants; this was an association only seen in the school year that had had the least exposure to the intervention, suggesting that it was due to chance rather than intervention participation (Ross et al. 2007). Overall, at the end of the trial 14 percent of males (average age 19) and 45 percent of females (average age 18) tested positive for HIV, herpes, gonorrhea, Chlamydia, syphilis, and/or Trichomonas; the latter was only tested in females (Helen Weiss, personal communication).

This book will describe young people's lives in rural Mwanza, with focus on typical sexual behavior, relationships and health in the absence of an intervention program. As such it will primarily draw upon qualitative data collected from *MEMA kwa Vijana* control communities which did not participate in the intervention during the course of the trial. The companion volume to this book will draw on the findings presented here and additionally examine qualitative data from *MEMA kwa Vijana* intervention communities (Plummer, forthcoming). It will evaluate the process and impact of the *MEMA kwa Vijana* intervention in order to understand the trial results better, and to identify ways that adolescent sexual health interventions may be improved in the future.

STUDY DESIGN

This book is primarily based upon findings from participant observation, but it also draws upon data from in-depth interviews, group discussions, and simulated patient exercises. Data were usually collected by a team of two male and two female East Africans in their twenties, although staff turnover meant that six different young researchers were involved from the start to the end of the fieldwork. Participant observation took place for a total of 158 person-weeks in nine villages selected for their representativeness. The four main villages were visited by 1–2 researchers for approximately seven weeks per year for three years. Another five villages were also visited for participant observation, either in pilot studies for the main participant observation work or as socio-demographic complements to the four main villages. During participant observation visits, each researcher lived in a village household and accompanied young people in diverse daily activities (e.g., fetching water, preparing meals, going to market, farming, fishing, and socializing) and at special events (e.g., funerals, drumming/dancing events, video shows, and Christian and national holidays). Each evening, researchers spent 1–3 hours writing field notes in Swahili or English.

In addition to participant observation research, 161 formal in-depth interviews were conducted with 92 trial participants, including 76 who were randomly selected, 13 who were HIV-positive, and three who were pregnant in primary school. Seventy-one of those individuals or their family members were interviewed both at the beginning and the end of the study. A first series of eight group discussions involving *MEMA kwa Vijana* peer educators and other pupils focused on their experiences of the in-school component of the *MEMA kwa Vijana* intervention. A second series involved 21 group discussions and 50 follow-up in-depth interviews with out-of-school young men and women. This latter series addressed particularly sensitive topics, such as why girls have sex, or the nature of sexual activities. Simulated patient exercises consisted of trained rural young people visiting 19 *MEMA kwa Vijana* trial health facilities with scripted concerns about sexually transmitted infection symptoms and/or requests for contraception or condoms, in order to assess service quality. In-depth interviews, group discussions, and simulated patient exercises were conducted in Swahili or Sukuma, and were audio-recorded. Each of these HALIRA research methods will be described in detail in chapter 2.

DATA VALIDITY AND REPRESENTATIVENESS

The validity of research findings—or the extent to which they accurately reflect the reality on the ground—is a perennial concern for social scientists, particularly when self-reported information is involved (Caldwell, Caldwell, and Quiggin 1989; Catania et al. 1993; Hingson and Strunin 1993; Bulmer and Warwick 2000; Buvé et al. 2001; Weinreb 2006; Minnis et al. 2009). Self-reported information may be inaccurate due to poor recall, misunderstanding, or intentionally false statements made to be polite, to seek praise, or to avoid criticism or embarrassment (Catania et al. 1993; Brewer, Garrett, and Kulasingam 1999; Fenton et al. 2001; Turner et al. 2009). Validity can be especially problematic in the study of a highly sensitive topic such as sexual behavior, and particularly when it involves young people in sub-Saharan Africa (Huygens et al. 1996). For example, in two surveys one-year apart with 12–19-year-olds in Nairobi, Kenya, 49 percent of those who reported sex in at least one of the surveys gave inconsistent information about whether they had ever had sex, or the timing of their first intercourse, in the other survey (Beguy et al. 2009).

There are several reasons why such high proportions of adolescents may provide inconsistent sexual behavior reports in sub-Saharan Africa. First, unmarried adolescent sexual activity is typically condemned by adults, inhibiting disclosure; second, there is very little experience of nonjudgmental research, so study neutrality and confidentiality may be doubted; and third, poor education can contribute to misinterpretation of questions or inaccurate responses, such as age estimates (Binson and Catania 1998; Cohen 1998; Singh et al. 2000; Cowan et al. 2002; Wijsen and Tanner 2002; Mensch, Hewett, and Erulkar 2003). In sub-Saharan Africa, as elsewhere in the world, adolescents tend to underreport sexual behaviors in surveys, due to what they believe will be socially desirable to the interviewer, or for fear of punishment. However, in some cases sexual behaviors may be overreported, for example, if boys want to exaggerate their sexual experience, or if intervention participants wish to report a promoted activity, such as condom use (Catania et al. 1990; Agnew and Loving 1998; Devine and Aral 2004). These issues all create enormous challenges for researchers attempting to collect honest and accurate data.

Most research on young people's sexual behavior in Africa relies upon self-reported information in formally structured surveys, or less often, semi-structured in-depth interviews or focus group discussions (Gallant and Maticka-Tyndale 2004). Quantitative surveys involve directly asking the same questions of a large number of people, and recording their responses numerically so that the data can be easily analyzed using statistical methods. An advantage to interviewing large numbers of people is that the results are more likely to be representative or generalizable, that is, they are more likely to reflect the total population and not specific subgroups (Bulmer and Warwick 2000). However, the large number of structured interviews involved in survey research means that topics are usually only addressed superficially.

Qualitative research such as in-depth interviews or focus group discussions also involves asking respondents direct questions, but those questions may be open-ended and semi-structured, and responses are given in a narrative form. Qualitative interviews usually take longer than survey interviews, giving the respondent more time to develop rapport and trust with the interviewer. Topics can thus be explored in more depth and complexity than is possible in surveys, which can be particularly important for sensitive, private, and sometimes complicated topics such as sexual behavior (Ankrah 1989; Huygens et al. 1996; Agadjanian 2005).

However, qualitative research usually cannot be done on a large scale, specifically because it is less structured and more intensive and time-consuming than quantitative research, so qualitative findings usually cannot be assumed to be representative (Bulmer and Warwick 2000). In addition, most qualitative studies of young people's sexual behavior in rural areas of sub-Saharan Africa have involved group discussions and/or secondary school students (e.g., Vos 1994; Nzioka 2001; Nyanzi et al. 2001). Group discussions may overestimate socially stigmatized behaviors, because respondents are typically asked to reflect on what they believe is happening in their communities, rather than their own behavior (e.g., Luke 2003; Longfield et al. 2004; Neighbors et al. 2006). Furthermore, as already noted, only about one-quarter of young people in sub-Saharan Africa reach secondary school (Palmer et al. 2007), and secondary students are not likely to be representative of other youth because they are relatively wealthy, educated, and have different ways of thinking about the future.

Participant observation—when researchers live and work among members of a target population for an extended period of time—is a qualitative method that provides an alternative to methods that rely solely on self-reported information. Participant observation can reduce self-reporting biases because the data come from researchers' observations of everyday life and their informal conversations with people. Respondents may present themselves in inaccurate ways that they perceive to be socially desirable when completing questionnaires or participating in formal interviews, but they are less likely to maintain this over a long period of time in their normal social environment. By living with the people they are studying, and joining in their daily activities over weeks and months, researchers can see how people present themselves differently in different social contexts. In the HALIRA study, for example, participant observation researchers often found that young people initially concealed their sexual relationships but subsequently disclosed them once a good rapport had been established through shared activities and empathic conversations.

Given the private nature of sexual behavior, participant observation in the literal sense (that is, direct observation of sexual activity) has very rarely been used as a research method. However, some aspects of sexual behavior, such as sexual negotiation, can be easily observed and sometimes overheard simply by living and interacting in a community (e.g., Desmond et al. 2005). This can allow for a more complex study of social interactions and provides helpful insight into sexual and reproductive health and practices. For example, in a study in rural Ghana, Bleek (1987, 316) learned a great deal about abortion by what he observed before and after abortion procedures. He comments: "Although I never witnessed an abortion, I learned much about their causes and consequences. I *saw* these causes and consequences."

Similarly, in a discussion of anthropological work conducted in Mwanza, Tanzania, Pool (1997, 70) commented:

> The usefulness [of participant observation] is based on the assumption that much relevant and interesting information, particularly regarding topics which are delicate, taboo or hidden, is more likely to surface in informal contexts than in a formal interview setting; and to get that information you have to be there.

Historically, participant observation has usually taken the form of one re-searcher living in a single village for one or more years. This allows for the collection of valid, in-depth information that can be contextualized through a detailed knowledge of a particular community. However, when only one re-searcher and location are involved, the representativeness of the findings may be quite limited. Recognizing this, we took an innovative approach in designing this study's length, geographic range, and researcher differences to maximize the representativeness of the participant observation data collected. The six young fieldworkers represented different sexes, ethnicities, linguistic skills, and education levels. The nine selected villages and seventeen host house-holds were typical of the range of socio-demographic conditions within rural Mwanza, that is, primarily agricultural or fishing, entirely Sukuma or multieth-nic, and dispersed/remote or larger villages. This study design does not ensure perfect generalizability, but we believe it is a practical and balanced approach that resulted in both valid and unusually representative qualitative data about sensitive behaviors. Indeed, a formal comparison of data collected from par-ticipant observation, in-depth interviews, survey questionnaires, and biological markers in the *MEMA kwa Vijana* trial found that participant observation was the most useful method for understanding the nature, complexity, and extent of youth sexual behavior (Plummer, Ross, et al. 2004).

COMPLEXITY, CONTRADICTION, AND AMBIVALENCE

A key theme that cuts across many of the chapters in this book is that rural life is contradictory in ways that have serious implications both for the HIV epidemic and for sexual health intervention effectiveness. For example, we found that single young women were considered respectable if they did not engage in sexual relationships, and yet they were often tacitly expected to exploit sex for material gain, and were sometimes disparaged for not doing so. Similarly, social ideals specified that school pupils should be sexually abstinent, but restrictions on sexual activity were informally relaxed at festi-vals, sometimes even for school pupils. Such inconsistencies contributed to common but highly secretive sexual relationships among young people, and sometimes led to ambivalent reactions to them when they became public.

Social scientists have long recognized that the ways in which individuals present themselves in social life are often contradictory (Goffman 1959; Ewing 1990; Helle-Valle 2004). As anthropologist Katherine Ewing (1990, 251) noted:

In all cultures people can be observed to project multiple, inconsistent self-rep-resentations that are context-dependent and may shift rapidly. At any particular moment a person usually experiences his or her articulated self as a symbolic, timeless whole, but this self may quickly be displaced by another, quite different "self," which is based on a different definition of the situation. The person will often be unaware of these shifts and inconsistencies and may experience wholeness and continuity despite their presence.

In anthropological work in Botswana, for example, Helle-Valle (2004, 201) found that traditional kinship and marriage coexisted with widespread extramarital sexual relationships. He explained:

> Different social contexts involve different rules and taboos associated with sex. . . . But in the daily life and the pragmatic ways of much African sociality this sexual multiplicity is not seen, and often not reflected on by participants themselves. . . . By framing different practices in different settings people manage to live lives that appear as rather ordinary and uncomplicated but which owe their smoothness to the extent the participants manage to frame sociality in practical ways.

Presenting oneself in different ways in different contexts is probably common to all people and all human societies, but the degree of inconsistency, the circumstances in which it occurs, and the extent to which it is regarded as desirable or problematic, varies. In rural Tanzania, we found that some people maintained seemingly contradictory roles in different social contexts, often without undermining their credibility amongst other villagers. Two things that often seemed essential for such contradictions to be accepted were that the individuals involved were discreet, and no one was believed to be harmed directly. For example, one young single mother in our study lived with her parents but snuck out at night to have sex outdoors with the father of her child, even though he was publicly acknowledged in that role and was on polite terms with her parents. Her ongoing sexual relationship while living in her parents' home was an "open secret," but her attempt at discretion made this tolerable. When attempts at secrecy or discretion were unsuccessful, and apparent contradictions were discussed publicly, then community members often had ambivalent responses even when disapproval was voiced. However, when someone was believed to have been malicious in their contradictory behavior, for example, by injuring others through suspected theft or witchcraft, this was seen as an unacceptable violation and sometimes was met with severe punishment.

These issues have implications for HIV-related behavior and research. For young people in our study, the highly secretive nature of sexual relationships meant that relationships were not reinforced through social recognition and there was little scope to develop intimacy through nonsexual contact, which contributed to short relationship durations, high levels of partner change, and concurrency. For research, understanding the different ways that villagers presented themselves in different social contexts—particularly as related to sexual behavior—helps to explain why questionnaire surveys provided data of limited validity.

BOOK OVERVIEW

There has been great concern about young Africans' sexual risk behaviors in recent decades, but few studies have attempted to examine their motivations and experiences in depth, from their own, often diverse and unique perspectives (Wijsen and Tanner 2002). One goal of this book is to describe rural young people's perspectives on their lives and sexual behavior. Towards that end, in the main chapters we draw heavily on interview quotes and participant observation conversations. In addition, there are three series of case studies placed at intervals throughout the book which describe individual young people's lives in depth. These case studies consider each young person's family and school background, socio-demographic activities, and sexual relationship history, and the particular ways in which they managed conflicting social and sexual norms and expectations in their lives.

Another goal of this book is to present the study's findings in a way that is clear and useful to people from a wide range of backgrounds. As the outcome of a rigorous, multidisciplinary research project, we hope that specialists in social sciences, public health, and areas studies will find this book valuable. Towards that end, we have tried to provide detailed evidence for our conclusions and to contextualize them within the broader academic literature throughout the book. In offset boxes, we have also highlighted some of the challenges we encountered while trying to collect reliable and valid data.

In addition, we would like the material presented here to be accessible and useful for program developers, policy makers, government officials, undergraduate students, and interested members of the general public in East Africa and elsewhere. We have thus tried to write this book in clear language that avoids academic jargon. When it has been necessary to use specialized terms which might be unfamiliar to the general public, we have explained them upon introduction.

In the next chapter (chapter 2) we will describe the study's background, design, and individual methods, as well as the process of the research in detail. The book's general findings then begin with an overview of village life in chapter 3, which addresses material conditions, occupations, social relationships, social events, supernatural beliefs, and health beliefs and practices. In chapter 4, we describe features of village life that specifically involve young people, including school conditions and children's general relationships with their parents, peers, and teachers.

Chapter 5 examines the sexual norms and expectations affecting young people in rural Mwanza, contrasting those which discourage sexual activity, such as school pupils' abstinence, women's sexual respectability, and the appropriate context for discussing sex, with those that encourage sexual activity, such as the perceived inevitability of sex, the notion of sex as a female resource, the masculine esteem gained through sexual experience, and the relaxation of prohibitions at festivals.

Between chapters 5 and 6, the first case study series examines the lives and premarital sexual histories of five typical young people, from prepubescence through unmarried young adulthood. Chapters 6 through 8 then address unmarried young people's sexual behavior, moving from the broad, macro-social level to the interpersonal, micro-social level. Chapter 6 describes three common relationship types and typical sexual relationships for preadolescents, school pupils, and unmarried young adults, before addressing overarching issues, such as emotional intimacy, concurrency, and sexual mixing patterns. Chapter 7 describes sexual negotiation, including material exchange for sex and sexual coercion, while chapter 8 addresses common sexual practices.

Between chapter 8 and 9, the second case study series describes the family and school backgrounds, socioeconomic activities, and sexual relationship histories of four young people who married and/or divorced during the course of our study. Chapter 9 then examines the process of marrying and how young couple's relationships changed once they married. This is followed by chapter 10, which explores young women's attitudes towards and experience of contraception, fertility protection or promotion, reproduction, and abortion.

Chapter 11 then describes beliefs about the causes of sexually transmitted infections and their biomedical and traditional treatment in rural Mwanza, with a special focus on HIV/AIDS. Between chapters 11 and 12, the third case study series describes the lives and experiences of two HIV-positive teenagers: a boy who was probably infected since infancy, and a girl who was probably infected during adolescent sexual activity. In the final chapter (chapter 12), we will review our findings on the social, economic, and cultural context of young people's sexual behavior. Specifically, we will discuss factors which may be barriers to, or facilitators of, sexual risk reduction.

NOTE

1. At the time of the research, the exchange rate was Tanzanian Shillings (Tshs) 1,000 to US $1.20. The official minimum monthly wage was Tshs 30,000, but many laborers made far less than that.

Chapter Two

Research Methods

Social science publications often focus on research findings and provide only a superficial description of the research process, making it difficult to fully assess the study's quality, or to appropriately adapt its methods elsewhere. There is also a tendency to highlight successful aspects of the research and to ignore the difficulties encountered, preventing discussion of lessons learned. In this chapter, we will describe the research methods used in this study, including some of the complex, real-world challenges we encountered during the research process, and the ways we tried to resolve them.

This chapter begins with an overview of the Health and Lifestyles Research (HALIRA) Project and describes its staff, training, and capacity-building. The bulk of the chapter is then devoted to describing each qualitative method in detail. A formal methodological comparison found that participant observation was the most useful method in collecting valid and meaningful sexual behavior data within our study (Plummer, Ross, et al. 2004). Participant observation was thus the main source of data used in this book, and it is the method that is described in greatest depth here.

AN OVERVIEW OF THE HALIRA PROJECT

Early in the *MEMA kwa Vijana* trial the principal investigators recognized that it would be useful to conduct detailed qualitative studies of trial participants' lifestyles and sexual behavior, to better contextualize, interpret, and understand trial results. Ideally, such qualitative research would precede and inform initial intervention development, but funding for the HALIRA Project was not obtained until the first year of intervention development was completed and baseline trial data had already been collected. Prior to beginning

23

fieldwork, the HALIRA proposal was approved by the Tanzanian Medical Research Coordinating Committee and the London School of Hygiene and Tropical Medicine Ethics Committee.

The HALIRA Project began in April 1999. From April to September, HALIRA staff were hired and trained, and research protocols and instruments were designed, pretested, and piloted. The main fieldwork then took place in Missungwi, Kwimba, Sengerema, and Geita Districts of Mwanza Region from September 1999 to August 2002. This primarily involved participant observation, in-depth interviews, group discussions, and simulated patient exercises. Figure 2.1 shows the locations where qualitative research was conducted relative to the trial intervention and control communities.

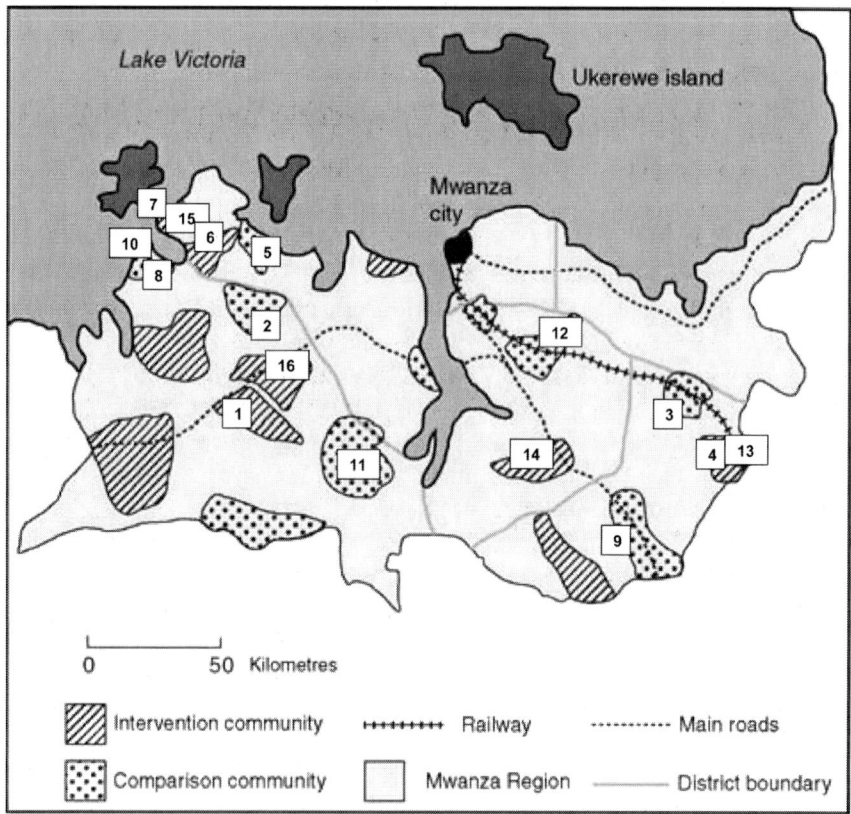

Figure 2.1. Mwanza Region, Tanzania, showing *MEMA kwa Vijana* trial intervention and control communities, and locations of HALIRA fieldwork. In-depth interviews were conducted and simulated patient exercises attempted in all 20 trial communities. Villages numbered 1–9 = participant observation; 10–12 = young adult group discussions; 13–16 = pupil group discussions.

The HALIRA Project had three British principal investigators: David Ross (a clinical epidemiologist), Richard Hayes (a statistician), and Daniel Wight (a social anthropologist), the last of whom led the design and supervision of the project. Daniel Wight had previously conducted a participant observation community study and qualitative research on young men's sexual behavior in Scotland. He had also developed a theoretically based, teacher-delivered sex education program there, and led its process and impact evaluation in twenty-five schools. His involvement in African research began in Uganda in 1992. He started collaborating on research in Mwanza in 1997, and he was 41 years old when the HALIRA Project began. During the HALIRA fieldwork, data analysis and write-up, he was employed by the Medical Research Council in Glasgow, UK and he spent approximately one month per year in Mwanza to support the ongoing work there. At the time of this writing, Daniel Wight is the Leader of the Sexual Health and Families Program of the UK Medical Research Council Social and Public Health Sciences Unit.

Mary Plummer was the *MEMA kwa Vijana* Social Science Coordinator from 1999–2002. In that position she was responsible for codesigning, coordinating, and managing quantitative and qualitative social science research within the trial, including the HALIRA Project. She is a US citizen who, prior to joining HALIRA, had lived and worked in urban and rural Mwanza Region for three years. When she started working with HALIRA she was 33 years old and had a bachelor's degree in sociology and a master's degree in botany from a field naturalist program. At that time, she also had more than a decade of professional experience as an HIV/AIDS educator, curriculum developer, and program evaluator in the United States, Germany, and Tanzania. During the HALIRA fieldwork and most subsequent data analysis and writing, Mary Plummer was employed by the London School of Hygiene and Tropical Medicine. In the same period she completed her PhD, which compared the validity of *MEMA kwa Vijana* trial biological marker, face-to-face questionnaire, and assisted self-completion questionnaire sexual behavior data with those collected by HALIRA in-depth interviews and participant observation. Mary Plummer is currently working as an independent consultant based in Dar es Salaam, Tanzania.

HALIRA fieldwork was conducted by two university graduates (hereafter referred to as "graduate researchers") and at any given time two Sukuma-speaking secondary school graduates (hereafter referred to as "Sukuma researchers"). Gerry Mshana, a 27-year-old Tanzanian, began his HALIRA position with a master's degree in international relations. Joyce Wamoyi, a 25-year-old Kenyan, began hers with a bachelor's degree in environmental studies. Zachayo Shigongo, Halima Abdallah, Kija Nyalali, and Neema Busali were Tanzanians in their early twenties when they joined the project.

These six HALIRA researchers were all employed by the Tanzanian National Institute for Medical Research during the study.

BUILDING A MULTILINGUAL RESEARCH TEAM

The integration of three languages—Sukuma, Swahili, and English—within the research project posed challenges. The principal investigators and research coordinator were all native English speakers. At the start of the study, none of the principal investigators spoke Swahili or Sukuma, and Mary Plummer only had an intermediate command of Swahili. As the national language, Swahili is spoken by many villagers in large, multiethnic villages and towns in Mwanza, but most remote villages had almost exclusively Sukuma populations and few villagers in such areas understood Swahili well. The original HALIRA proposal thus called for two young Sukuma-speaking university graduates to collect qualitative data. The project advertised these positions locally, regionally, and nationally, and offered exceptionally good salaries, but nonetheless could not recruit such applicants. Most fluent Sukuma speakers had been raised in rural Mwanza, where the quality of formal education had been very poor in the decades preceding the study, even in comparison to other Tanzanian schools. As a result, the vast majority of fluent Sukuma speakers did not attend all seven years of a Swahili-speaking primary school and then gone on to English-speaking secondary school, let alone to highly competitive Swahili- or English-speaking universities.

Given these challenges, the original research plan was modified and Gerry Mshana and Joyce Wamoyi, the two most promising Swahili-speaking applicants, were hired instead. During their first months conducting participant observation and in-depth interviews, these graduate researchers were able to collect some valuable data, but they were clearly constrained by their inability to follow Sukuma conversations or to formally interview villagers who spoke little Swahili. It was thus decided to additionally hire two outstanding Sukuma speakers from the pool of 1998 *MEMA kwa Vijana* survey interviewers, Zachayo Shigongo and Halima Abdallah. Both had demonstrated exceptional critical thinking and interview skills during the surveys. These Sukuma researchers had lived in rural Mwanza for part of their childhoods, but not in the villages where HALIRA research was conducted.

The HALIRA Project faced similar linguistic challenges when hiring transcription and translation staff. Swahili and Sukuma field books and interview cassette tapes were to be transcribed verbatim and then translated into English for most analyses. The bilingual (Swahili-Sukuma) transcriber and trilingual translator positions were widely advertised locally, and many dozens of applicants participated in a series of language skills examinations. These showed that by far the most capable Sukuma-English translators were in their late 50s or older. One of these individuals had worked in a low level secretarial position and thus knew how to type, but most did not, and none had prior experience with computers. These extraordinary trilingual individuals were amongst a small minority of their generation who had been educated in English during the British colonial period, prior to national independence in 1961. The colonial and postcolonial history of Mwanza Region will be described more in the next chapter.

Sukuma is a tonal language; for example, a simple word such as "*nda*" can mean pregnancy, head, or lice, depending on the tone used when the word is spoken. There is virtually no history of the Sukuma language in written form to assist in standardizing tones and spelling (Gleason 1961; Abrahams 1967; Wijsen and Tanner 2002). At the time of the study, we were only able to locate one brief English-to-Sukuma dictionary that had been produced by the African Inland Mission church, probably in the mid-1900s. It was superficial and much of the terminology was out-of-date. The HALIRA Sukuma translators thus worked with the Sukuma field researchers and transcribers to develop a standardized way of writing Sukuma and translating it into English.

RESEARCHER ATTRIBUTES, TRAINING AND CAPACITY-BUILDING

Social science data collection requires varying levels of skill and training, depending on the methods. Survey questionnaires generally follow exact question and answer options, so survey interviewers may only need minimal training and independence to collect data well. In contrast, qualitative research methods—and particularly in-depth interviewing and participant observation—require some analysis during data collection in order to direct further investigation. In addition, to carry out participant observation well, researchers should be able to empathize with their informants and critically reflect on their own cultural perspectives (Pool and Geissler 2005).

In high income countries, qualitative methods are usually conducted by local graduate or doctoral researchers. In low income countries anthropological research has historically been carried out by highly educated foreign researchers who have learned the local language as an adult. For Swahili and a few other African languages this can involve formal study at an academic institution prior to fieldwork, but for most African languages, such as Sukuma, linguistic training typically is limited to the anthropologist's experience while immersed during fieldwork. In either case the researcher is unlikely to become fully fluent in the language, as noted by Wijsen and Tanner (2002, 5):

> [The Sukuma language] has a total of eighteen tenses, including six present tenses, and twelve linguistic tones. Furthermore, there are regional, sub-regional and even individual variations in the use of this grammar. . . . There are not many outsiders who have an understanding of this complexity semantically, except possibly a few missionaries who spent many years in Africa, but certainly not anthropologists who usually remain only for a brief period of time.

In practice, anthropologists have often informally relied on local, untrained translators in their data collection, or hired junior or lay researchers to collect additional data independently. For example, in her 1965–1967 anthropological study of the Sukuma, Varkevisser (1973) employed fourteen secondary school girls to conduct participant observation in Sukuma homesteads across Mwanza and neighboring regions over a series of school vacations. Varkevisser acknowledged her research assistants' contributions in her book, but many of her contemporaries relied on similar assistance and did not make this explicit in their research publications. Qualitative social science research practices in sub-Saharan Africa are shifting. Collaborations between senior foreign and junior local qualitative researchers are being made more explicit (e.g., Price and Hawkins 2002; Kaler 2004a; Watkins and Swidler 2006; Parikh 2007; Francis and Hemson 2009; Sommer 2009), while local researchers are gaining higher level degrees and increasingly leading their own social science projects.

Anthropological data collection by different types of researchers have different advantages and disadvantages. Someone from a similar background to that of the study participants has an intimate social knowledge even before the research begins. If they are fluent in the local language, they also have the potential to engage with informants in subtle and complex conversations. However, if their research skills are limited, or they lack the training to constantly question their familiar culture, they may not recognize and pursue relevant issues as they arise. A local researcher may also find it difficult to ask "naïve" questions that study participants think have obvious answers, since people are generally more willing to explain taken-for-granted aspects of their lives to "outsiders," such as those from different countries or ethnic groups.

In this study the field team combined many of the advantages and disadvantages outlined above. As native Swahili speakers from Kenya and urban Tanzania, the graduate researchers were "partial" outsiders who brought analytical skills from other disciplines to their work. The Sukuma researchers had quite limited training prior to being hired by the project, but they were highly intelligent and personable young people who brought an intimate understanding of local culture and language.

The field researcher training included: detailed discussions of the research objectives and key methodological texts; formal and informal seminars on specific research methods; pilot field research for each method alone or with senior researchers; debriefings partway through and immediately after fieldwork; instruction and detailed feedback on writing field notes, compiling data summaries, and drafting summary reports; individualized mentorship; and collective development of a qualitative data coding frame. Over the three years of data collection, the field researchers were closely supervised and their ability to analyze data and generate new research questions improved with each round of fieldwork. Three of the researchers stayed for all three years of field work. This continuity was important, since the trusting relationships they built during participant observation and in-depth interviews in the first year of research allowed them to reestablish rapport easily on subsequent visits, and gave them a deeper understanding of the transitions that young people experienced in the interim. The first two female Sukuma researchers (Halima Abdallah and Kija Nyalali) left the HALIRA Project for university after its first and second years, respectively, but they returned to work for it during their university vacations.

Developing the HALIRA team's research capacity was an important project objective and was actively pursued throughout the study and beyond. Each researcher was encouraged to participate in every stage of the research process, not only at a level reflecting their prior training and experience, but also in ways that promoted new skills development. The two graduate researchers were employed for an additional one to two years beyond the fieldwork, during which they received more training and held new responsibilities in budgeting, management of support staff, data processing, data analysis, and drafting publications. During the research and afterwards, field researchers were encouraged and assisted in obtaining higher education placements and funding. Their achievements in this area are notable, as each field researcher has earned one or two higher degrees since the project ended.

PARTICIPANT OBSERVATION

Participant observation usually involves researchers living with those they are studying and participating in their activities for an extended period of time. As discussed in chapter 1, anthropologists have traditionally lived in a single village for one or more years. While the resultant findings may be highly valid for that particular community, they may not be typical of the broader population of interest and they will be shaped by the specific characteristics of a single researcher. In this study, we attempted to maximize representativeness by conducting participant observation in a number of carefully selected sites. In addition, during any period of fieldwork there were four field researchers of different gender and ethnicity collecting data, reducing the chance that findings were strongly influenced by one individual's characteristics. By collecting data at systematic intervals over an extended period of time, we also attempted to identify and monitor trends.

Prior to participant observation, researchers received permission to conduct research from regional, district, ward, and village-level elected and appointed officials, as well as the heads of household where the field researchers were to live. In addition, early in their village stay, field researchers usually participated in public meetings in which they explained that they were studying the health and lifestyles of village youth. In the meetings and one-to-one contacts afterwards, researchers answered any questions people had about the research.

Village and Household Selection

Nine villages were visited for participant observation for a total of 158 person-weeks. One pair of representative intervention and control villages was selected for participant observation in each of three districts. These included a pair of large, primarily Sukuma, roadside villages near a gold mine (1 and 2); a pair of remote, dispersed, and almost entirely Sukuma villages (3 and 4); and a pair of large, multiethnic roadside fishing villages near Lake Victoria (5 and 6) (figure 2.1). Specific characteristics of these villages, the host households for participant observation, and the number and lengths of visits are detailed in table 2.1.

Village pairs 1 and 2 and 3 and 4 were visited for approximately two months per year for three years. Villages 5 and 6 were each only visited once for approximately two months due to researcher time constraints, although another village (7) with similar characteristics was visited by other researchers for one visit later in the study period. The remaining two villages (8 and 9) were used for one-week participant observation pilot and training visits. Village 9 was visited by each new researcher being trained, accompanied by an experienced researcher.

Upon first arriving at a village, participant observation researchers enlisted the support of village authorities to identify households of *MEMA kwa Vijana* trial participants where they might live. Each researcher requested to stay with a typical family, that is, one that was not unusually wealthy, educated, religious, or otherwise distinct. They also took into consideration the characteristics of the other participant observation host families in order to achieve a demographically representative range of households. Researchers usually visited three to four households before selecting one. Pairs of researchers

Table 2.1. Description of Participant Observation Villages and Households

Village number	Number annual visits (Total person-weeks)	Village characteristics* Months visited: Seasonal events	Village facilities	Head of household characteristics** (Number in household)***	Number informants in MEMA kwa Vijana trial****
1	three (35)	• Large, roadside villages, approximately 6 km from gold mines. • Water sources mainly unprotected hand-dug ponds. • Vast majority Sukuma. Minorities included Sumbwa, Rongo, Ha, Nyamwezi, and Nyaruanda. *Dec.–Jan.:* —*Weeding crops, end cultivation, start of some harvesting.* —*Christmas and New Year*	One law court, 8 shops/kiosks, two mills, two storage facilities, one bar, and two churches.	Poor farmer, monogamous couple (8) Very poor farmer, Protestant widow (8)	21
2	three (36)		One government health facility, 15 shops/kiosks, one mill, three storage facilities, one bar, two churches, and a mosque.	Kiosk owner, political leader, farmer, monogamous Protestant couple (18) Poor farmer, divorced female (9)	24
3	three (25)	• Remote villages with dispersed populations; neighboring villages were on main roads or railway line.	Three seasonal kiosks, one storage facility, and two churches.	Poor farmer, alcohol brewer/seller, monogamous couple (14) Poor farmer, polygynous couple (9)	17
4	three (27)	• Cattle important to economy. • Water sources mainly 1–2 protected wells per sub-village, built by charities. • Almost 100 percent Sukuma.	Several kiosks, one mill, one storage facility, and two churches.	Very poor farmer, previously polygynous couple (8) Kiosk owner, alcohol brewer/seller, political leader, farmer, Nyakyusa Seventh Day Adventist widow (6);	26

(continued)

Table 2.1. Description of Participant Observation Villages and Households (*continued*)

Village number	Number annual visits (Total person-weeks)	Village characteristics* Months visited: Seasonal events	Village facilities	Head of household characteristics** (Number in household)***	Number informants in MEMA kwa Vijana trial****
		June–July: —Harvesting and selling crops. —Relaxing, socializing and ngoma (drumming-dancing) celebrations **Bulabo** (Christian Eucharist) and Saba saba (*Farmer's Day*)		Traditional healer, farmer, polygynous Muslim husband and wives (12)	26
5	one (7)	• Large, roadside villages on or near Lake Victoria. • Many involved in fishing economy.	Over 30 shops and kiosks, two mills, two storage facilities, 4 churches, and a mosque.	Teacher, kiosk, and bar owner, farmer, polygynous Sukuma/Zinza couple (7)	—
6	one (7)	• Water sources included the lake, deep wells, protected deep ponds, and/or unprotected seasonal shallow ponds.	Many shops and kiosks, one mill, two cement buildings, two storage facilities, and 4 churches.	Retired teacher, farmer, monogamous Protestant couple (4)	—

7	one (10)	• Majority Sukuma ethnicity. Minorities included: Zinza, Jita and Kerewe; also some Haya, Luo, Rundi, and Nyaruanda. Villages 5 and 6: *July–Aug.* Village 7: *April–May (Easter)* Village 8: *June (pilot)*	Many shops and kiosks, two mills, several bars and video halls, three guest houses, two churches and one mosque. Private church facilities (an air strip, a dispensary, schools).	Poor fisherman, farmer, monogamous couple (14) Poor fisherman, farmer, monogamous Kerewe couple (8)	13
8	one (1.5)		One law court, a police post, 15 shops and kiosks, three mills, one storage facility, one bar/video hall, and one guest house.	Government employee, landlord, monogamous couple (11)	—
9	three (9)	• Remote village with dispersed population. Roads impassable in rainy season. • Cattle important to economy. • Water source was seasonal river that flowed during rainy season, and in which people dug unprotected ponds in dry season. • Almost 100 percent Sukuma. *March, June, Oct., Dec. (pilots)*	One storage facility, three seasonal kiosks.	Poor farmer, monogamous couple (6) Poor farmer, polygynous couple (10) Tailor, farmer, polygynous husband, and wives (9)	17

*In all villages, most villagers engaged in farming cotton, cassava, maize, sweet potatoes, peanuts, cow peas, millet, and/or sorghum. In all villages, many families also kept cattle.
**Heads of household were Sukuma and Catholic, unless otherwise noted. "Polygynous couple" signifies that another formally recognized wife lived in another household.
****Number in household was total number over 2–3 visits, so this could be greater than the number present at any one point in time.
****Villages 5, 6, and 8 were only visited in 1999 by one researcher each. At that time, information was not collected on whether informants were also *MEMA kwa Vijana* trial participants.

lived in different households within the same village, and they almost always returned to live in those same households on subsequent visits to the village.

Researchers usually found their hosts to be welcoming, gracious, and helpful throughout their stay. This is illustrated by comments the male Sukuma researcher made about one of his host households in a summary report:

> The family that I stayed with was very poor. For example, when I arrived, I learned that they did not have flour for *ugali* [a stiff porridge staple made of maize, or maize and cassava mixed], so I had to buy one bag of maize flour. Another example is the sleeping place. The family of eight did not even have one bed, so they spread their bedding on the floor, as I did with the mattress I brought with me. I always saw each of my hosts wearing one set of clothes, without ever changing them. Despite the very harsh conditions, the family lives with mutual understanding and respect. Family members were very cooperative with me and with each other. [PO-01-I-1-3m]

Researcher Integration into Villages

The researchers were generally welcomed as guests by their hosts, but they contributed to households by paying for some basic staples, helping in chores, and writing or reading as requested by their semiliterate hosts. The researchers did not pretend to be villagers, but they sometimes altered their appearance and habits to avoid stark differences. For example, female researchers did not wear trousers during fieldwork, because this was very uncommon in rural areas.

During the first days of a first visit to a participant observation village, fieldworkers found that local people were often cautious with them, treating them politely but with some reserve. The levels of curiosity and wariness about researchers varied within and between villages. Within a few days of familiarity, however, villagers usually seemed to become comfortable with them and even to take their presence for granted. The Sukuma researchers were particularly successful in quickly and effectively integrating into households and villages. They could easily follow and participate in informal discussions and exchanges, which were often in Sukuma, and this was very important in quickly building rapport with villagers. Being in their early 20s, they were also several years younger than the graduate researchers and sometimes were mistakenly perceived to be even younger. For example, one female Sukuma researcher was only asked to pay a child's fee at some large social events, as if she were a dependent teenager.

Most village households consisted of an immediate family and one or more extended family members who came from within and beyond the village, including young people who might join a household for some months or years.

The Sukuma researchers' backgrounds were so similar to other villagers that they were treated very similarly to such young people and others in the household of their age and gender. Of all of the researchers, the female Sukumas seemed the least likely to be perceived as guests within households and villages, and they were readily expected to participate in the routine menial tasks expected of other girls and young women. As one of the female Sukuma researchers described in a summary report:

> The more days went by, the more close my relationship with villagers became, especially with young people. I think it is because I was always with them in their discussions and their daily activities, so I became familiar to them. In the beginning, they wanted me to just sit idly while they worked, and they were surprised when I joined them in their work. They thought I could not do rural activities like digging up or pounding cassava, carrying water, speaking Sukuma, or curtseying when greeting an old person. [Sharing in their activities] made it easy for me to collect data, because after becoming acquainted with me, young people told me about their sexual relationships, and those of their peers. [PO-01-C-2-5f]

The graduate researchers were not absorbed into households and villages in the same way as Sukuma researchers. Neither graduate researcher was a member of a local ethnic group nor spoke a local language other than Swahili, and the female graduate researcher spoke Swahili with a Kenyan accent. These attributes, combined with the graduate researchers' somewhat older, urban identities, always indicated that they were visitors to the area, even after they built rapport with many villagers and learned basic Sukuma terminology. Graduate researchers assisted in some daily chores within households and farms—particularly the female researcher, since domestic work was largely done by women—but this was less frequent and was not taken for granted in the same way that it was for Sukuma researchers, particularly the females. Nonetheless, there were times when the graduate researchers' identities as urban, professional "outsiders" seemed advantageous. Villagers could be particularly patient and detailed with them when explaining beliefs and practices which they might have felt were self-evident to others of a similar background.

Participant observation researchers began and continued their fieldwork by accompanying the young people in their households in their normal daily activities outside of school. These activities included work, such as cultivating or harvesting crops, cattle herding, running errands (for example, grinding flour at a mill, or buying fish at Lake Victoria), and for women only, domestic chores such as peeling and pounding cassava, cooking, and collecting water and firewood. Researchers also accompanied young people during their leisure

time, such as when they strolled and mingled in the village center in the evening, talked with their family over meals, attended choir practice, or, usually
for boys and men only, played soccer, netball, or traditional board games. Over
time, young people in the host household and others that researchers met in the
course of daily activities were befriended, informally interviewed, and accompanied to social settings, such as markets, weekly church services, weddings,
funerals, video shows and *ngoma/**mbina*** (drumming/dancing events), as well
as celebrations related to Christmas, Easter, ***Bulabo*** (the Christian Eucharist
holiday), and *Saba saba* (the July 7th national holiday).

Informants

During the three years of fieldwork, the participant observation researchers
identified a total of 927 informants of various ages. The term "informant"
is used here to mean anyone for whom information was documented; the
amount of information varied from very brief (for example, someone was
seen playing cards) to detailed and lengthy. In the villages which were only
visited by one researcher in 1999, information was not collected on whether
informants were also *MEMA kwa Vijana* trial participants. In the remaining
six villages, 118 of the informants were trial participants.

   Most informants were aged between 14 and 25 years. Fieldworkers tried
to engage with as wide a range of young people in each village as possible,
by intentionally getting to know different networks, both formal (such as
different religious groups) and informal (such as groups with "respectable"
or "badly behaved" reputations). However, the research priority was to
build trusting relationships with teenagers, particularly *MEMA kwa Vijana*
trial participants, and in some situations this meant discouraging other relationships from becoming too close or too public. For example, the female
graduate researcher was old enough that she might have easily developed
close, peer-like relationships with the parents of her teenage informants,
but she specifically tried to avoid this because she felt it might inhibit those
informants from confiding in her. In another example, upon returning to one
village the male graduate researcher learned that two young men associated
with his host household had developed negative reputations as womanizers.
To avoid developing a similar reputation by association, he reduced his public contact with them. Sometimes adolescents did not associate with each
other or disliked each other, such as children in a religious host family who
disapproved of young people who attended video shows. In such instances,
researchers tried to be diplomatic in meeting different individuals at different times, and being polite and respectful of all of them. If questioned about
perceived alliances, fieldworkers explained that they needed to get to know

as many different kinds of young people as possible in order to do their work well, while also stressing that anything anyone told them was confidential.

Pairs of researchers often lived several kilometers apart from one another, and developed distinct and only occasionally overlapping informant lists. For a given visit, each researcher typically had twelve to fifteen key informants with whom they spent a great deal of time and discussed adolescent sexual heath issues in depth. This usually included several household members, several other adolescent *MEMA kwa Vijana* trial participants, several single or married young adults in their late teens or 20s, and several 30–60-year-old villagers who engaged in activities of interest such as health services, traditional medicine, and teaching. Most of these people continued to be key informants in subsequent visits when new key informant relationships were also developed.

In the early years of participant observation, it was sometimes difficult for researchers to spend much time with *MEMA kwa Vijana* trial participants other than those in their host household, because many trial participants were still in primary school during the day. Even when they were out of school, it was not always easy to establish close relationships with them since it was unusual for people in their twenties to seek out youths of the same sex who were five to ten years younger to socialize with them. In addition, social division of the sexes was strongly established in rural areas. When researchers attempted to engage with the opposite sex, this was often interpreted as a kind of sexual negotiation. Researchers thus mainly spent time with older, out-of-school youth of the same sex, although they established relationships with trial participants whenever possible.

Data Collection and Recording

Participant observation data collection was guided by a detailed list of research topics. This guideline addressed broad aspects of village life, such as main economic activities, social divisions, kinship relations and illness treatment beliefs and practices. It also focused on young people's social lives, such as youth interactions while working within *rika* (youth peer groups), carrying out chores, or attending sport, video or *ngoma* events. It additionally addressed characteristics of youth sexual culture, such as how young people negotiated sexual encounters, or managed ongoing sexual relationships.

Researchers collected sexual behavior data in multiple ways. The following examples were listed by the female graduate researcher after one visit:

> I accompanied my host family members to the paddy field to harvest rice. Two of the daughters were members of the church choir, so they sometimes invited fellow choir members to assist them harvesting rice. While with that group

comprised of both sexes, I was able to observe how they relate to each other in public. I also assisted some of my informants to harvest cotton, where I learned they were free to talk about sex and other topics with fellow girls, but they would never mention a word of such topics in the presence of their parents. I went along with several of my informants to get water and had informal conversations about their lives. When I went to the herding fields with one of my informants, I learned from her about sexual activities which take place there, and I was also able to observe other people who come to herd. . . . By visiting the girls and their visiting me, opportunities arose that enabled us to discuss their sexual lives. When it was difficult to talk about their personal issues due to the presence of other family members, we went for a walk. . . . I also accompanied different girls to the local market, the nearest village center, and the large market three hours walk away, where they went on errands or for a stroll. While with them I observed different men try to seduce them. I also saw male vendors try to seduce the girls when they went to purchase a certain item from them. While at the large market, I too was approached by three different men who tried to seduce me. . . . I also attended ***Bulabo*** and *Saba saba* celebrations . . . where youth hang out until dusk and meet other youth from neighboring villages. They strolled up and down the market and asked one another for "*Halleluya*" gifts [money a boy/man gives a girl/woman on a holiday that is typically reciprocated with sex later]. [PO-00-C-3-2f]

Each researcher frequently witnessed couples discussing plans to meet for sex later, or an intermediary negotiating sex for a third person. Researchers were also sometimes present when young people prepared for, or returned from, sexual encounters. For example, in some villages, female researchers shared a room and a mattress with young women who snuck out of the house late at night to meet boys or men for sex at a prearranged times. Similarly, researchers observed young men within their households preparing for clandestine sexual encounters at night, such as when a young man explained that he carried a mat with him each evening to use when having sex in fields.

At all times, researchers carried a small notebook so that they could discreetly jot down notes soon after an event or a discussion of interest. These jottings facilitated recall and accuracy when researchers wrote lengthier notes in a larger notebook each day for one to two hours. These field notes were entered as a series of short segments identified by number, codename of person, place, date, and time. Several measures were taken to prevent villagers reading confidential information in these notebooks: confidential codes were used in place of informant names; the researcher always kept the master code list on him/her; the notebooks were locked inside a suitcase when not in use; and the graduate researchers wrote in English, a language that was rarely spoken or understood in rural Mwanza. Sukuma researchers instead wrote their participant observation field notes in Swahili.

Researchers conducted five Swahili and three Sukuma group discussions during participant observation visits, as well as sixteen Swahili and seven Sukuma formal individual interviews. For some of these, informants agreed to be audio-recorded. Informants usually spoke much less freely in the formal, recorded interviews than they did in informal discussions. The resultant cassette tapes were locked in the suitcase during field work.

Researchers did not take photographs during the first eighteen months of participant observation because of the possibility that this might draw undue attention to them. At the time, cameras of any kind were rare in rural Mwanza. During the last eighteen months of research, however, each pair of participant observation researchers carried one 35 mm camera with them, which they occasionally used to document typical aspects of village life. When not in a public setting, researchers requested verbal permission of their subjects before taking photographs. They offered to send a copy of photographs back to those subjects after the field work ended, and most people requested this. Fieldworkers were discreet in their photography, and during their two-month participant observation visits each pair of researchers only took forty photographs on average.

Each two-month participant observation visit included a day-long debriefing meeting in Mwanza City with the research coordinator and other field researchers mid-way through and immediately after the participant observation ended. After each visit was completed, field researchers also wrote a summary report in English or Swahili, and compiled a list of all informants mentioned in their field notebooks, with a twenty-five-word profile of each. These meetings and reports were used to assess the research process, identify and resolve problems that had arisen, evaluate the nature and quality of the data already collected, and revise the approach to subsequent data collection accordingly.

A saturation approach was employed for collection of data on general topics. For example, if sufficient socio-demographic information had been collected about a village on a previous visit, researchers did not seek out or record additional socio-demographic data in subsequent visits unless important changes occurred. In contrast, researchers attempted to document all observations or discussions related to reproductive and sexual health and behavior throughout their participant observation research, including any mention of *MEMA kwa Vijana* or other sexual health interventions.

Problematic Perceptions of Researchers

Generally the participant observation research proceeded smoothly and the researchers developed friendly and pleasant relationships with villagers.

Sometimes villagers initially misunderstood the fieldworkers' relationship, research, or affiliation, such as when a research pair was assumed to be married, or they were mistaken to be health care providers or *MEMA kwa Vijana* trial survey staff. When such misunderstandings were voiced, fieldworkers were usually able to quickly correct them. Occasionally, fieldworkers encountered more serious problems in how they were perceived or treated in the field. The two most important examples are described below.

The graduate researchers visited the first two participant observation villages (5 and 6) alone in 1999, before the Sukuma researchers had been hired. In order not to draw attention to themselves, the researchers arrived using public transportation and brought a minimal amount of gear, including a kerosene lamp, an insecticide-treated mosquito net, notebooks, and a lockable suitcase. However, this informal entrance proved confusing and even suspicious for some villagers, who had only known development and research staff to arrive in project vehicles. Villages 5 and 6 were large, multiethnic fishing villages with sizeable trade centers. Illegal activity such as theft, production of bootleg alcohol, and bribery of government representatives were fairly common, and sometimes led to police raids. Some of the villagers thus suspected that the researchers were government or police spies, particularly after a police raid occurred in the female graduate researcher's village during her visit. The fieldworkers could refute such suspicions when they were voiced openly, but often they heard of distrust second- or third-hand, and found it more difficult to address. In his summary report, the male graduate researcher elaborated on this:

> The exact dimension of the problems and barriers caused by this perception cannot be known for sure. This is partly due to the practice that people do not face you and state any doubts they have about you, but they ask the people they see are close to you. I got a sense of the constraints caused by these rumors when I started doing formal interviews and found them somehow frustrated. Even the one I did with an informant who was very close to me was awkward. [PO-99-I-6-1m]

To prevent a similar occurrence in subsequent participant observation visits, researchers arrived in a HALIRA Project vehicle, worked in pairs with at least one Sukuma speaker, and arranged formal, public introductions very soon after their arrival. In other villages, researchers occasionally learned that isolated individuals (particularly those involved in illegal activities) were suspicious that the researchers might be investigating crime, but this rarely seemed a broader concern and usually was easily resolved with direct discussion. In fact, when two Sukuma researchers later conducted participant observation in a similar multiethnic fishing village (7) most residents seemed quite disinterested in their arrival and work, specifically because those villagers were accustomed to a variety of people traveling through the village for different purposes.

The second example of problematic interactions in the field occurred when villagers aggressively pursued sexual relationships with fieldworkers. Each researcher had multiple experiences of villagers of the opposite sex trying to negotiate sex with them. This was relatively infrequent and indirect for male researchers, usually involving young women trying to enlist female researchers or other villagers as intermediaries to arrange a sexual rendezvous. In contrast, in most villages each female researcher experienced many direct and indirect approaches from different men to seduce them. These rarely seemed to relate to the researchers' study of sexual behavior, but were instead an expected part of normal life amongst young people in villages. It is however possible that the researchers were perceived as particularly desirable sexual partners because they were new to the village, urban, and relatively affluent.

Researchers generally had little difficulty fending off such proposals, but occasionally a villager was persistent and an intervention was needed. During one participant observation visit, for example, a young man in a host household employed multiple strategies while pursuing a sexual relationship with a female researcher, including declaring to her and others that he wanted to marry her, ignoring her clear refusal to have a sexual relationship, repeatedly refusing to leave her bedroom until late at night, entering her room as she slept, moving his belongings into that room, and napping on her mattress during the day. When she appealed to the heads of her household, they agreed to ask the young man to stop, but the behavior continued. She then arranged a formal household meeting to discuss the issue with the male researcher present. This went well and afterwards the heads of household supported her more strongly, and the young man left her alone.

Researcher Health and Safety

Participant observation researchers' health and safety were a great concern because fieldwork living conditions were often harsh and there was little privacy. HALIRA paid for routine medical examinations and appropriate vaccinations (e.g., rabies) and treatments (e.g., schistosomiasis), but this was not sufficient to fully protect the researchers' health. As already discussed, in early participant observation visits researchers brought very few supplies with them. During those visits, all of the researchers suffered water-, sanitation- and/or mosquito-borne infections, in some villages they were very hungry for much of their stay, and individual researchers encountered problems with bedbugs, lice, leeches, snakes, and scorpions. The researchers' welfare was a higher priority than their conspicuousness in the villages, so with each new participant observation visit they brought additional materials to address newly identified problems, often sharing those resources with their host families. By the third year, their fieldwork supplies included a water filter, water purification tablets, antiseptics and sterilizers, sugar tablets, emergency food supplies, insecticides, a mattress, bedding, pepper spray, rubber boots, a local snake bite identification and treatment book, a first aid kit, medications for common conditions (e.g., pain relief, allergies, diarrhea, worms, malaria), and copies of *Where There is No Doctor* (Werner, Thuman, and Maxwell 1992) and *A Comprehensive Guide to Wilderness and Travel Medicine* (Weiss 1998), almost all of which were luxury items in village households.

The extent to which researchers used these items varied between households. For example, female household members were responsible for the household's water and in some homes they routinely boiled it for drinking, while in some they offered to boil and filter it specifically for a resident male researcher. In other households, however, this was not done, or the female researcher was expected to do it for herself. This was challenging given other commitments, so in those cases the researchers used purification tablets and then filtered the water.

Pepper spray was only added to supplies after a drunken man threatened to rape one of the female Sukuma researchers when she was alone with two 3–4-year-old children in her host's house. Her account follows:

> In the morning while I was writing field notes the children came into my room and said, "A drunken man is coming." Then I heard his voice calling from the front door, and I could tell he had been drinking alcohol. Suddenly he was at the door of my room and he began saying, "I have come to rape you" in Sukuma. I grabbed a heavy iron that is used to pound grains. After seeing that, he asked if we had any beer that we could give to him. We told him that there was no beer, and he left. [PO-00-I-4-4f]

Fortunately, the researcher escaped that encounter without physical harm, but her experience highlighted the fieldworkers' vulnerability. Male researchers also felt vulnerable to violence during nighttime events at which drunkenness was common. Researchers were instructed to avoid situations which might be dangerous, but this could not always be predicted. Researchers thus began to carry pepper spray discreetly, to use only as a last resort if they could not otherwise escape a dangerous situation. In fact, pepper spray was only used once, when a male researcher lay down on his mattress on the floor to sleep one night, and a spitting cobra rose up beside his head. He quickly used the pepper spray to disorient the snake, and soon afterwards he arranged for a door to be built for the family's home to reduce the chance of a snake entering again.

Researchers occasionally paid for minor materials or construction such as this when it resolved a specific concern they had about their safety, hygiene, or privacy. Other examples include having a pit toilet dug for a household that had no toilet, having a blind built to screen outdoor bathing, or placing a plastic tarp on the ceiling over a mattress to reduce leakage during rains. Researchers were encouraged to be assertive so that their basic needs were met, even if this went against normal practices in the household. For example, some families did not have their first meal until 3:00 p.m., and those meals were very simple and particularly small for females. Some researchers resolved their hunger in such situations by buying an earlier meal in the village center.

The emotional challenge of living in harsh conditions with very little privacy also needs to be acknowledged in any discussion of researcher health and safety. This study preceded the widespread use of cell phones in sub-Saharan Africa, so participant observation researchers usually spent several weeks in rural areas with little or no contact with anyone in their personal or professional support networks. Anticipating that this might be challenging, researchers were strongly encouraged to reflect upon their experiences and to work through difficult feelings they might experience in personal diaries. These were purchased expressly for their private use and were not read by any colleagues. The researchers later reported that they did indeed use their diaries for this purpose and found them helpful. Importantly, researcher isolation was greatly reduced when they started visiting villages in pairs after the first few participant observation visits. All of the researchers were grateful to have a colleague nearby, particularly when they encountered challenges during fieldwork.

IN-DEPTH INTERVIEWS

An in-depth interview usually involves an interviewer asking a respondent a series of open-ended questions based on a broad topic guideline. The interviewer tries to create an intimate and trusting setting during the interview, encouraging the respondent to carefully reflect and honestly answer questions even if they address sensitive or difficult topics. The respondent is encouraged to describe their particular world view in their own terms. The semi-structured nature of this approach allows respondents to raise unanticipated issues within a topic, which can then be explored in-depth (Smith and Morrow 1996; Price and Hawkins 2002). As discussed in chapter 1, in-depth interview findings are generally considered to be less representative but more accurate and meaningful than survey interviews (Parker, Herdt, and Carballo 1991; Konings et al. 1995; Smith and Morrow 1996; Messersmith et al. 2000; Larsen and Hollos 2003).

Interview Guide and Protocol Development

The HALIRA interview guides were initially drafted in English, translated into Swahili and Sukuma, back-translated into English, and then edited to promote conceptual equivalence in all three languages. They were further modified based on pilot study findings and tailored to the specific interview series. Pilot interviews were conducted from April to September 1999, both to train researchers and to improve the interview schedule and protocol. These interviews were conducted with twenty-six *MEMA kwa Vijana* trial participants randomly selected from a range of schools. An additional fourteen pilot interviews were conducted with other rural youth, teachers, and village authorities.

In the course of the pilot interviews, some problems were identified. First, some respondents spoke little or no Swahili, even though they were in the upper years of Swahili language primary schools. This highlighted the need for Sukuma-speaking interviewers. Second, some respondents had substantial difficulty clearly recalling an earlier age (e.g., age at first sex), the timing of events (e.g., first sex with different partners), or estimating accurate summaries or frequencies (e.g., number of partners). This led to a new technique to help clarify reports. If a respondent mentioned a sexual partner, the researcher might do a simple sketch of that individual with one or two identifying characteristics, such as shirt color, a fish (for fishermen), or a book (for school boys). A sequence of partners could then be drawn and referred to throughout the interview. This process allowed for revisions. For example, if the respondent corrected herself to report a partner prior to the first one mentioned, the new one would be added at the beginning of the series of drawings, or the order of partners could be rearranged. While this technique seemed to improve the accuracy of some reports, inconsistencies in estimated age and the other variables mentioned above continued to be a great problem in all of the research methods used in the study, as is illustrated by box 2.1. The problem of frequent large errors in age-related data has also been documented in other studies which have scrutinized age estimates in sub-Saharan Africa (Cohen 1998; Żaba et al. 2009).

BOX 2.1. ESTIMATING AGE AND TIME PERIODS

Inconsistent estimates of age, school year, and calendar year were a common problem for data collection in all research methods used in this study. For example, there were frequent differences between the pupil ages listed in school registries and the ages pupils reported during enrolment for the *MEMA kwa Vijana* trial. Reported age for both males and females was usually higher, and increased with the age of the pupil, with an average difference of 3 months at age 13 years, rising to 15 months at age 16 years (Todd et al. 2004). Reported age was what was used in all trial analyses.

In general, math skills were very rudimentary in rural areas, and birthdates and absolute ages were not concepts that villagers often thought about or valued. As the anthropologists Wijsen and Tanner (2002, 29–31) noted:

> Sukuma society is not based on clocks and calendars. . . . As time is not built into their thinking as a necessary foundation for statements, the Su-kuma's sense of time is very elastic. . . . Thus it is necessary to examine how they treat different events which occur in sequence.

In our study, for example, a few in-depth interview respondents said that they did not know their month or year of birth, or how old they were. Also, individuals often provided substantially different estimates of the timing of an event within and between interviews. It was not unusual for this to involve inconsistencies of two or more years, even within a recent time period. Below we will draw upon excerpts from two interviews conducted with a young man named Makoye to illustrate these common inconsistencies.

During the first *MEMA kwa Vijana* survey in late 1998, Makoye reported that he was 16 years old and in Year 5, which was consistent with his report in his first in-depth interview on March 2, 2000, that he was born in 1982 and was 18 years old and in Year 7. In his second in-depth interview with the same interviewer on March 3, 2002, Makoye said that he was 20 years old at the beginning of the interview, but he referred to himself as 21 years old later in the interview. He consistently reported that he had repeated Year 4 in school, which would have meant that he was both 14 and 15 during the two years when he was in Year 4.

(continued)

Makoye's estimates about the timing of his sexual relationships were more difficult to interpret. In his first interview, he reported that the first time he had sex he was in his first year of Year 4, suggesting that he had been 14 years old. In his second interview he instead reported that he first had sex in his second year of Year 4, suggesting that he had been 15 years old. However, in the course of the two interviews he sometimes referred to himself as having been 12, 13, 16, or 17 years of age when describing that same, first sexual encounter. For example, in his first interview:

I: How old were you when you first had sex?

R: Twelve years old.

I: Twelve?

R: Yes.

I: And what was your class year?

R: I was in Year . . . I was still in Year . . . in Year 4.

I: Year 4?

R: Yes.

I: Mh, before you repeated, or after you had repeated?

R: Before I repeated. [II-00-I-75-m]

And in his second interview two years later:

I: In which class were you [the first time you had sex]?

R: I was in Year 4 when I had sex for the first time.

I: Year 4?

R: Yes. . . .

I: Was it the first time you were in Year 4, or the second?

R: The second. . . .

I: How old were you?

R: At that time I was about 16 or 17 years old.

I: About 16 or 17 years old?

R: Yes. [II-02-I-275-m]

(*continued*)

Makoye's estimates involving earlier calendar years were similarly confusing. For example, he and the researcher had the following exchange in 2002, during his second interview:

I: Can you remember what year it was when you had sex for the first time?

R: It was last year, 2001, there in my village.

I: That was when you had sex for the first time?

R: Yes.

I: You didn't have sex before that time?

R: I had sex another time in the year 2000.

I: 2000?

R: Yes.

I: And another time before that?

R: I didn't have another lover. . . .

I: But when we spoke in 1999, I remember that you told me that you had already experienced sex?

R: 1999?

I: Do you remember that you had already started? Or how was it?

R: It is true that in 1999 I had started.

I: In which class were you?

R: I was in Year 4 the first time I had sex.

I: In Year 4. It was which year, ninety-what?

R: It was in ninety- . . . [long pause]

I: In the year 2000, you were in Year 7?

R: Yes.

I: So in 1999, you were in Year 6?

R: Yes . . . and in 1997 I was in Year 5, so I first had sex in 1996. [II-02-I-275-m]

Even after this long process of clarification, Makoye missed one year (1998) in his final calculation. It is possible that Makoye was not fully

(continued)

engaged in the interview, so he did not pause to reflect accurately until he was questioned closely, or that he intentionally wished to mislead the interviewer by reporting a more recent sexual debut. In fact, it was not unusual for in-depth interview respondents (particularly females) to report a later age and school year of first sexual experience in the second series of interviews than they had reported in the first. This inconsistency tended to go in one direction, suggesting it involved recall and/or social desirability biases. In addition, however, Makoye's inconsistencies seemed to reflect a pronounced—but not uncommon—difficulty in accurately calculating time in terms of absolute age and calendar years.

Respondent Selection

After completion of the 26 pilot in-depth interviews with *MEMA kwa Vijana* trial participants, HALIRA researchers conducted a total of 161 formal interviews with 92 other trial participants (table 2.2). This included 73 interviews in 1999–2000, 69 interviews with those same respondents or a family member again in 2002, and 19 additional interviews with different trial participants in 2002. In-depth interview respondents were drawn from all *MEMA kwa Vijana* trial communities. Most respondents were randomly selected from the general population, but some were selected because they were pregnant or they had a preliminary HIV-positive test result. To reduce the possibility of bias, interviewers did not know the reason why any in-depth interview respondent was selected. The selection process is described in detail below, after a description of testing and treatment for sexually transmitted infections within the *MEMA kwa Vijana* trial surveys.

In the first of the *MEMA kwa Vijana* surveys in 1998, trial participants who were 14 years old or older were asked to provide urine samples which were subsequently tested for HIV, Chlamydia, gonorrhea, and for females, pregnancy. An intravenous blood test would have enabled more rigorous HIV testing, but this procedure was considered too invasive for the young study population. In a second survey 18 months later, participants provided urine specimens and finger-prick blood specimens, while in a third survey 18 months after that they provided urine, intravenous blood, and (for females) vaginal secretion specimens, the latter collected by self-administered swab. The later survey specimens were tested for HIV, herpes, Chlamydia, gonorrhea, syphilis, Trichomonas, and/or pregnancy. In each survey, trial participants also saw a clinician who asked him or her about signs and symptoms of illness, and treated those with a suspected sexually transmitted infection and/

Table 2.2.   In-Depth Interviews with *Mema kwa Vijana* Trial Participants, by Series, Selection Status, and Sex

Year	Interview Series	Number of Respondents Interviewed					
		Randomly Selected*		Confirmed HIV-positive		Pregnant in 1998	
		Male	Female	Male	Female	Female	Total
1999	Pilot	13	13	0	0	0	26
1999–2000	Series 1	29	34	2	5	3	73
(2002)	(Series 2)**	(29)	(33)	(1)***	(3)***	(3)	(69)
2002	Series 3	4	9	1	5	0	19
1999–2002	Total	46	56	3	10	3	118

   *Randomly selected respondents in the three series are defined as: (1) pairs randomly selected from the same class in a school that had no HIV-positive trial participants (n = 27); (2) individuals randomly selected from the same school and class as a trial participant who had a preliminary positive HIV or pregnancy test result (n = 33); and (3) respondents who were selected for interview because of a preliminary HIV-positive result, but who subsequently were confirmed to be HIV-negative through a series of later tests (n = 16).

   **The second interview series involved re-interviewing all respondents from the first series who could be located and who agreed to participate.

   ***Two HIV-positive respondents from the first interview series died before the second series took place. Two semi-structured interviews were instead conducted with a guardian or parent for each of them.

or schistosomiasis. After each survey, participants whose specimens tested positive for a curable sexually transmitted infection were visited and treated at a later date.

In all surveys, participants were asked if they wanted to know their HIV status, and those who did received pre-test counseling and had a separate intravenous blood specimen drawn and sent to Mwanza City for testing according to the national guidelines at the time of that survey. Those individuals received their HIV test results from a counselor locally within six weeks. Trial participants were not informed of their HIV status based on their preliminary survey test results, because those tests had a higher rate of false positives than the tests used for voluntary counseling and testing services. For example, of the 9,283 trial participants who provided urine specimens for HIV testing in the 1998 survey, 23 had preliminary HIV-positive test results (Todd et al. 2004). However, later testing of those specimens and/or other specimens provided at later surveys determined that only eight of those 23 were in fact truly HIV-positive (Plummer, Ross et al. 2004). To have 15 false positive results in a sample of 9,283 individuals suggests that the urine HIV test had a greater than 99.9 percent specificity, which is the ability to identify people who are truly negative. While this is considered a very high level of accuracy for population-based research, the possibility of receiving a false positive result was unacceptable at an individual level, so no trial participants received HIV results based on those tests.

The first series of HALIRA in-depth interviews took place in 1999–2000. These involved pregnant, HIV-positive and randomly selected pupils. One percent (32/4149) of the female participants in the 1998 survey tested positive for pregnancy, and three of them were randomly selected for this interview series. Twenty of the 23 participants who had preliminary HIV-positive results were also randomly selected for interviews, of whom 7 (2 males and 5 females) were eventually determined to be truly HIV-positive (table 2.2).

During analysis and in this book, those respondents who were initially selected because of an HIV-positive test result, but who later were confirmed to be HIV-negative, are included with those who were randomly selected from the general population. Specifically, in the first series of in-depth interviews, respondents were considered to be "randomly selected" from the general population if they were selected in one of three ways: (a) pairs randomly selected from the same class in a school that had no HIV-positive trial participants in 1998 (n = 27); (b) one individual randomly selected from the same school and class as each trial participant who had a preliminary positive HIV or pregnancy test result in 1998 (n = 23); and (c) respondents who were selected for interview because of a preliminary HIV-positive result in 1998, but who subsequently were confirmed to be HIV-negative through a series of later tests (n = 13) (table 2.2).

In that first interview series, most respondents were found at school and the remainder in their homes. Of the 74 individuals who were initially selected, eight of those who were randomly selected were either not found (7) or refused to participate (1), resulting in 89 percent compliance. Randomly selected alternates were used for seven of the eight missing people; the eighth alternate was excluded after he was found to be using another child's name in school.

The second series of in-depth interviews involved reinterviewing respondents from the first series (table 2.2). In the 2 to 2½ year interim, most respondents had left primary school and had begun their lives as independent adults. This included some who had married and moved to another village (mostly women), and some who were working in occupations that involved travel, such as fishing, mining, or trade (mostly men). Field researchers made intensive efforts to interview every original respondent, to minimize the chance that particular types of individuals might be excluded from repeat interviews. One randomly selected woman refused to be reinterviewed, one HIV-positive woman could not be located, and two HIV-positive youths (one male, one female) had died. In the event that a respondent had died, researchers then interviewed a close family member using a special interview guide.

For the third series of in-depth interviews, respondents were selected based on their preliminary HIV test results from the 2001–2002 survey at the end of the trial (table 2.2). At the time of selection, 26 (3 male and 23 female) survey participants had results which suggested they had become HIV-positive since the 1998 survey. All three of those males and seven of the females were randomly selected for in-depth interviews. An additional three males and seven females were randomly selected for interview from the same school and class lists as those respondents. However, one of the HIV-positive men could not be located for interview. In addition, one man and two women in this series with preliminary HIV-positive results were ultimately found to be HIV-negative after later testing, so only 6 of the 19 people interviewed in this series were truly HIV-positive.

Final, confirmatory HIV test results were not available until approximately one year after all fieldwork ended. At that time HALIRA staff learned that, of the total of 29 respondents who had been selected for one of the interview series because they had a preliminary HIV-positive test result, only 13 (45 percent) were truly HIV-positive.

Interview Content and Process

For the first two series of in-depth interviews, researchers travelled in same-sex pairs of one graduate researcher and one Sukuma researcher. For the third series, one male and one female Sukuma researcher travelled independently. Verbal consent was obtained from all respondents prior to interviews, and again immediately prior to the use of a tape recorder. For respondents who were still in school and/or living with their parents, verbal consent was also obtained from a head teacher and/or a parent.

The interviewers tried to spend one to two hours building rapport with respondents prior to interviews, taking walks with them, playing games, telling jokes, and sharing a snack with them. In the first and second series of interviews the research pairs did this with their two respondents together, which allowed them to identify which youth might most benefit from being interviewed in Sukuma. There was no occasion when both youths said that they would be unable or uncomfortable participating in an interview in Swahili, which would have required recruiting another randomly selected, Swahili-speaking youth. In the first series, 45 (62 percent) interviews were conducted in Swahili, and 28 (38 percent) in Sukuma, compared to 46 (67 percent) in Swahili and 23 (33 percent) in Sukuma with the same respondents in the second series. In the third series, the Sukuma researchers conducted 9 (47 percent) interviews in Swahili and 10 (53 percent) in Sukuma with the new set of respondents.

Interviews were conducted away from home, school, and work settings, usually in an isolated, outdoor, shaded area where there was little chance of interruption or eavesdropping by passers-by. They usually took two hours. Respondents were first asked general background questions about their home life, family, school experiences, friendships, and paid and unpaid work. They were then asked their opinions about young people being sexually active, and about their own sexual experiences. Young people who reported they had never had sex were asked about their attitudes and decisions related to this. In the first series of interviews, respondents who reported experience of sex were then asked in-depth questions about their first sexual experience, including the circumstances that led up to it, how it was negotiated, character-istics of their partner, and the nature of any ongoing sexual relationship that resulted from it. They were also asked about other partners, and to estimate their total number of partners and sexual encounters. However, discussion of these topics was sometimes constrained by limited time. The latter part of the interview usually focused on respondent opinions and experience of preg-nancy, contraception (including condom use), abortion, circumcision, health care, and HIV/AIDS, and other sexually transmitted infections.

The second and third series of interviews addressed many of the same topics that were discussed in the first. New questions included those related to the respondents' older age and experience, such as end of primary school, start of secondary school, work, marriage, and/or children. These interviews did not focus on first sexual experience, unless respondents had reported never having had sex in their first interviews. Respondents were instead asked to describe the circumstances surrounding their last sexual experience. They were also asked questions to elicit information on broader behavior pat-terns, such as their experience of one-off encounters and concurrent partner-ships. For intervention participants, the final portion of the interviews focused on their experience of the *MEMA kwa Vijana* intervention.

Many in-depth interviews were awkward and respondents reticent, only answering questions with a few words and rarely making expansive con-tributions, particularly in the first interview series when respondents were still primary school pupils. These interviews rarely functioned as qualitative research is intended to, allowing respondents to describe their world from their own perspectives and not according to a structure and themes imposed by the researcher. Much of these interviews was devoted to establishing basic information, such as whether a respondent had ever had sex, and then to un-derstanding the circumstances surrounding his or her first sexual experience or relationship. Attempts to ascertain broader sexual behavior patterns were often superficial. Reports about frequency of sex or total number of partners sometimes changed within the course of the interview. In-depth interview respondents' reluctance to talk probably related to multiple factors, including: rarely, if ever, having been interviewed or asked to describe their lives in narrative form; the status difference between themselves and their interviewers; lack of trust in research confidentiality, particularly amongst school pupils; and for young women, the importance of discretion given stigma associated with premarital or extramarital sexual activity.

For a total of eleven pilot in-depth interviews or in-depth interviews in the first formal series, respondents were asked if they would like to identify a close, same-sex friend to participate in the interview with them. Paired interviews were attempted to see if young people were more comfortable or honest talking about sensitive issues in the company of a close friend. This seemed to be effective in a few cases in which truly close friends were selected, as respondents seemed to relax and openly discuss sensitive issues that they had already shared with one another. In a number of interviews, however, researchers found the respondent selected someone who was only a casual friend, and this did not become clear until the interview was well underway. Such paired interviews became uncomfortable when the respondents were asked about sexual behavior. Given the difficulty of identifying close friends in advance of the interview, this paired interview approach was rejected.

All interviews were audio-recorded. After each one, field researchers wrote a brief process report, describing their interactions with the respondent before, during, and after the interview, and any unusual events that occurred related to it.

BOX 2.2. COMPARING DATA FOR ONE
INDIVIDUAL ACROSS RESEARCH METHODS*

From 1998–2000 there was only one person in the *MEMA kwa Vijana* trial, Susana, from whom sexual behavior data were collected using five research methods: biological tests, face-to-face questionnaire survey, assisted self-completion questionnaire survey, in-depth interview, and participant observation. Susana was 16 years old and in Year 5 of primary school when she participated in the first surveys in 1998. In those surveys and the subsequent ones 18 months later, she reported that she had never had sex, and she did not test positive for any sexually-transmitted infections or pregnancy.

In between the 1998 and 2000 surveys, a HALIRA researcher conducted a Sukuma in-depth interview with Susana and participant observation in her village soon afterwards. Susana reported having had

(continued)

sex in both her in-depth interview and during participant observation. However, her in-depth interview was awkward, with only rare free-flowing or expansive contributions on her part. In addition, the quality of the information collected in it was poorer than that collected for her in participant observation.

In her in-depth interview, Susana reported that she lived with her grandmother and some of her younger siblings in a mud brick, thatch roofed house. She said that her mother did not live in her village, but her father, his second wife and their child lived there in a separate household, where he brewed and sold local beer. Susana reported that she herself farmed her own cotton and cassava, and that she sold the latter to her father to use in making alcohol for sale. In the dry season, she said she also sold peanuts. Susana reported that she used the money she earned to buy food for her family and her own school supplies, but she hoped to save enough money to buy a bicycle, to make it easier to carry water for domestic use. She reported sharing farming responsibilities within a *rika*, and she said that farming was the only activity that they did together. In her interview, Susana reported that she did not attend local video shows or discos.

During the interview, Susana first denied having ever had sex, but afterwards said she had had one sexual partner only, a Year 5 pupil who farmed cotton and maize and sold sugar cane. Later in the interview, Susana admitted to having had another sex partner, a Year 6 pupil who herded cattle and brewed local beer, but she said that she had only ever had sex with those two partners three times in total. At the very end of the interview, however, Susana mentioned having had sex one time with a third sex partner, a Year 6 pupil who farmed and sold chickens. When asked, she described different aspects of these relationships in detail, such as when a sexual encounter was arranged (en route to fetch water from a well), where they had sexual encounters (at night at the boy's home, or at her home when others were away), and what her partners gave her for a sexual encounter (body lotion or Tshs 500–1,000 ($0.60–1.20), which she used to purchase sandals, body lotion, and a pen).

The interviewer met Susana again three weeks later on the first day of the researcher's participant observation research, because Susana happened to be an immediate neighbor of the researcher's household. During participant observation, the researcher and Susana shared chores

(continued)

and attended activities such as video shows, *ngoma*, and Easter celebrations together. The researcher observed that much of what Susana had reported in the interview about her home life was true, including living with and supporting her grandmother and some of her younger siblings. In addition, the researcher learned that Susana's home life was difficult. On more than one occasion, she observed Susana's grandmother drinking heavily or passed out from drunkenness by the side of the road. The researcher also witnessed a shouting argument between Susana and her grandmother, because Susana had taken money for the family's food which her grandmother had intended for alcohol.

Both the in-depth interview and participant observation data suggest that Susana obtained money and food for her family through a range of farming and small business activities. During participant observation, Susana and others also reported that she exchanged sex for money and materials in order to support her family. While Susana seemed to work hard and to devote much of her earnings to her family, she also used them for entertainment and treats, such as spontaneously buying snacks for her girlfriends, including the researcher. Contrary to what Susana had reported in her interview, her *rika* was also an *ngoma* group, and she participated in public performances as a dancer. In addition, although Susana had denied attending video shows in the interview, she regularly attended them during participant observation.

The participant observation findings also suggest that, in her formal interview, Susana substantially underestimated her total number of sexual partners and the number of times she had ever had sex. During participant observation, Susana reported that she had three ongoing sex partners: Maisha and Kazimili, who were 25-year-old members of her *rika*, and Nasibu, who was about 30 years old and owned a kiosk in the village center. None of these individuals was the same as any of the sexual partners Susana had mentioned in her in-depth interview approximately one month earlier. Excerpts from the researcher's field notes follow:

> Susana said that during the rainy season she farms with her younger brothers and sister. She said she earns money for her personal use by selling tomatoes, and she uses the remainder of the money to buy salt or kerosene, or to grind grain. She said she also gets money by making love with boys, who are Maisha and Kazimili. . . . She said she and her younger siblings are all given body and cooking oils free from her lover,

(continued)

Nasibu. She said Nasibu has promised to marry her after she completes school. She said she had made love with Nasibu eight times right in the house where she lives with her grandmother. She said she sleeps with her sisters, who are still young. She said that in order for them not to tell their grandmother, she gives them sweets or sugar canes. [PO-00-I-4-4f]

Comments to the researcher by Maisha, Kazimili, and Nasibu, and the researcher's observations of Susana's interactions with them, supported Susana's comments during participant observation. In addition to these relationships, the participant observation researcher repeatedly observed Susana engaging in negotiations which young women often had with men to obtain something in exchange for sex—for example, payment to enter a video show, or "*Halleluya*" money given on Christian holidays.

*Material in this box was adapted from: Plummer, M. L., D. A. Ross, D. Wight, J. Changalucha, G. Mshana, J. Wamoyi, J. Todd et al. 2004. 'A bit more truthful': The validity of adolescent sexual behavior data collected in rural northern Tanzania using five methods. *Sexually Transmitted Infections* 80(Supplement 2):ii49–56.

COMPARISON OF SURVEYS, IN-DEPTH INTERVIEWS, AND PARTICIPANT OBSERVATION

A formal comparison of the research methods used in HALIRA and the *MEMA kwa Vijana* trial found that the in-depth interviews produced more valid sexual behavior data than the surveys (Plummer, Ross, et al. 2004). For example, of six female in-depth interview respondents who had sexually transmitted infections in 1998, only one reported ever having had sex in any of the four surveys between 1998 and 2000, while five reported it in their 1999–2000 in-depth interviews. Nonetheless, the in-depth interviews were fraught with inconsistent reports. Box 2.2 summarizes data collected from one young woman to illustrate the relative strengths and weaknesses of the different methods.

Participant observation found there was a powerful culture of secrecy surrounding young people's sexual activity, helping to explain the many inconsistencies seen in the three formal interview methods, and suggesting that sexual behavior findings from those methods may have been serious underestimates, particularly for females. This point is illustrated by an exchange that the Sukuma male researcher witnessed while out walking with two male *MEMA kwa Vijana* trial participants:

> Japhet interrupted Godfrey and told him to be truthful, and not to hide his lovers like he is used to, when the reality is that he is experienced and has many lovers. Godfrey said that at least he is a bit more truthful than Japhet, who, when answering *MEMA kwa Vijana* [survey] questions, said that he had never ever had sex, when he is actually an expert in these matters. Japhet in turn asked Godfrey why even Godfrey had said [in the survey] that he had only had sex once, when he too is an expert and has a child by now. . . . Japhet said that he answered the *MEMA kwa Vijana* questions by claiming he had never had sex even once, because he thought that the teachers might follow-up on those who have lovers and expel them from school. [PO-00-C-3-3m]

GROUP DISCUSSIONS

Group discussions are intended to give study participants more influence over the research process than might occur during individual interviews. Researchers facilitate group discussion in a semi-structured way, using open-ended questions to prompt participants to engage with one another (Bernard 1995; Mack et al. 2005). Ideally, group discussions are more inductive than in-depth interviews, allowing free-flowing informal exchanges that lead to the emergence of new issues which were not previously identified by the researchers (Madriz 2000).

There are essentially two kinds of discussion groups: those composed of strangers and those of preexisting social groups. A possible advantage of group discussions between strangers is that they may not take their fellow participants' views for granted and so may clearly explain their opinions and experiences (Bloor et al. 2001). They may also be more comfortable expressing sensitive views because they do not have existing roles and relationships to maintain with other group members. Groups of existing friends or acquaintances, on the other hand, are less artificial and mirror real life, because participants tend to present themselves to each other in much the same way that they do in everyday life. They also may remind one another of shared experiences, or challenge one another if statements seem inconsistent with their prior knowledge of each other (Bloor et al. 2001).

The HALIRA Project conducted two series of group discussions during the three years of field work. First, discussions were held with intervention school pupils and peer educators in 1999, to address their impressions of the *MEMA kwa Vijana* school curriculum, and particularly peer education. Second, in 2000 a series of discussions were held with same-sex groups of

out-of-school youth to better understand particularly sensitive sexual topics that had been difficult to investigate through other research methods.
All group discussions were audio-recorded, and researchers wrote detailed
summary reports on each series at the end of fieldwork.

Group Discussions with Primary School Pupils

The *MEMA kwa Vijana* primary school curriculum included a training course
for pupil peer educators, who were taught to perform scripted dramas and otherwise support the teacher-led curriculum in class. Pupils from two schools in
each of the four study districts were randomly selected for one peer educator
and one general pupil group discussion (figure 2.1). In total, four male and four
female group discussions were held with six to eight pupils or peer educators,
sampling pupils in each year of the curriculum (Years 5–7). Head teachers and
pupils gave verbal consent for the group discussions. Same-sex pairs of one
graduate researcher and one Sukuma researcher led each discussion, following a semi-structured question guide. Pupils were provided with a snack and
chatted with researchers for 5–10 minutes before discussions, which were held
away from the school, usually outdoors or in an empty building. The discussions were planned and implemented in collaboration with the *MEMA kwa
Vijana* intervention staff, as part of their ongoing, internal process evaluation.

All pupils were asked about material covered in their *MEMA kwa Vijana*
classes (such as the content of what they had learned; what they liked or
disliked; what was clear or confusing); how they felt about teachers teaching
them sexual health information; and their perceptions of the peer educators'
role and the dramas themselves. The peer educators were additionally asked
about any benefits or challenges of being a peer educator, including skills
development and personal behavior.

These discussions generated some useful information about the pupils'
experiences and perceptions of the intervention, but they did not flow easily,
and the researchers found it difficult to facilitate an open dialogue between
participants. Rather than participants discussing topics between themselves,
these sessions were effectively group interviews in which the researcher
asked questions which specific individuals answered in turn.

Group Discussions and In-Depth Interviews with Young Adults

Following the first year of fieldwork, a series of 3–4 discussions and follow-
up in-depth interviews were conducted with each of six groups of out-of-
school young people, to explore sensitive sexual topics which had been particularly difficult to investigate through participant observation or in-depth
interviews. Generally, group discussions are used to examine broad social

norms, not intimate, personal experiences, or sensitive behaviors (Madriz 2000; Mack et al. 2005). This sub-study was thus designed so that general opinions would be explored in group discussions and salient issues that warranted further, private exploration, could be followed-up through individual interviews with participants afterwards.

Three villages were selected to represent different types of rural settings: multiethnic lakeside fishing/farming, multiethnic interior farmland near a mine, and almost entirely Sukuma interior farmland (figure 2.1). The team of four researchers spent one week in each village. During the first few days they developed rapport with young villagers in public areas, such as markets and sports fields. The researchers tried to select and recruit preexisting same-sex groups of friends for discussions, in order to maximize group participants' confidence in discussing sensitive issues amongst themselves, and to minimize the artificiality of the interaction. Over the final two or three days, same-sex researchers then facilitated three to four two-hour discussions with a male and a female group on the following topics.

The first discussion explored girls' motives for sex, including affection, pleasure, coercion, and a desire or need for gifts or money. The second discussion investigated beliefs and practices related to pregnancy prevention, suspended pregnancy (a widely reported belief during participant observation), and induced abortion. The third discussion addressed the range, frequency, and contexts of specific sexual practices, including intentional lubrication or drying of the vagina; foreplay; vaginal intercourse; anal intercourse; oral sex on a man or a woman; male and female homosexuality; and masturbation. The fourth discussion examined condom use and beliefs about the causes and treatment of sexually transmitted infections.

The groups consisted of nine to twelve young people aged 15 to 27 years, with mean group ages of 18–21 years. In two villages, the female groups were mainly single young women engaged in petty trading or farming, while in the third village they were mainly primary school girls or recent primary school leavers. Most of the male respondents were farmers, fishermen, or cattle herders, although some petty traders and primary and secondary school students also participated. After each discussion, facilitators held 15–30-minute individual in-depth interviews with two to three participants. These interviews were fairly brief and unstructured and focused on one or two specific topics which had arisen during the group discussion. In total, 21 discussions and 50 follow-up interviews were conducted.

The group discussions with young adults generally proceeded very well. Participants usually entered into lively discussions, and respectfully questioned and challenged each other based on their mutual familiarity. The facilitators were generally able to curtail individuals who dominated discussions by re-directing questions to less talkative members, and they sometimes interviewed those individuals afterwards. Overall, this set of discussions was very effective in collecting information on highly stigmatized practices (such as anal intercourse), even when they were infrequent or illegal (such as induced abortion).

Three innovative aspects of this group discussion protocol contributed to its success. First, the two or three days that researchers spent socializing with young people was very useful in identifying friendship groups and in building a trusting rapport before the formal research began. Second, conducting individual in-depth interviews immediately after the group discussions enabled researchers to follow-up on salient, personal information that could not be satisfactorily explored in the discussion. These interviews also allowed participants to explain themselves further in private, after the researchers had already demonstrated that they were sympathetic and nonjudgmental. Third, having three to four discussions with the same groups allowed confidence and mutual respect within a group to develop incrementally. It also provided opportunities for respondents to build and expand upon comments made in earlier discussions when new, relevant topics came up, allowing for more complex explanations.

SIMULATED PATIENT EXERCISES

In simulated patient (also called "mystery client" or "dummy patient") exercises, trained local community members visit health facilities in the assumed role of clients, and then report on their experiences to researchers afterwards. Simulated patients generally are not expected to undergo clinical examinations, so this method is best used to assess the quality of clinical interactions (Boyce and Neale 2006). Simulated patient research is more objective and less biased than some other methods, such as clinician interviews or formal observation, because clinicians may not report or follow their normal practice in such conditions (O'Hara et al. 2001). However, one limitation of this method is that it usually depends on simulated patient recall of what they experienced, and memory can be inaccurate (Baddeley 1979; Leiva et al. 2001; Joel et al. 2004; Boyce and Neale 2006; Colvin et al. 2006; Oraby et al. 2008).

In 2000, HALIRA researchers collaborated with the *MEMA kwa Vijana* intervention team to conduct a process evaluation of the youth-friendly health services component of the intervention. Simulated patient exercises were attempted by trained rural young people in twenty trial health facilities. Approximately six months before these exercises took place, all intervention and control health facilities were informed of, and agreed to, the possibility of such visits. All health workers were subsequently reminded of this possibility by a letter from the Regional Medical Officer. In each of the ten intervention and ten control communities, a health facility was randomly selected for a simulated patient visit.

The simulated patients were selected from 84 young applicants from a Sukuma village outside of the study area, based on their confidence, recall, creativity, acting skills, and youthful, rural appearance. Two male and two female 15–17-year-olds were trained to present themselves at health facilities as patients seeking condoms, contraception, or advice about a possible sexually transmitted infection. In case they were challenged, each simulated patient carried letters from the Regional Medical Officer and the *MEMA kwa Vijana* Director explaining their role in the exercise. In addition, a clinically-qualified supervisor was present in a nearby guesthouse when the simulated patient visited a health facility, and could be called on if necessary.

Three scenarios were developed for the simulated patient exercises. In the sexually transmitted infection scenario, the adolescent told the clinician that he or she had had sex with someone two days earlier, and then heard that the person had a sexually transmitted infection, so was concerned about exposure. If the clinician requested an examination, the adolescent was instructed to decline because there were no symptoms. In the condom scenario, the adolescent requested condoms, and at some point during the consultation asked whether new condoms have holes in them, as rumored. In the contraception scenario, a female adolescent requested birth control, and if given options, said that she preferred oral contraceptives. If the clinician requested to examine her, the adolescent was instructed to decline, saying that she was menstruating.

One health facility was closed, so no simulated patient exercise was conducted there. Simulated patients carried a tape-recorder to discreetly record clinical consultations. Three visits did not result in usable recordings, because one health facility did not have condoms available for a condom request and two recordings were inaudible. Immediately after each exercise, a field supervisor debriefed the simulated patient using a semi-structured questionnaire. At the end of the field work, the senior field supervisor wrote a summary report.

The simulated patient exercises generally proceeded well. The scripted scenarios provided adequate, plausible reasons for adolescents to obtain sexual health services from clinicians without an examination, although in a couple of instances the adolescents had to repeatedly refuse to be examined. The trained young people acted out their scenarios well, and came up with appropriate responses when they were asked unexpected questions, such as those about their sexual partners. None of the clinicians seemed to suspect that an adolescent was a simulated patient, although several clinicians seemed suspicious of the adolescent's motivations for other reasons. For example, some clinicians were concerned that girls might have requested contraception to abort an existing pregnancy. The simulated patient transcripts were very useful when compared to debriefing questionnaires and the summary report.

DATA PROCESSING, ANALYSIS, AND WRITE-UP

For the formal HALIRA analyses, participant observation field notes and recordings of in-depth interviews, group discussions, and simulated patient exercises were transcribed verbatim in their original Sukuma, Swahili, or English. Sukuma and Swahili transcripts were then translated into English. The quality of transcription or translation was randomly assessed for almost half of all documents by having a second transcriber or translator review them for accuracy. The full English language qualitative dataset consisted of 4.9 million words, 54 percent of which were trial participant in-depth interviews, 24 percent participant observation field notes, 13 percent young adult group discussions and follow-up interviews, 6 percent participant observation group discussions and in-depth interviews, 2 percent pupil group discussions, and 0.3 percent simulated patient exercises.

A coding frame of thirty-two broad categories was developed to organize the data by theme within NUD*IST 4, the Non-numerical Unstructured Data Indexing Searching and Theorizing Computer Program Version 4 (QSR International Pty Ltd, Melbourne, Australia). Sample transcripts from different research methods were used to pilot test and finalize the coding scheme. Five graduate researchers coded different sections of the dataset after each received training that included an evaluation of inter-coder reliability and resolution of differences.

Over twenty broad and sometimes overlapping sexual health topics were selected for analysis, such as cultural norms, school experiences, first sexual experiences, and concurrent partnerships. Analysis took place using a thematic and grounded theory approach to generate hypotheses. Hypotheses were then tested against the data through repeated readings of the transcripts and discussion with other HALIRA researchers. For analysis of most topics, data organized under relevant NUD*IST codes were summarized within 1–3 dozen pre-identified themes, as well as themes which emerged during analysis. Additional analysis then often included: comparison of findings with field summary reports; direct searching of the original transcripts using key roots or words; and/or reading all data for people mentioned within particular incidents or topics. This latter step was often critical to obtain a nuanced and full understanding of individuals and the particular contexts of their behaviors.

Analysis of the topic "school experiences" provides one example of the process described above. Data which had been organized under NUD*IST "schools" and "peer education" codes were summarized under thirty-three pre-identified themes, such as "teaching methods," "pupil likes/dislikes of teachers/school," and "teacher-community relationships." New themes which emerged from the data were also coded, such as "mandatory pregnancy examinations." In addition, every mention of certain individuals in the participant observation data was reviewed, such as teachers who were reported to have had sexual relationships with pupils.

The massive scale of the combined HALIRA dataset meant it was not feasible to analyze it in its entirety for some topics. Usually the entire participant observation database was analyzed for all topics, but when analysis of a topic was particularly subtle, complex, and time-consuming, it was occasionally restricted to a pre-selected portion of the participant observation dataset. For example, a detailed analysis of the "cultural norms" topic was only conducted with the Sukuma researcher's participant observation field notes, since the Sukuma researchers documented villagers' conversations whether they were in Sukuma or Swahili. In that case, the detailed findings were then compared to all field researchers' summary reports and other data sources to assess their generalizability.

Data from in-depth interviews were also analyzed for most topics. Data from other methods were analyzed when the dataset was particularly relevant to the topic and time allowed. Sometimes analysis of a different dataset involved a different protocol. For example, the simulated patient transcripts were so brief that they could be read repeatedly in their entirety. Based on those transcripts and the simulated patient debriefing questionnaires, measures of the quality of clinical consultations (e.g., confidentiality, respectfulness, privacy, and service) were ranked independently by two individuals: first by the Assistant Intervention Coordinator (Bernadette Cleophas-Mazige), who was also the senior field supervisor for the simulated patients' study, and then by Mary Plummer, who conducted the assessment blinded to the intervention or control status of the health facilities. There were few discrepant rankings, and for those Mary Plummer again reviewed the relevant transcripts and debriefing questionnaires before deciding a final rank.

In addition to the clinician above, six HALIRA staff compiled data summaries, conducted preliminary analyses, and/or drafted reports on some subjects addressed in this book or its companion volume: Caroline Ingall (contraception; induced abortion; boys' first sexual experience), Tom Ingall (condom use; *MEMA kwa Vijana* schools component evaluation), Gerry Mshana (sexual activities; illness causation beliefs and treatment practices), Kija Nyalali (number of lifetime partners), Joyce Wamoyi (sexual activities; material exchange for sex), and Zachayo Shigongo (sexual activities; number of lifetime partners). The authors closely guided these individuals' work, and conducted additional analyses on those topics as well as all analysis for the remaining book topics.

The use of multiple researchers and research sites, and the extraordinarily large size of the dataset, helped contribute to highly valid and unusually representative qualitative findings. However, these benefits came with challenges. Unlike traditional anthropology, many researchers generated data and no individual was intimately familiar with all of it at the start of the analysis, which made that process highly complex. The scale of the dataset also made it very difficult and time-consuming to manage, both for individual researchers and for the NUD*IST 4 software that was available when we began the study. NUD*IST 4 was sometimes useful in organizing, sorting, and searching data. However, on many occasions we needed to revert to systematically analyzing the dataset in individual word documents, because NUD*IST 4 was either too slow or unable to process requests within the large dataset. Attempts to upgrade to a newer qualitative data analysis program (e.g., NVivo Versions 6 and 7, QSR International Pty Ltd, Melbourne, Australia) did not resolve these issues.

For this book Daniel Wight wrote chapters 5, 7, and 12, as well as most of the findings section of chapter 3, and the introduction and discussion sections of chapter 8. He also read and commented on the remaining chapters, and contributed passages to some of them. Mary Plummer wrote all of the remaining chapters, chapter sections, and case studies. She also substantially revised and expanded each of Daniel Wight's chapters, and edited the completed book manuscript.

USE OF DATA IN THIS BOOK

In this book words in *non-bold italics* are Swahili, while words in ***bold italics*** are Sukuma. In Tanzania there are seven Standards, or years, of primary school and six Forms, or years, of secondary school. In this book, to make the total years of schooling clear to readers who are unfamiliar with this system, primary school level is referred to by "Year" (such as "Year 7"), and secondary school level is referred to by both "Form" and "Year" (such as "Form 2, the equivalent of Year 9"). "Informants" refers to those who provided information during participant observation, "respondents" to those who provided information in in-depth interviews, and "participants" to those who provided information through group discussions, unless otherwise specified.

Excerpts from participant observation field notes or summary reports are a researcher's reconstruction of what was said or observed previously. Informant and respondent names have been replaced with pseudonyms. In in-depth interview excerpts, "I" refers to the interviewer and "R" to the respondent; in group discussion excerpts, "F" refers to the facilitator and "P" to the participant; and in simulated patient excerpts, "HW" refers to the health

Table 2.3. Examples of Transcript Codes

Code	Explanation
PO-02-I-4-1m	2002 participant observation notes from intervention village no. 4, written by male researcher no. 1.
II-99-I-52-f	In-depth interview no. 52 conducted in 1999 with a female intervention participant.
GD-00-C-10-2f	Group discussion no. 2 conducted with female participants in control village no. 10 in 2000.
GDII-00-C-12-4m	In-depth interview no. 4 conducted with a male group discussion participant in control village no. 12 in 2000.
SPE-00-I-21-7f	Simulated patient exercise in intervention village no. 21 conducted in 2000 by female simulated patient no. 7.

worker and "SP" to the simulated patient. After each excerpt, references in brackets first indicate method, year, trial intervention/control status, and village number. In addition, researcher number and sex are indicated for participant observation and simulated patient excerpts, while group discussion or interview number and sex are indicated for other methods. Examples are provided in table 2.3. Most photographs used in this book were taken by the field researchers during participant observation, except for one that was taken by an author during fieldwork.

In this book the themes discussed in each chapter generally reflect findings recorded on multiple occasions and usually in multiple villages, although space only allows for one or two illustrations. Where a field note excerpt or quote represents an unusual finding, it is identified as such.

CONCLUSION

In this study we found several innovative techniques and methods to be useful for collecting valid and representative information on sensitive behaviors of young, rural Africans. These novel approaches include: participant observation by diverse researchers in multiple, representative sites over an extended period; informally building rapport with local people for several days prior to conducting a series of group discussions with them; conducting individual in-depth interviews immediately after a group discussion to follow-up on personal issues; and recording simulated patient exercises to maximize data accuracy and detail. In contrast, one of the greatest challenges our study faced was the collection, processing, analysis, and write-up of an extremely large qualitative dataset. We thus recommend that any researcher wishing to adapt these methods for applied research only do so on a smaller scale.

Chapter Three

Village Life

To understand young people's sexual culture and behavior it is first neces-sary to understand their wider social context. In this chapter we will briefly review historical, anthropological, and socio-demographic literature related to Mwanza Region and the Sukuma[1] people before presenting our findings on general village life during the study period. Many of the topics addressed in this chapter could easily be the focus of books in their own right, so this is neither intended as a systematic literature review nor as a comprehensive ethnography of rural Mwanza. Instead, we will describe the main features of village life here, while in the next chapter we will consider aspects of village life which specifically affect young people, such as parent-child relationships, peer relationships, and school experience. These two chapters are intended to provide a broad context for our findings on young people's sexual behavior, which is the main focus of this book.

A BRIEF HISTORY OF MWANZA REGION AND TANZANIA

The geographic area known as Mwanza Region today overlaps with a 50,000 km^2 area historically identified as ***Usukuma*** or Sukumaland, which mainly consisted of many small, Sukuma chiefdoms (Abrahams 1967). Sukumaland bordered chiefdoms of the closely related Nyamwezi to the south, the Ha and Sumbwa to the west, and the Zinza and Haya to the northwest (Abrahams 1967; Mafeje 1991). This area underwent many political and social changes in the last two hundred years. During the nineteenth century, Arabs, Indians, and Europeans entered the area as traders, slavers, explorers, and missionar-ies. Germany colonized the area from 1890–1917 and during that period a se-ries of public health and ecological disasters devastated the local population, including epidemics of smallpox and jiggers in the human population, and an epidemic of Rinderpest that destroyed 90 percent of the cattle population (Birley 1982). German rule was followed by British rule from 1918–1961, when influenza, sleeping sickness, relapsing fever, and other epidemics continued to affect human and cattle populations severely (Birley 1982; Wijsen and Tanner 2002). Large portions of land were abandoned during some of these epidemics, sometimes due to forced relocation by the colonists. Many areas subsequently were cleared of wild vegetation and reclaimed for human habitation, contributing to a landscape that is often treeless, overgrazed, and prone to soil erosion (Birley 1982).

Many other changes took place in the Mwanza Region during the colonial period, including the building of all-weather roads and a railway to the Indian Ocean, the development of markets for livestock and agricultural produce, and the introduction of cotton as a major cash crop (Abrahams 1967). A very limited number of hospitals and dispensaries were established in rural Mwanza during the colonial period, but the few villagers who used biomedical services typically also sought treatment from indigenous practitioners as well (Abrahams 1967; Varkevisser 1973). The German and British colonists ruled Mwanza Region by military force and indirect power. Some Sukuma chiefs were able to maintain their formal titles but they became administrative agents of the central government, enforcing laws and collecting taxes (Abrahams 1967; Bessire and Bessire 1997).

After national independence in 1961, the chiefdom system largely was abolished and locally elected councils were established under the new one-party, socialist state (Abrahams 1967). From 1973–1976, the national government implemented a rural modernization campaign commonly referred to as *"Operesheni Vijiji"* ("Operation Villages") that required massive numbers of people who lived in remote areas to relocate to government-designated rural centers. One of the goals of this campaign was to provide better social, economic, medical, and educational services to rural residents. However, the campaign was not popular, and some uncooperative residents were forcibly moved after their homes were burnt down (Stroeken 2001). The program had other unintended negative consequences, for example many villagers needed to travel long distances every day to farm and herd their cattle (Lawi 2007). The villagization campaign was thus stopped, and by the mid-1980s many abandoned rural homes had been reclaimed by their former residents, or new ones.

In recent decades Tanzania has shifted away from socialism and moved towards democracy. In the 1980s the national government began to allow private entrepreneurship and other forms of economic liberalization, which has contributed to industrialization, urbanization, improved communication systems, and a generally more globalized economy. In the early 1990s Tanzania became a multiparty state, although it has remained dominated by one party, *Chama Cha Mapinduzi* (CCM) (The Revolutionary Party of Tanzania). Since independence, Swahili and English have both been official national languages. Swahili is the language of instruction in primary school and it is widely spoken across the country. Only a small minority of Tanzanians speak English fluently, but it is the country's commercial language and the official teaching language for most subjects in secondary school and higher education institutions.

During the colonial period, large gold and diamond mines were opened in rural Mwanza and neighboring Shinyanga Region. One of these had its own airport, lake port, and hospital and employed 150 Europeans and over 2,000 local men, but it was closed at the time of national independence because of disputes over distribution of profits (Wijsen and Tanner 2002). During the latter half of the twentieth century, mining continued in the area on a relatively small-scale and private basis, drawing people from elsewhere in Tanzania and neighboring countries and usually involving artisanal miners who lived in scattered, mobile, and poor communities (Clift et al. 2003). In 1999–2000, however, large multinational mines were reestablished in Mwanza and Shinyanga and these drew large populations of migrant male mine workers from surrounding communities, as well as female sex workers and women who worked in the service industry (Desmond et al. 2005). HIV and other sexually transmitted infection rates have been relatively high in those areas. For example, a 2003–2004 survey found that 8 percent of males and 7 percent females aged 15–49 years in the general population in rural Mwanza were HIV-positive (TACAIDS, NBS, and ORC Macro 2005; NBS and ORC Macro. 2005). However, research with a similar age group in mining areas three years earlier found that 42 percent of female food and recreational facility workers, 18 percent of other local women, and 16 percent of local men were HIV-positive (Clift et al. 2003).

The nature and scale of fishing practices in rural Mwanza also changed dramatically near the end of the twentieth century. In the 1950s, a massive, meaty fish called Nile perch was introduced to Lake Victoria to strengthen commercial fishing stocks, and by the early 1980s its population had exploded (Witte et al. 1992; Lowe-McConnell 1994). As a result the fishing industry expanded substantially and began exporting fish to elsewhere in Africa and Europe. Fishing became much more lucrative for local men, and lake shore farmers and occasional fishermen began to work as full-time fishermen, while many men migrated to the area to do the same, creating large, multiethnic, and relatively affluent fishing villages along the lakeshore. Research conducted during the 1990s found that HIV prevalence within the sexually active population in such villages was 10 percent, compared to 3–5 percent in other rural villages (Schapink et al. 2001). During that period large fishing camps were also established on remote shores and islands. These camps had primarily male populations supported by small numbers of female service workers and sex workers. Research in the 1990s also found these settings to be high risk, as 9–10 percent of men and women in fishing camp islands had symptoms of sexually transmitted infections, compared to 1 percent of men and women on the mainland (Schapink et al. 2001).

At the time of our study, Sukumas were estimated to be the largest ethnic group in Tanzania, with 5–6 million people or 13–20 percent of the total population (Levinson 1998). Mwanza Region had a population of almost three million people, 90 percent of whom were Sukuma (United Republic of Tanzania 1997; National Bureau of Statistics and ORC Macro 2004). The region consisted of seven districts (including the four study districts), each subdivided into approximately 20 wards, with each ward being further subdivided into 5–9 villages. The village was the basic government administrative unit. Eighty percent of the region was rural, and most of the urban and non-Sukuma populations were concentrated in Mwanza City, the second largest city in Tanzania with an estimated population of 385,000 residents (United Republic of Tanzania 1997; National Bureau of Statistics and ORC Macro 2004). Members of most rural Mwanza households spoke Sukuma as a first language, particularly in remote areas; many children only began to learn Swahili in primary school (Bessire and Bessire 1997). Rural Mwanza remained very poor: in 2002, for example, 98–99 percent of households in the four study districts did not have electricity, and 70–94 percent used a pit latrine as a main toilet facility, while almost all the rest had no toilet facilities (National Bureau of Statistics and ORC Macro 2004).

Sukuma History and Social Relationships

Very little is known about the origins of the Sukuma people, although some recorded oral histories suggest that the ancestors of today's Sukumas first arrived in Sukumaland as hunters around 1500 A.D. (Abrahams 1967; Wijsen and Tanner 2002). Finding the area largely uninhabited, these immigrant peoples are believed to have eventually become well established as both farmers and cattle keepers. Sorghum and bullrush millet were the main food crops in the early twentieth century, but these were later replaced by maize and cassava, which required less labor and returned higher yield per acre (Varkevisser 1973; Wijsen and Tanner 2002). Rice and cotton also became increasingly important as cash crops (Abrahams 1967).

Cattle ownership traditionally has been central to Sukuma social and economic life as a primary measure of wealth, an insurance against famine, and the most established means of major exchange. For example, the Sukuma bridewealth custom primarily involved a man's family giving a woman's family cattle around the time of their marriage (Cory 1953). In 1967, 50 percent of households in Sukumaland were estimated to own cattle (Abrahams 1967). Anthropological research in the twentieth century documented many other important economic activities amongst rural Sukumas, including fishing, beer brewing, shopkeeping, and craftwork such as tailoring, carpentry, and bicycle repair (Abrahams 1967; Varkevisser 1973).

Traditionally, all adults in Sukuma villages belonged to one of three social groups, depending on their age, gender, experience, and contribution. One group consisted of young men and unmarried young women who were responsible for communal physical activity, such as digging wells. A second group was made up of married women who were responsible for brewing beer and preparing feasts for the neighborhood. The third group consisted of older, married men who made a contribution and were initiated into a group that presided over neighborhood agreements and disputes (Juma 1960; Abrahams 1967; Varkevisser 1973; Stroeken 2001).

Social control was maintained in villages and neighborhoods in several ways. Abrahams (1967) reported that ostracism was the main way that offenders were punished, and Varkevisser (1973) said that it was the most severe sanction that could be brought to bear against an offender. Stroeken (2001, 292) however suggested that fines were the most common form of punishment:

> [Sukuma people] maintain an ambiguous relationship to community norms, on the one hand heavily fining any violation of agreements and on the other hand willing to negotiate the rules during meetings in a ternary practice bordering on plain detachment and irony. . . . Paying fines preserves the integrity of the household head . . . as opposed to reprimand or moralization which do not tally with Sukuma culture.

In addition, village elders sometimes meted out punishments involving physical repercussions. In the early 1980s increased social disruption and crime in rural areas, and inadequate assistance from urban police and judicial systems, led to the creation of a new association of village-level crime control (Abrahams 1987; Wiijsen and Tanner 2002). This was initiated and led by local elders, but largely consisted of young men called ***sungusungu***, a term that literally means "poison" in Sukuma and a cooperative but aggressive kind of ant in Swahili. Initially ***sungusungu*** groups had a limited range of responsibilities within a few villages, and government authorities were wary or ambivalent towards them. Within a few years, however, most Mwanza villages had their own, local *sungusungu* group that worked together with village elders and collaborated with government authorities in a range of cases related to theft, property disputes, debt, witchcraft, and adultery (Wijsen and Tanner 2002; Paciotti et al. 2005).

Within families and villages, Sukuma men traditionally have held considerably more power than women (Cory 1953). Marital traditions contributed to this, including the common practice of a man's family paying a woman's family substantial bridewealth around the time of their marriage, and the practice of a young woman moving from her parents' home to her husband's parents' home upon marrying. During the colonial period, Cory (1953) documented many different types of marriage, including some forms of elopement, but almost all involved an exchange of wealth of some kind either before or soon after marriage. In Varkevisser's (1973) study from 1965–1967, only 16–18 percent of marriages were "free," in that no bridewealth was given to the woman's family around the time when the couple married, although wealth may have been exchanged at a later date. She found that some women's parents were disappointed not to receive bridewealth in such instances, but others were pleased, as this meant they could claim the grandchildren from such unions as part of the maternal home and clan. In addition, 18 percent of children in Varkevisser's (1973) study were born out-of-wedlock and were raised by their maternal grandparents, and these children were also considered to be part of their maternal clan.

During the twentieth century, bridewealth typically consisted of 10 cows but could range from about 3–17 cows (Cory 1953; Varkevisser 1973). Customary law restricted chiefs and other wealthy men from paying more than 17 cows in bridewealth, to reduce the chance that affluent men had multiple wives when poor men were unable to marry one (Cory 1953). This total number of cows exchanged in bridewealth represented a series of smaller payments which entitled a husband to sexual access to his wife, to move her to live and work at his homestead and farm, and to claim any offspring as his descendants, including keeping them after divorce if they were already weaned (Cory 1953; Varkevisser 1973). Bridewealth payment thus typically took place in stages, and usually it was understood that a certain amount would remain outstanding long-term, as this served as a kind of insurance enabling parents to intervene if a couple encountered difficulties. For example, if a young husband physically abused his wife, her father might threaten to demand the remaining bridewealth if he did not start treating her better.

Gender segregation has been fundamental to Sukuma culture historically, with men and women sharing few work or social activities in daily life (Abrahams 1967). Heavy work typically was done by men, while repetitive domestic tasks and most everyday agricultural work were done by women (Abrahams 1967). Usually, meals were segregated within a household, with men and boys eating together outside around a fire (***kikome*** singular, ***shikome*** plural) in the evenings, while women and girls ate near the cooking area (Varkevisser 1973). In her 1965–1967 anthropological research, Varkevisser (1973, 80) described how Sukuma marriages were based on what anthropologists refer to as an "avoidance relationship," that is, a relationship characterized by authority on one side and respect and obedience on the other. She explained:

> Part of a wife's obligation to obey her husband and never contradict him in the presence of her children entails respect manifested through formal avoidance: husband and wife do not eat together, they do not touch each other except as a specific prelude to sexual intercourse, they seldom set off in each other's company to attend a feast or a funeral in a neighborhood at which the presence of both is required.

Several anthropologists have noted that divorce was fairly common amongst the Sukuma historically. Describing the late colonial period, Abrahams (1967) commented that, regardless of whether marriages had involved bridewealth payment, a large majority of Sukuma 50-year-olds had experienced at least one divorce, and often more. Despite the relative power that men held over women in traditional Sukuma marriages, divorce was often initiated by wives, suggesting that Sukuma women had more choice to leave unsatisfactory marriages than was the case in many other patriarchal societies (Varkevisser 1973).

Other Characteristics of Sukuma Culture

Anthropological research in the twentieth century highlighted how cooperation, reciprocity, hospitality, and humor were highly valued within Sukuma culture. Varkevisser (1973) noted, for example, how Sukumas preferred to engage in agricultural work in groups rather than individually, unlike some other local ethnic groups. She described many different types of farming groups which either hired themselves out for pay or alternated between members' farms in turn. Importantly, many groups which worked for pay ultimately shared their earnings with others outside the group. For example, young men typically used the majority of their group's revenue on a feast of meat and beer which they shared with other villagers, including the people who had hired them (Varkevisser 1973).

Other researchers have similarly found Sukumas to be exceptionally generous. For example, Paciotti and Mulder (2004) found that, if Sukuma participants were given a choice to share money with other Sukumas, they typically gave away more than half of the money, even if the recipient was a stranger, unlike members of another ethnic group in the study who were not as generous (Paciotti and Mulder 2004). Paciotti and Hadley (2003, 431) suggested that Sukumas consider sharing with other Sukumas to be mandatory, because it is "disgraceful to act like a hyena and take too much," and because those who fail to share can expect to be punished.

However, some anthropologists have argued that, given the historical unpredictability of the environment in Sukumaland, the chronic nature of hunger, and the ever-present focus on subsistence, Sukuma culture has been characterized by reciprocity rather than generosity. Wijsen and Tanner (2002, 129) argued:

> The problem in the Sukuma social environment is that there is very little sharing unless there are advantages to be gained by such behavior or that it is part of an ongoing and finally [*sic*] balanced network of reciprocities. A Sukuma might well argue that charity is something which the well-to-do can afford but that is not something which a subsistence farmer can indulge in when his own and his family's future is by no means assured.

Historically, music, dance, humor, and storytelling have been an integral part of Sukuma life, work, and entertainment (Mirambo 2004). Many individuals and social groups have semiformal, joking relationships involving horseplay and verbal banter (Abrahams 1967). Farming groups have often used song to ease their agricultural work, and some performed and competed publicly in celebrations after the harvest (Gunderson 2001). For most of the twentieth century, the main form of entertainment in rural Mwanza was such *ngoma* competitions (Cory 1953). In the 1960s, for example, small *ngoma* events with local drumming-dance groups were hosted weekly in some villages, while in others they only took place as large events with traveling performers between June and August, after the main harvest (Varkevisser 1973). These events typically involved two *ngoma* groups performing simultaneously on opposite sides of a performance ground, competing in magical medicine, skill, and outlandish behavior to draw the largest audience. In addition to drumming, dancing, and singing, *ngoma* performers attempted to draw a crowd's attention by appearing "wild, powerful, and dangerous" (Stroeken 2001, 305): dressing in striking costumes, engaging in acrobatics, acting out exciting mini-dramas, and using moveable figurines to enact shocking sexual scenes. As Bessire (2005, 44) explained: "Separated by the confines of the dance space, [*ngoma*] dancers can sing racy lyrics, make the dance figures perform lewd gestures, or mimic sexual acts, and in general express artistically what they could not in daily life."

Traditionally, Sukuma religious beliefs were diverse. They included belief in a benevolent God; potentially punitive ancestral spirits (***masamva***);

taboos (***migilo***) common to all or to specific clans and life circumstances; and good or malevolent magic, such as witchcraft (*uchawi* or ***bulogi***) (Tanner 1956a; Tanner 1956b; Tanner 1957; Tanner 1959; Varkevisser 1973). Generally, Sukuma culture has distinguished between aspects of life which are ***mhola*** (literally "cool," implying peace, purity, or wholeness) and ***nsebu*** (literally "hot," implying disruption, impurity, or evil, such as witchcraft) (Varkevisser 1973; Stroeken 2001). Historically, individual or local interpretation of specific Sukuma religious beliefs have varied considerably (Wijsen and Tanner 2002). For example, Varkevisser (1973) found that descriptions of a single Sukuma ritual could be radically different even within the same neighborhood.

Sukumas traditionally associated illness and misfortune with active, supernatural agents, such as dissatisfied ancestral spirits or a malicious witch, but this did not rule out the possibility of natural causes, as has also been found elsewhere in sub-Saharan Africa (Schoepf 1992b). For example, in Sukumaland as in Botswana and Zambia anthropologists have documented beliefs that evil spirits prompt an illness even though its immediate cause is believed to be an accident or unclean water (Tanner 1956b; Ingstad 1990; Yamba 1997). Traditional healers (*waganga wa kienyeji* or ***bafumu***) such as diviners or herbalists usually have been consulted to determine whether ancestral spirits or witchcraft caused a problem, and to resolve it through ritual and traditional medicine (Tanner 1957). If a Sukuma person did not practice appropriate behavior in honor of an ancestor, it was believed that ancestral spirits could exact revenge in the form of illness, sterility, mental unrest, cattle death, or poor harvests.

Misfortune or illness resulting in death, however, usually was attributed to witchcraft rather than ancestral intervention (Varkevisser 1973). Witchcraft involved a person intentionally and maliciously using magic or supernatural power to cause harm to another. Typically, the witch was believed to be someone close to the victim, who knew them well and might envy them (Abrahams 1967; Stroeken 2001). Individuals who were unusually successful or proud were believed to risk others becoming envious and using witchcraft against them, or alternatively, risked being accused of witchcraft themselves (Varkevisser 1973). Stroeken (2001, 297) stipulated that Sukumas are extraordinarily generous specifically to counteract this possibility of envy and witchcraft, commenting that: "the Sukuma's well-tried method of dissolving envy [is] sharing."

In reviewing the existing literature in the late 1960s, Varkevisser (1973) concluded that witchcraft accusations had increased amongst the Sukuma in the prior decades. Since then, Mwanza Region and neighboring Shinyanga have had far higher rates of killing of people accused of witchcraft than anywhere else in Tanzania (Wijsen and Tanner 2002). A number of factors may have contributed to this phenomenon, including the replacement of chiefs by a more distant and less responsive national government, and how forced relocation in *Operesheni Vijiji* may have increased social tensions and competition for limited resources (Mesaki 1994; Stroeken 2001). A third possible factor unique to the region was the growth of commercial cotton farming during the twentieth century, and the divisive effects of the uneven distribution of wealth from that crop (Wijsen and Tanner 2002).

At the time of this study, the Sukuma people were the largest ethnic group in Tanzania. However, their social and economic power within the country did not reflect their size, as they remained a relatively poor and underrepresented group within the government (Stroeken 2001). The Sukuma are widely considered to be more culturally conservative than most Tanzanian ethnic groups, and relatively indifferent or resistant to foreign education and religion. For example, relatively few Sukumas had converted to either Christianity or Islam by independence, and postindependence they were slower to adopt the national language, Swahili, than most other ethnic groups (Iliffe 1979). However, research in rural Mwanza in the late twentieth century highlighted some important changes within Sukuma culture, including that young people had begun to value cattle and farming less, and housing and trade more, than had prior generations (Madulu 1998).

In the next section we will describe our study's findings on the general features of village life in rural Mwanza from 1999–2002, including male and female occupations, material living conditions, social relationships and events, supernatural beliefs, and illness beliefs and practices.

FINDINGS

Most of our study's villages had a population of 2,000–3,000 residents, although one on a large road had a population of more than 7,000. Each village consisted of 5–8 sub-villages (*kitongoji* singular; *vitongoji* plural), and each of these consisted of about 50 family compounds or homesteads. One Village Chairman reported, for example, that his village consisted of eight sub-villages, 315 families, and 2,405 people. Outside of that village's center, homesteads were typically 100–300 meters apart, and the distance from one *kitongoji* to another was 1.5–3 km.

In our study, households varied widely in their number of occupants, ranging from just a few members to 25 or more, although most households had 6–8 adults and children. Family obligations meant that many households expanded as necessary to host the head of household's siblings, nieces, nephews and in-laws. Household size also varied because some men and a small number of women immigrated for work; most young women moved from their parent's household and to their husband's upon marrying; and many children moved between households or to a distant school depending on family or schooling needs.

Farming and Cattle Keeping

With the exception of some fishing villages, agriculture was the core of economies in our study villages, and most families grew a mix of subsistence and cash crops. The agricultural calendar and routines thus dominated village life. The main crops grown for household use were: maize, sweet potatoes, cassava, sorghum, millet, bananas, bambara nuts, peanuts, beans, and lentils. Many older villagers reported that more cotton had been cultivated when they were younger, but by the time of the study less was cultivated because the cotton price had fallen while the cost of insecticides and fertilizer had risen. Rice, on the other hand, was widely reported to be the most important food cash crop, followed by maize and cassava. Some young entrepreneurs also had businesses growing tomatoes, but only where they could be readily irrigated. Farmers of cash crops complained when good harvests led to an abundance of produce and resulted in lower prices

Many families in study villages owned their own land, typically several acres or more made up of different *mashamba* (cultivated plots; singular *shamba*). It was not uncommon for young people to have land which they cultivated separately from their parents and to sell the produce for themselves, but they often required parental permission when they worked on their own *shamba* rather than the family's. Villagers considered the minority of farmers who owned more than ten acres to be wealthy, and that amount of land typically provided a good income from cotton, maize, and other cash crops. Only a small minority of families in our study were landless, usually because they were relative newcomers to a village or because they had experienced misfortune. Such families rented or borrowed land to cultivate, or resorted to daily farm laboring.

Almost all cultivation in study villages was still done by hand. Typically hoes were used both to break up the soil for planting and for subsequent weeding. A very small minority of farmers used ox-drawn ploughs, either their own or hired. There were no tractors in any of the study villages. The main cultivation season took place during the long rainy season, from February to May. At that time, almost everyone in farming households worked from dawn until dusk on their *mashamba*; even many pupils were required to stay home to help, so absenteeism was much higher during that period. Conversely, in the dry season after the main harvest, from June to September, there was little farming work. During that period, men had a lot of free time and women had fewer agricultural demands competing with their domestic work.

In the study villages, cattle continued to be highly valued for the security and status associated with them. In one inland village, a researcher estimated that 30 percent of families owned at least one cow, and the majority of those families owned from one to nine cows. Villagers who owned more than 10 cows were regarded as affluent, and those with more than 50 were considered to be very rich. Only two villagers in that village owned more than 100 cows. In general in the study villages, owning a large number of cattle was far more prestigious than being a large landowner or a successful cultivator, and profit from commercial crops was often invested in cattle. Cattle in our study villages were usually only sold or bartered in exceptional circumstances, for instance, to acquire land, pay bridewealth, or cope with an emergency such as a health crisis. Few parents sold their cattle to pay for their children's school fees, and there were many instances of parents allowing their children to drop out rather than do so.

Cattle were owned by the heads of household, usually older men, but typically 5–8-year-old boys herded them. Most of these boys had not yet attended school or had dropped out; because of the long days involved in cattle-tending, some cattle herders never attended school. Some of these boys were family members, and the chore of cattle-herding passed from one son to another as each became old enough for the responsibility but not so old that he needed to begin school. Other cattle herders were not family members, but were relatively poor boys who were paid a very small wage, or who only received food and shelter in exchange for their labor.

Other animals that were widely kept were goats, chickens, and muscovy ducks, although none of these had the symbolic importance of cattle. As children grew older, they sometimes were given a few such small animals of their own. For example, in the 1998 *MEMA kwa Vijana* assisted self-complete questionnaire survey, 31 percent of boys (average age 16 years) and 22 percent of girls (average age 15 years) reported that they owned farm animals themselves.

Other Occupations for Men

In our study villages, opportunities for nonagricultural livelihoods varied considerably according to the village's proximity to roads, urban settlements, fishing villages, or mines. In general, the further villages were inland and away from main roads, the fewer nonfarming occupations there were, and the poorer the population. In those villages, nonagricultural work was also often limited to the dry season, when farmers had more free time away from their fields. An important exception to this was remote villages near mines, where there were relatively diverse and numerous nonagricultural livelihoods year-round.

Some of the large study villages had permanent shops, but most relied on small kiosks for the sale of manufactured products and several other items. The number of kiosks in each village center varied considerably and fluctuated over time, some being short-lived. More kiosks appeared after the harvest when farmers had more money. Even the most remote villages had one or two small kiosks, although some were only open in the evening, once their owners had completed their own agricultural work. Kiosks generally were owned and run by young men and typically stocked limited quantities of cooking oil, sugar, wheat flour, rice, candy, cookies, *dagaa* (a small fish similar to whitebait), soda, soap, body oil, kerosene, matches, or bicycle spare parts. They also usually provided basic medicines such as antimalarials (e.g., choloroquine or sulfa drugs), headache tablets (e.g., acetaminophen or aspirin), and antibiotics (e.g., co-trimoxazole) (figure 3.1). Some larger villages had a specialized pharmacy kiosk that sold additional medications, but the vendors in such shops rarely had any pharmacological training.

Most villages also had a weekly market, either in their village center or that of a nearby village. Petty trade was a common occupation, pursued primarily by young men who sold products either by running a market stall, hawking in the village center, or staffing a more permanent kiosk or shop there. In our study, petty traders typically saved or borrowed a small amount of capital to buy stock and then gradually built up their businesses, usually sticking to one or two products. Agricultural products included rice, cassava, maize, sweet potatoes, oranges, tangerines, bananas, tomatoes, onions, millet, beans, peanuts and sugar cane. Near to Lake Victoria, fresh fish could be bought for resale the same day, but trading in dried fish happened across the region. The

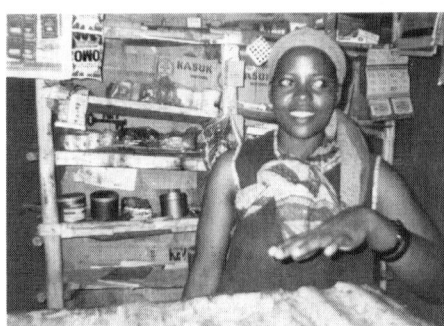

Figure 3.1. A woman in a village kiosk with a child on her back. Materials for purchase include aspirin, antimalarial drugs, laundry soap, and body oil.

heads and skeletons of large fish from fish factories in Mwanza City, a by-product of the fish-fillet export trade, were transported for up to two days by bicycle to be sold for fish stews. On a larger scale, a few men traded in cattle, buying at cattle markets and selling to urban butchers. Nonagricultural items of trade were obtained from nearby towns or Mwanza City, such as clothes, utensils, soap, body oil, bicycle parts, condoms, cooking oil, or fish.

Other livelihoods for men in our study included selling wood, burning charcoal, brick making, house building, carpentry, transportation of heavy items, bicycle taxi driving, and bicycle repair. All men were expected to be able to construct and repair houses within their own homestead, but some also hired themselves out to do so. In one village there were three blacksmiths who made a variety of iron items such as hoes, axes, spears, ox-plough shears, machetes, and sickles.

Adolescent boys were expected to help farm during the cultivation season, and younger boys sometimes had domestic responsibilities. Generally, however, adolescent boys had more free time than adolescent girls and could use that time to work for pay. In the 1998 assisted self-completion questionnaire survey, for example, 62 percent of boys reported that they sometimes earned money from work, compared with 38 percent of girls. During the cultivation season, both boys and girls could earn about Tshs 500 ($0.60) per day hiring themselves out from about 7:00 a.m. until 6:00 p.m. as part of a farming team. In many families, boys and girls were expected to begin paying for some of their basic needs before they reached their teen years, and increasingly to meet those needs themselves during their teens, including clothing, underwear, soap, body oil, and school fees and supplies. For example, a 16-year-old girl explained that she needed to pay for her own school fees:

> *R:* I am now in Year 7, but I have not yet paid my school fees. . . . I will do so when I harvest and sell my cassava. [My father] says, "I can't pay for such old children. You have to be independent." He only pays when you begin Year 1. But once you know how to farm, he does not pay at all. [II-99-I-54-f]

In all of our study villages, a small proportion of young men migrated to towns or Mwanza City, usually to work as casual labor. Young people were often attracted by what they perceived as a *kisasa* (modern) way of life and potentially lucrative occupations in urban areas. Sometimes such moves were planned in advance, but often they were sudden decisions in response to a relative who offered a job or simply a place to live while the youth sought work. Young men sometimes left their village for months or years in pursuit of such work. Returnees or visitors from town were of high status in rural areas, but villagers often had exaggerated expectations of the wealth that could be accumulated in the city, and this prevented some poor migrants from returning to their villages.

In study villages close to Lake Victoria, a large proportion of the male population engaged in fishing. Some local men fished individually using hooks, but most worked in groups using nets. Those nets often had holes smaller than the 4-inch legal limit that was mandated to prevent the loss of juvenile fish important to the future fish stock. Fishermen feared being caught and imprisoned by a fisheries officer, so they hid this practice by fishing at night and selling their haul early in the morning. During the day most of these fishermen were able to relax, mend their nets, and prepare their vessels for the night. Boys got involved in fishing from as young an as age six, and some school pupils set their nets in the evening and brought them in the following morning before school.

In addition to those individual fishing practices, some local men worked for the fishing companies in remote camps. These men were often away from their villages for days or weeks at a time. Alcohol consumption and drunkenness were reported to be high at fishing camps, and men in those sites were rumored to engage in unlawful and dangerous behavior. For example, researchers heard multiple reports of women and boys at fishing camps being sexually assaulted; this will be described further in chapters 7 and 8. No researcher visited a fishing camp, however, so no participant observation data were collected in those settings.

Most people in fishing villages engaged in a limited amount of agriculture, but the fishing villages in our study differed from typical agricultural villages in multiple ways. For example, the populations were much more mobile, and far more money was in circulation. They were typically larger than remote, inland villages, and they were also more ethnically heterogeneous, so that Sukumas were sometimes in the minority in the village centers, although they were still the largest ethnic group overall. These villages were less interknit and provincial than inland villages, and they experienced more crime.

Within our study there were also two inland villages that were approximately 20 kilometers away from large, multinational gold mines, and a third village that was farther away from a smaller diamond mine. A minority of men in those study villages tried to find casual work in those mines, while a few others worked in smaller, artisanal gold mines in the area. Some of these men stayed at a mine for extended periods, while others travelled in and out on a daily or weekly basis. Men who worked in mines for extended periods were said to return to their home villages at intervals with extremely large sums of money, ranging from Tshs 100,000 ($120) to Tshs 2,000,000 ($2,400). These men were often rumored to spend their money fairly quickly on women and alcohol in their villages, before returning to mines to earn more money.

In most villages, the only salaried workers were the Village Executive Officer, school teachers, and health facility staff, if there was a health facility nearby. All of these positions typically were held by men. In most villages there were also usually 5–6 individuals who maintained a large enough traditional medicine[2] practice for this to be their main occupation. These traditional healers were also usually, but not exclusively, men.

Finally, in several study villages there were indigenous microcredit schemes comprised of people of the same clan and those they married. Each member contributed an agreed sum to this scheme, and the funds were used to help members in economic difficulties. A loan would be given at an agreed rate of interest, such as 20 percent.

Other Occupations for Women

Adolescent girls and women had far fewer options than boys and men for paid work in rural Mwanza. If they were not in school, girls spent almost all of their waking time engaged in farming or domestic chores (figure 3.2) which left them little time for leisure activities or paid work. However, even if they had had time, most of the occupations above would have been considered men's work and thus inappropriate to pursue.

If they had time available and parental permission, adolescent girls could hire themselves out as farm labor at a similar rate to that described above for boys. In addition, many young women who did domestic and farm work for most of the week prepared food items to sell at the weekly market, or to hawk in the village center in the evening. A minority of women also engaged in petty trade as described above for men, and a small minority migrated to larger towns or Mwanza City to work in recreational or food facilities, or in domestic service. However, after marrying, young women typically reduced

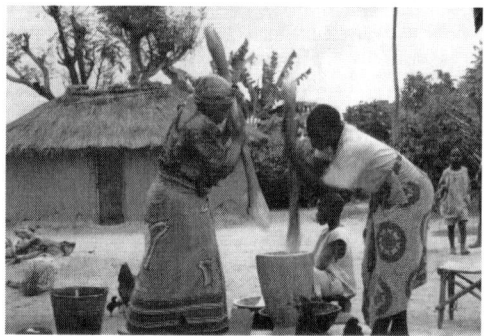

Figure 3.2. Two young women pounding dried cassava while a girl sieves cassava powder in the background. Such powder was used to make the most common food staple, a stiff porridge (*ugali*).

or stopped such external economic activities in order to focus entirely on domestic work and subsistence farming for their husbands' households.

In our study, most village centers had food stalls where meals typically were provided during the evening. A minority of women in study villages staffed those food stalls, sometimes working in pairs on alternate days, serving items such as roasted peanuts, *vitumbua* (fried rice cakes), *mandazi* (doughnuts), *chapati* (flat, unleavened bread), *uji* (maize- or millet-based porridge), sugar cane, or *tangawizi* (a hot ginger drink). Women could earn as much as Tshs 1,000–2,000 ($1.20–2.40) per day running such a food kiosk. Their customers were almost entirely men. Women rarely ate at food stalls, and then usually were accompanying male customers.

In all villages, brewing and selling *pombe* (home-made beer) made from sorghum or millet was an important occupation for some women, particularly unmarried or separated women, who could earn Tshs 1,000–2,000 ($1.20–$2.40) per day doing this. It was technically illegal to brew or distil alcohol without a license, but in practice these activities were so common and accepted that little effort was made to hide them. Some *pombe* was used in traditional Sukuma ceremonies. However, most *pombe* and homemade distilled alcohol known as *moshi* (literally "smoke") or *gongo* (literally "club") were sold in or near the compound where they were made, either in small quantities for individual consumption or large quantities for social events. Larger villages sometimes had a bar where a few young women worked as waitresses selling bottled beer.

In several study villages there were also externally funded microcredit schemes specifically to assist women's economic activities. In such programs, a group of women collectively guaranteed each other for small loans from a development nongovernmental organization, following the model of the Bangladeshi Grameen Bank.

Living Conditions

Most residents in study villages lived in homesteads consisting of two or more houses built of wattle and mud walls, or occasionally fired brick walls. These homes had thatched roofs and no internal doors, and sometimes also no external doors. In some villages, about one half of houses had corrugated tin roofs, but these were typically only found amongst wealthier households close to the village center, and they were very rare in other villages. Most households had pit latrines, but many were not used because they were in poor condition, in which case people relieved themselves in fields nearby instead.

Small children typically slept in the same room as their parents. Older children and adolescents of the same sex within a homestead usually shared a sleeping room, either within their parents' house (mainly girls) or in a free-standing house in the same compound (either boys or girls). An important rite of passage for many young men in their late teens or early twenties was to build their own **maji** or *geto* (from the English "ghetto"), a one-roomed hut within their parents' homestead. All household members slept on the earth floor, on a reed mat, sacking, cattle hide (especially girls), or a homemade mattress stuffed with cotton. People usually shared one sheet between two or three individuals. A few homes had a bed with a metal frame, but only very wealthy households had wooden beds.

Village men generally wore western style shirts or T-shirts and long trousers. Women typically wore simple dresses or a blouse and a *kanga* (a colored, patterned cotton cloth with a border and message) wrapped around the waist like a long skirt. The majority of villagers wore some kind of footwear, often flip flops or open sandals made from car tires, but in the poorest villages most people went barefoot, especially in the rainy season when paths were submerged or muddy. Young people had two to three sets of clothes, one for working, a neater set for public places and, if at school, the required uniform. Many could only wash their clothes once a fortnight or less frequently due to lack of soap or water. Some primary schools insisted that pupils wear shoes, in which case pupils often struggled to buy second-hand pairs or borrow them from relatives. Soap was highly valued, as was body oil, which villagers considered essential to prevent unhealthy and unattractive dry and cracked skin. Girls and women used old cloths for sanitary towels.

Most households in study villages did not own a bicycle, although many could borrow or hire one, which was very important for transportation, particularly of water. Few households had a radio at the time of our study, although perhaps one in ten young men did. Mobile telephone services did not yet reach rural Mwanza at the time of our study. The only service available was thus provided at public telephone offices in large rural towns, so very few villagers had ever used a telephone.

In the wet season, most women in our study villages walked 1–2 kilometers to fetch water for their household's drinking, cooking, and washing, often from a shallow pond dug where there was a high water table. Sometimes they walked twice that distance in the dry season. Girls and women typically carried water by hand as well as a bucket or a different vessel balanced on top of their heads. Firewood used for cooking was generally collected two or more kilometers away from homesteads.

Meals usually were segregated in households in our study (figure 3.3). When breakfast was available, it typically consisted of *ugali* or another form of carbohydrate, such as roasted maize, sweet potatoes, or cassava. However, many families did not eat breakfast, and it was not unusual for a

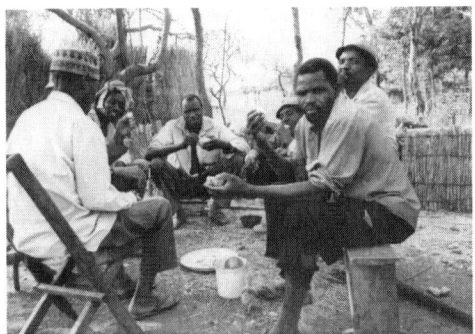

Figure 3.3. A head of household eating potatoes with other male villagers.

family to only eat two meals per day, one around 3:00 p.m. and the other at about 8:00 p.m. Typically these consisted of *ugali* and some kind of *mboga* (a vegetable side dish that sometimes included beans, fish, or rarely meat), depending on affluence and proximity to Lake Victoria. Food was scarce in the cultivation season and then many families lived with hunger as a part of daily life and only had one meal in the evening each day. Girls and women were especially likely to be hungry when food was scarce as they generally received smaller portions of food than boys and men. A male researcher described this dynamic in one of his host households: "If the men are still hungry when they finish eating their *ugali* or *mboga*, they just take more food from the women's portion, sometimes leaving the women without any food until the next meal" [PO-02-I-1-3m].

Demand for alcohol, primarily *pombe*, fluctuated considerably with the agricultural cycle in inland villages, being at its lowest during the cultivation season and highest after the main harvest, when more money was available and men had more time to socialize and drink. Alcohol use was more common year-round in fishing villages, where men's incomes were relatively high and steady. In every village there were individuals—mostly men—who were known for drinking heavily and being drunk in public in all seasons. In one remote village, for example, villagers complained that most male teachers and village leaders were drunk during working hours, and these reports were supported by researchers' observations.

Social Relationships

Village administration was led by the elected Village Chairman, who was assisted by the government-employed Village Executive Officer. In our study villages, these positions were almost always held by men. Village leaders sometimes held meetings for an entire village or *kitongoji* adult population, at which men and women sat separately and a variety of issues were addressed, such as local bylaws and crime. Government police had no presence in most study villages, although they were involved in intermittent crime control in some of the larger villages. Most study villages instead had a *sungusungu* group that followed the instructions of the Village Executive Officer, the Village Chairman, and local elders.

Local conflicts such as property disputes, marital discord, or rape accusations were sometimes resolved through a process called *kusuluhisha* (to conciliate, mediate, or make peace), involving villager leaders and/or elders hearing out an issue and making a perpetrator apologize, sometimes with the payment of a fine. The *sungusungu* sometimes also used threats or intimidation to ensure payment of legal and customary fees and fines, such as funeral contributions required of the relatives and neighbors of a deceased person. Theft was considered to be a very serious crime, and the *sungusungu* sometimes punished people believed to be guilty of theft or other serious offenses with beating or caning.

Beyond the center of villages, homesteads generally were dispersed widely, but people knew the kinship status of most of their fellow villagers and were well informed about their lives. The convention of Sukuma greetings helped to maintain this familiarity. A person's grandparents were mentioned in the course of daily greetings, especially if the people involved did not know one another, and married women were referred to by their parents' names, thus reinforcing lineage identity. Conventional greeting also involved inquiring about the well-being of close kin and those in the household. In this way, news of births, deaths, or other significant events could thus spread throughout a village in a day. If collective action was required, such as attending a funeral or shared construction work, it was also announced by someone moving through the village blowing a whistle or ringing a bell. Such conventional greetings, interest in other villagers' affairs, and general cooperation between villagers were more prominent in the more remote study villages. In fishing villages and those close to large roads, which were usually more densely populated and had a greater ethnic mix, inhabitants were less communally minded.

The main formal divisions within villages were religious. In the 1998 assisted self-completion questionnaire survey, 77 percent of school pupils reported that they were Christian, 13 percent said they had no religion, 9 percent reported they were Muslim, and 1 percent said they followed a traditional religion. Amongst Christians about one-half were Roman Catholic and one-half Protestant, the latter mainly of African Inland Church, Pentecostal (several different sects), and Seventh Day Adventist faiths. Rural Muslims instead were Sunni of varying sects. Religious belief and practice varied greatly, from those who rarely attended church or mosque to a small minority who prayed everyday and attended services more than weekly. While most villagers identified themselves as Christians or Muslims, almost all maintained traditional beliefs and practices which contradicted Christian or Muslim theology, as will be discussed later in this chapter. Villagers generally cooperated with each other without regard to religious affiliations. It was rare to hear religious affiliation being mentioned in general conversation, and when it did it was incidental and not a source of tension or conflict between people of different religions. Usually everyone participated in celebrating major holidays, including Christmas and Easter, irrespective of religion.

In some villages, membership in political parties intermittently divided the population, particularly around elections for the Village Chairman and national elections. At the time of the study, the CCM continued to be the dominant political party in rural Mwanza as in most areas of Tanzania. In some study villages, everyone in an official role was a CCM member, but some minor opposition parties were represented in others. While political arguments could be heated around elections in rural Mwanza, they were rarely socially divisive, and they did not prevent normal cooperation between villagers.

Important informal social divisions in our study villages were based on wealth, respectability, and moral judgment. Most informants said that the men accorded the most respect in villages were the wealthy (in terms of money, cows, or land), the successful farmers, the teachers, and the village leaders. However, if a relatively rich man was believed to flaunt his wealth and be arrogant or scornful of poorer families, he might be widely resented and disliked. More generally, villagers who lived peaceably with their neighbors, behaved well, worked hard, and brought up their children to be respectful were highly regarded. Sharing food, clothes, or advice about farming and other issues was also highly esteemed. Anyone visiting a household when food was being served would be invited to join the meal and it was considered insulting to refuse. Sharing food was also a central part of funerals and weddings. However, each village had internal hostilities, resulting from quarrels over particular concerns, such as farm boundaries, seducing others' spouses, and accusations of theft or witchcraft. Men rumored to be thieves were strongly disparaged and severely punished if caught. For women, sexual respectability was extremely important. Those who were perceived to be faithful to their husbands had much better reputations than single or separated women; this will be discussed more in chapter 5.

Relations between the sexes in rural Mwanza is a topic that will be addressed in almost every chapter of this book, so our findings on this will only

be introduced briefly here. We found that most productive and social activities in rural Mwanza continued to be segregated by gender with the exception of very young children's activities. Men were generally more socially
and economically powerful than women. As already described, men had
more access to paid employment and they generally owned the land and the
cattle. About half of young women entered their first marriages with parental
consent and an advance agreement about bridewealth, and lesser elopement
or pregnancy fines were often paid in the remainder, which continued to
give fathers a strong economic interest in their daughters' sexual relationships. Young women still typically moved to their husband's family home
upon marrying, including moving to an entirely unfamiliar village in many
cases. Within their new households, young wives were expected to be hard-
working and to follow the wishes of their husbands and in-laws. Any man
in a household generally had greater authority than resident women and was
responsible for major decisions. It was unusual for men to use physical force
to assert their will over their wives, but this did happen on occasion, typically
with heavy drinkers.

Relations between the sexes will be discussed in detail later in the book,
including unmarried young people's sexual relationships (chapter 6), the impact of the division of labor and coercion on those relationships (chapter 7),
and young people's marital relationships (chapter 9).

Social Events

During evening hours some villagers, primarily young and adult men, strolled
and mingled in the village center, and some men regularly met to drink *pombe*
together in the home of a beer brewer or at a bar. Attending weekly markets,
church, funerals, weddings, video shows, discos, holiday celebrations, or
ngoma events were the main events at which people met informally outside
of work. With the exception of Christian or Muslim events, men were more
likely to drink alcohol and become intoxicated than normal at the social gatherings above, as were a small minority of women.

In most villages, a video show was hosted by traveling business men from
approximately 8:00 p.m. to 1:00 a.m. on market days or holidays. Attendance
typically cost Tshs 100 ($0.12). A diverse range of videos were shown, such
as East African music videos, Chinese action films, and American pornogra-
phy, the latter typically shown late at night. Videos were often accompanied
by an interpreter who loosely and sometimes quite inaccurately translated the
non-Swahili content into Swahili and Sukuma, including exaggerating sexual
content and exchanging sexual comments about the video with male audience
members. Video shows mainly were attended by married and unmarried men,

but a small number of unmarried girls and women also attended them, usually in the company of a man.

Discos were also held in many study villages during participant observation visits, although they were less common than video shows, and seemed to draw fewer participants. Discos took a number of forms, including all-night events which took place in village centers on holidays, private events at weddings, and semipublic events held in private homes as a way to generate money. Young men were most likely to host these latter discos, in order to earn money for major expenses, such as bridewealth. Discos usually took place outside, mainly were attended by village men, and were hosted by a traveling disc jockey who brought a small group of female dancers (*msela* singular, *basela* plural) as part of the entertainment. Typically, a male villager paid Tshs 100 ($0.12) to have the song and dance partner of his choice, unless someone else bid more money, in which case the lower bidder effectively was "benched" (*kubenchiana*). The highest such bid that a researcher observed during participant observation was Tshs 800 ($0.96). A winning bidder then danced for that song with his friends and his chosen *msela* within a circle of onlookers. Men might also pay for sex with those young women, and *basela* were rumored to have several partners a night during a disco. In our study, both discos and video shows were held most frequently in fishing villages, where they typically were more crowded and involved more cash flow than in other villages.

Ngoma events continued to be important social occasions in most of the villages in our study, particularly those in remote, almost entirely Sukuma settings. Unlike video shows and discos, *ngoma* events were attended by large numbers of male and female villagers of all ages, particularly before dark. Small *ngoma* events were sometimes held in a village center on a weekly market day, while large events took place on holidays and after the main harvest. For example, in one remote, inland village the *ngoma* associated with the *Saba saba* holiday lasted an entire week. During that week, two *ngoma* groups danced on opposite sides of a large, cleared area every afternoon from 3:00 p.m. until late at night. Villagers were allowed to observe the performances for free during the week, but adults needed to pay Tshs 100 ($0.12) and children Tshs 50 ($0.06) on the final night of the competition, as the most exciting performances typically took place that night. *Ngoma* performers claimed to use traditional medicine to draw a crowd and to repel magical attacks from the other *ngoma* group. Performers often wore elaborate body paint and costumes, and used many means to draw a crowd's attention, including athletic dancing, creative songs, drama, and snake handling. At each event, an organizing committee determined the winner by judging which of the two groups attracted the biggest crowd.

Supernatural Beliefs

As already discussed, the majority of people in our study identified themselves as Christian or Muslim. Both Christians and Muslims commonly referred to the power of God to direct their lives and determine their exposure to misfortune. This could either be expressed positively, demonstrating faith in a divine plan, or negatively, indicating powerlessness and an inability to avoid misfortune. Belief in God's power occasionally involved active attempts to solicit his protection or intervention, most obviously by praying, but also by other means, such as wearing rosary beads or sleeping with a bible under one's pillow.

Ancestral Beliefs

Although most villagers identified themselves as Christian or Muslim, most of them also held traditional beliefs and practices which contradicted those religions. Very few villagers felt a conflict about such pluralistic beliefs. It was widely believed that one's ancestors influenced one's life, either through protection from illness, injury, or malicious forces, or by withdrawing protection and actively causing harm if they became angered. Ancestral spirits were sometimes believed to object to certain modern practices, such as sending children to school or abandoning traditional house designs. They particularly were angered by direct harm to their lineage, for instance, when a pregnancy begotten by a descendant was aborted, which will be discussed in chapter 10.

Many homesteads had ancestral shrines, which were frameworks of woven branches in conical shapes that stood two to four feet above the ground. Two shrines representing maternal and paternal lineages typically were built in the center of a household compound. Respect for ancestors was expressed through rituals of pouring milk or local brew on such shrines. Some villagers also wore metal bangle amulets that had been given to them by traditional healers to promote harmony with their ancestors and protect them from harm.

Witchcraft

Belief in the effectiveness of traditional medicine was widespread in rural Mwanza, as was the belief in the possibility of witchcraft. A small minority of devout Christians believed that both traditional medicine and witchcraft were derived from the devil and thus were evil, but the vast majority of villagers distinguished between witchcraft as evil and traditional medicine as either ineffective or beneficial.

Witchcraft beliefs were strongest in the longer-settled and more exclusively Sukuma districts. For example, in two such villages Sukuma researchers attended village-wide crime-reduction meetings at which leaders held a vote to identify witches. However, witchcraft beliefs were also common in other study villages, including amongst Christian and Muslim leaders and non-Sukuma teachers. Witchcraft was particularly linked to envy: some villagers who accumulated wealth or other advantages feared that envious people might bewitch them, and people who experienced misfortune sometimes believed that they had been bewitched by others who envied them.

In most study villages there were a few individuals—usually older women—who were reported to be witches by many of their fellow villagers. Those who lived alone particularly were suspect because, it was reported, they did not want others to observe their witchcraft, a belief that made single old women particularly vulnerable. In one village, one of the researchers was warned by the 35-year-old senior wife in her household: "My child, do you think here in the village there is a decent old woman? Few, [because] every one of them is just a witch" [PO-02-I-4-5f]. Concern about being labeled and stigmatized as a witch led some older women to be careful not to draw attention to themselves. For example, a married woman in her 40s explained why she only provided traditional medicine to her family:

> She said that personally she doesn't help people who are not her close relatives. She doesn't do so because, she said, if it becomes widely known that you treat [people], then people from outside will also come to seek help. And if you help them, then eventually you will be maliciously accused of being a witch. [She continued] that witches might change her medicine, and instead of curing people it will harm them. [PO-02-C-3-3m]

Traditional healers often played an important role in diagnosing witchcraft and thus perpetuating witchcraft beliefs. In many recorded accounts, a person or a person's child first suffered from an inexplicable illness and sought treatment from a traditional healer, who then established that the cause was sorcery. Sometimes the client was invited to identify who might want to harm them, but sometimes the traditional healer proposed a name, possibly based on familiarity with village relationships and who might be in conflict with the client. In one example involving a polygynous man and his two wives:

> The first wife says that she does not like the second wife, because the second wife is a witch and once made a traditional medicine in order to kill her and marry her husband. She learned she had been bewitched after becoming seriously ill and going to see a traditional healer, who told her that the other woman had bewitched her. [PO-02-C-2-6f]

Most villagers seemed to believe in traditional healers' abilities to identify witches, although occasionally people voiced suspicion that traditional healers used their knowledge of local animosities to make such claims. For example, doubt was expressed by an 18-year-old woman whose mother, a nurse, was reported to have died of AIDS: "[The young woman] said if she falls sick she will go to a hospital, because traditional healers are liars and tell patients that all diseases they suffer from are a result of witchcraft" [PO-99-I-1-2f].

Participant observation researchers found that villagers' concern not to provoke envy sometimes seemed to inhibit entrepreneurial activity. For example, some successful businessmen reportedly disguised their wealth or moved out of their village for fear of being bewitched. In almost all villages there were also reports of individuals or families that recently had fled the village either because they thought themselves the victims of witchcraft or because they were accused of it and feared retribution. In one participant observation village, for example, a woman was accused of bewitching and killing a small child, and then was attacked by a group with machetes. After she recovered in the hospital, she did not return to her village for fear of being attacked again.

In our study, village authorities' responses to witchcraft accusations varied, sometimes taking the side of the accusers and sometimes the side of the accused. An example of the latter was reported by a 25-year-old man:

> My informant told me that two women had quarreled with a man, and the man then got scared that the two women would bewitch him. He decided to take the offensive and went to the first woman's home and intimidated her by pulling grass from her roof while telling her that if she did anything to him, he would kill her. After that he went to the second woman's house where he found her boiling water to cook porridge. He poured the boiling water on her but she did not get hurt because the water only reached her clothes. The two women went to complain to the village authorities. The man said he was drunk and did not remember doing any of it. After being interrogated and various people giving evidence he was found guilty. He was required to give two goats to the woman who he attacked while cooking, a sheep to the other one, and another two goats to the *sungusungu*. [PO-00-I-4-1m]

Illness Beliefs and Treatment

Beliefs about illness causation in rural Mwanza generally fell into five categories which were not mutually exclusive: natural/biological, chance, God's will, ancestral spirits, and witchcraft. Beliefs that illnesses had supernatural causes were particularly strong in remote villages, but they were not specific to any gender, age group, education level, or formal religion.

Most villagers believed it was normal to be periodically ill with malaria, diarrhea, or headaches. Many simply described illnesses as being caused by

"God's will," not because God specifically planned them, but because they are within God's control. Similarly, informants sometimes referred to illness as the result of chance or bad luck. For example, when a girl complained about the smell and appearance of a woman's abdominal swelling, another girl replied, "What do you expect her to do? She didn't ask for this illness, it just happened to her" [PO-01-C-2-5f].

Some illnesses were instead attributed to natural or biological causes, particularly among people with more formal education, such as village authorities, health workers, or teachers. For example, a Village Executive Officer said: "People were troubled by stomach diseases, since the water they were using was not very clean . . . these problems have greatly reduced, because people now have toilets, and clean water is more available" [PO-99-I-6-1m].

Illnesses were also occasionally attributed to ancestral displeasure. In one example, a male farmer in his 50s described how the death of his grandchild due to jaundice led him to actively seek ancestral protection:

> He said that a traditional healer told him they must build some shrines for the spirits, like those which were being built by our ancestors. They were told if they do so, the family illnesses will diminish, as the spirits will be close to them and will be able to protect them. [PO-01-C-3-3m]

Witches were believed to make others ill in a variety of possible ways, such as tricking their victims to drink or step on magical and/or contaminated materials. Witchcraft-induced ailments reportedly included "normal" illnesses which occurred with abnormally high frequency, such as diarrhea and malaria, as well as less common illnesses, such as foot or leg problems, convulsions, infertility, and mental illness. Villagers sometimes took special measures to prevent being bewitched in this way, such as wearing magical charms, drinking or bathing in traditional medicines, cutting protective incisions in their bodies, placing special objects in key places in their homes, or asking a traditional healer to perform protective rituals.

In our study, less commonly reported beliefs included that ill health can be caused by *majini* (evil spirits) or *wazungu* (white people). For example, a participant observation researcher heard a 30-year-old single mother and a married mother in her 40s discuss this latter belief: "One said that whites are cunning, because they manufacture dangerous drugs and body creams and export them all to Africa. She said that they are using the same trick to make women sterile by encouraging them to use family planning pills" [PO-00-C-3-2f].

Symptoms were very important in illness recognition, diagnosis, and treatment in rural Mwanza, and once symptoms resolved people generally believed that they were cured of an illness. The three major sources of treatment were home remedies (both western and traditional), traditional healers, and biomedical health care providers (officially at health facilities, or less frequently at the providers' homes). Treatment-seeking was pluralistic and opportunistic, depending on factors such as the perceived cause, nature, and severity of symptoms, and the proximity, cost, and perceived confidentiality of care providers.

Home Remedies

Most ill people first tried to diagnose and treat themselves at home, because this was relatively convenient, private, and cheap. Knowledge of traditional home remedies was often passed from generation to generation. Adults who claimed knowledge of an illness recommended that certain plants be harvested, processed, and then typically swallowed. However, depending on the condition being treated, medicine might also be placed on an incision, in a bath, on or in the genitals, or—in the case of a breastfeeding baby—on the mother's breast. Treatments sometimes required that specific practices be followed, such as walking backwards after drinking a medicine.

In addition to, or instead of, traditional home remedies, many people used western medicines bought at a kiosk. Those medicines were generally sold by the pill without a prescription, although many were not approved for over-the-counter use. The type and amount of pills used were generally decided by how much money the customer had, and anecdotal recommendations by the kiosk salesperson or anyone else who claimed to have familiarity with that medication.

Traditional Healers

If home remedies failed, villagers then sought treatment from a traditional healer and/or a health facility. People sometimes preferred a traditional healer to a health facility because of familiarity, trust, accessibility, expense, payment plans (e.g., credit or in kind), and the illness itself. Traditional healers were believed to successfully treat many naturally caused and witchcraft-induced illnesses, but medical providers were not believed to successfully treat the latter.

Researchers visited a number of traditional healers at their homes and workplaces during participant observation, and one researcher lived with a farmer and entertainer in his 40s who had recently started a business as a traditional healer. Traditional healers were respected and sometimes feared in villages. For example, some informants believed that if a bill went unpaid a traditional healer would make a person's illness return. A few traditional healers reported that they referred people who they could not treat to other traditional healers or to health facilities, and a small minority also reported a faith in Christianity or Islam.

Traditional healers reported learning their skills from older healers within their immediate family, by paying to apprentice with established healers for months or years, and/or through dreams. Traditional healers identified illnesses by diagnosing symptoms, dream interpretation, and/or performing rituals with special plants or animals. Treatment sometimes included rituals against what was believed to be the original cause, for instance, conducting a ceremony to appease a patient's ancestors, or casting a counterspell to harm a suspected witch. Treatment usually also involved ingestion or external application of processed wild herbs, bark, and/or roots. Some traditional healers also performed minor surgery, such as incisions in the skin for application of a medicine, or cutting off unwanted growths. Some had compounds in which they provided long-term care for patients.

Biomedical Treatment

Many ill villagers sought to be treated by people trained in western medicine, either as a complement or an alternative to a traditional healer's treatment. This was particularly common for villagers who lived near health facilities or who attended health facilities for other reasons, such as mothers whose children were being vaccinated. For more substantial biomedical treatment villagers attended more distant hospitals. A 19-year-old shop attendant gave the following example:

> He said that after failing to be cured through a traditional healer, a local boy's father decided to take him to the nearest health center [4 km away], but the staff there referred them to the mission hospital [13 km away]. He said that the boy underwent an operation there and his condition improved. To meet the treatment costs, the father had to sell some cows, so there are only two cows remaining in their homestead. [PO-99-I-6-1m]

Each government health facility served three to five villages, so they were located at district capitals or large villages along major roads. Private facilities such as the mission hospital described above were less common. Most travel in rural Mwanza took place on foot, so villagers often walked three to ten kilometers to visit a health facility. Sick people who could not walk were usually carried on bicycles for a fee, or on locally made stretchers. This could be very difficult during the rainy season if roads and pathways were impassable.

Most government health facilities were staffed by one or a few clinical assistants, health auxiliaries, nurses, and/or rural medical aids, who usually

had completed Year 7 of primary school and some additional medical training. Less frequently facilities also had a clinical officer who typically had
completed Form 4 (Year 11) and an additional two to four years of medical
training. Medical staff were centrally assigned to their village positions, and
many did not speak Sukuma. Medical care was mainly limited to the treatment of symptoms or the syndromic management of common illnesses, such
as fever, cough, bloody urine, and genital discharge.

Health facilities were frequently reported to have basic equipment and
medication shortages. During participant observation visits, there were several reports of children dying after being turned away from health facilities
for lack of supplies. A Village Chairman described problems he encountered
with his own child:

> He gave his child local medicines . . . but the condition continued to be very
> serious, so he took the child to the nearest facility [6 km east]. They did not have
> enough equipment . . . So he went to the district hospital [13 km west], where
> the equipment had also been stolen. . . . The next day he had to take the child to
> a different hospital [33 km away]. [PO-00-I-4-4f]

DISCUSSION

Rural Mwanza experienced tremendous political, social, health, and ecological changes in the nineteenth and twentieth centuries. Nonetheless, many
aspects of daily life in Sukuma villages had not changed radically by the
time of our fieldwork from 1999–2002. This finding was supported by those
of anthropologists whose combined worked with the Sukuma spanned fifty
years (Wijsen and Tanner 2002). The main economic activity at the time of
our study was farming, which was still almost entirely nonmechanized, and
life in most villages was dominated by the agricultural seasons. Fishing villages differed from purely agricultural villages in several important ways.
Largely due to economic opportunities they tended to be larger with much
more mobile populations. Consequently they tended to be more ethnically
diverse and less interknit and conservative.

Almost all villagers in our study were very poor. Most young people grew
up in very modest houses of simple construction, shared sleeping places with
their siblings, had only a few sets of clothes, and lived on 1–2 high carbohydrate meals per day. The traditional gendered division of labor persisted,
so women were responsible for most domestic work and spent most of their
waking hours engaged in household chores, farming, or petty trade. Men had
few domestic responsibilities and more leisure time, particularly during the

dry season. Men often worked in trades or other businesses where they were compensated monetarily. The influence of this economic imbalance on young people's sexual behavior will be discussed throughout this book, but most notably in chapter 7.

In the early twentieth century, almost all wealth in rural Mwanza was in the form of cattle and land. These mainly were owned by older men, who also made most of the important decisions within their communities and families. By the time of our study, older men still wielded considerable control over life in rural Mwanza. However, at a village level their informal political leadership required collaboration with elected and appointed government officials. At a family level, young people—especially young men—increasingly were independent of their elder's influence because of more opportunities to earn money than in the past. Fewer young couples obtained parental consent and advance agreement of bridewealth before they married, so parental influence in partner selection and the economic benefits of daughters' marriages seemed to have declined somewhat. Our findings on young people's decision to marry and their marital and extramarital sexual relationships will be described in chapter 9.

At the time of the study, *ngoma* continued to be a very important part of cultural life and entertainment in rural Mwanza. However, modern forms of entertainment such as video shows and discos had also become popular and common in rural areas, especially amongst young men. Video shows in particular gave villagers glimpses into a range of diverse cultural beliefs and practices from elsewhere in Africa and the world. At these and other social gatherings there were also far fewer sexual restrictions than typically found in daily life, which will be discussed further in chapter 5.

In the early twentieth century health care in rural Mwanza almost entirely consisted of traditional medicine, but use of biomedical health services increased gradually since then. By the time of our study, most villagers had used western medicine at some point in their lives, but traditional health beliefs were widely maintained. We found that traditional medicines were often a first course of treatment for health problems, whether the medicines were obtained at home, from other villagers, or from specialized healers.

When considering the cause of a health problem or other misfortune, ancestral displeasure was no longer a great concern for most villagers, and few villagers regularly maintained rituals in honor of their ancestors. Such beliefs may have diminished over time as Christianity and Islam became more established in rural areas. However, the possibility of bewitchment was a very active concern for villagers in our study and misfortune was readily attributed to it. Later in the book we will discuss our findings on specific traditional and biomedical health beliefs and practices, particularly as relate to contraception, abortion, and fertility (chapter 10), and AIDS and other sexually transmitted infections (chapter 11).

Some of the most notable changes in villages during the last century took place in the lives of children and young people, particularly after the introduction of formal schooling. In the next chapter, we will review the historical literature on children's lives in rural Mwanza, before considering children's experiences with parents, peers, and school teachers at the time of our study.

NOTES

1. Some contemporary writers in English refer to the Sukuma and Swahili languages and peoples by the terms that would be used within either language, e.g., **Basukuma** (the Sukuma people), **Kisukuma** (the Sukuma language), and *Kiswahili* (the Swahili language). This is not practiced for most other languages and peoples, e.g., when speaking English, the German people are not referred to using the German term "die Deutschen" and the German language is not referred to as "Deutsch." In this book we have thus adopted the conventional English practice of simply referring to the "Sukuma" and "Swahili" languages and peoples.

2. When we use the term "traditional" to describe our findings in this book we mean local, non-Western beliefs and practices that were reportedly handed down from prior generations. However, it is likely that some of these were more recently introduced, or had been substantially modified over time (Wijsen and Tanner 2002).

Chapter Four

Children's Relationships with Parents, Peers, and Teachers[1]

In this chapter we will build upon the broad aspects of life in rural Mwanza described in chapter 3 to examine children's experiences and relationships with their parents, peers, and school teachers. We will also describe the formal education system in Tanzania and general conditions within primary schools. We will first review the historical literature on these topics before describing our study's findings at the beginning of the twenty-first century.

HISTORICAL LITERATURE ON SUKUMA CHILDHOOD

During the twentieth century, several anthropologists described common features of Sukuma childhood. Cory (1953, 86), for example, described Sukuma mothers as typically having a gentle approach to parenting:

> Orders are given without sharpness, questions are put without menace . . . children are treated with understanding and their faults are readily pardoned. Small children and even those of more advanced age are seldom punished; at least not methodically as a measure of education. A child is punished usually only when an adult person has been provoked to short-lived anger. Examples of persistent ill-treatment of children are very rare and are looked upon by everyone as symptoms of madness. Children are regarded by their parents and families as an asset not a liability; only a madman will destroy or damage valuable property of his own.

Anthropologists usually have described Sukuma mothers as being most openly affectionate with their children in their first one to two years, before the children were weaned. By the time a child could walk, however, Sukuma mothers were described as having a more detached approach, and primary child care was often handed over to an older child, particularly as many mothers were pregnant again or had a newborn at that stage (Varkevisser 1973). Generally, anthropologists have described Sukuma parents and their older children as having an "avoidance relationship," similar to that described between husbands and wives in chapter 3. For parents and children, one of the fundamental taboos of such a relationship is to speak of sexual matters (Radcliffe-Brown 1950; Abrahams 1981; Van Eeuwijk and Mlangwa 1997; Baylies et al. 1999; Bujra 2000). As Varkevisser (1973, 76) noted: "A relationship of respect precludes joking. Any sexual allusion to or in the presence of a person to whom one owes respect is a misdemeanour."

Sukuma children traditionally have helped with chores from an early age, small girls often caring for infants and toddlers and small boys often herding livestock while their parents farmed (Cory 1953). In their spare time, small boys and girls engaged in imaginative play together, particularly a game that involved pretending to be adults, building huts, making clay cattle, cooking imaginary food, and going to bed as a married couple, as they saw their parents do in rooms they shared with them at night (Cory 1953; Varkevisser 1973). In her 1965–1967 study of Sukuma childhood, Varkevisser (1973) often observed small children engaged in fantasy play, rhyming, singing, and playing traditional board games, during which they demonstrated an ability to count to ten and perform basic calculations. By the age of seven or eight, however, Varkevisser (1973) found that girls were discouraged from playing with older boys, and their mobility and free time reduced substantially because they had many domestic responsibilities. In contrast, by 10 years of age boys typically refused to assist in most domestic chores, but they participated in men's responsibilities such as house construction. Both boys and girls participated in farming and were expected to meet some of their own basic needs by an early age. Varkevisser (1973, 228) explained:

> Parents encourage children at a young age to provide new clothes for themselves. As soon as their offspring can manage to manipulate tools effectively and to perform elementary agricultural operations, at the age of 9 or 10, many parents assign their sons and daughter a small patch of ground on which to grow cotton, so that the children can earn cash to cover partially the costs of their own attire.

Varkevisser (1973) found that older children were expected to provide for other basic needs as well, such as school uniforms, school fees, and a pencil or notebook. By the age of 12 (for girls) and 15 (for boys), children were able to fulfill the main work responsibilities of adult women and men, respectively. It was also not unusual for children to move between homesteads during their childhoods, in response to invitations from relatives who needed help or wanted company, such as grandparents, uncles or aunts, or older siblings (Varkevisser 1973).

In the early to mid-twentieth century, before formal schooling became common, 10–16-year-old Sukuma boys and 10–14-year-old Sukuma girls formed informal organizations which mimicked the structure and functions of the older social group of young men and unmarried young women described in chapter 3 (Varkevisser 1973). The main purpose of these younger groups was farming, but they also had elected leaders who organized feasts, maintained peace amongst the members, levied fines for late arrival or absences, and managed group funds. Varkevisser (1973) observed that these preteen to early teen groups had the educational benefits of teaching diligence, collective work, public speaking and the rules which governed behavior in neighborhood associations of adults.

As children approached puberty, the groups described above and less formal peer groups typically played an important role in challenging parental discipline. At that age, children continued to follow rules in the presence of adults, but they increasingly subverted some rules when adults were out of sight. Varkevisser (1973, 239) explained:

> Although [Sukuma children] remain duty bound to honor parental commandments as they grow older—no aggression, no sexplay, no destruction or theft of homestead property—transgressions become more or less institutionalized in some pastimes.

In the early 1900s, unmarried teenagers and young adults from different homesteads often slept within a large, same-sex room in one homestead, the young men typically housed independently and the young women often sleeping in the company of a grandmother (Cory 1953; Abrahams 1967). Early anthropologists reported that young people in these "dormitories" were allowed to pursue nighttime sexual relationships as long as they were discreet (Cory 1953; Abrahams 1967). By the 1960s, however, many unmarried girls and young women no longer slept in large numbers in a dormitory with a grandmother. Instead, the unmarried sisters and cousins in each household typically shared one room within the homestead. Nonetheless, discreet nighttime sexual liaisons for unmarried youth were still fairly common (Varkevisser 1973). At that time, young Sukuma women typically married by the age of 15 or 16 years, and most young men five years later.

A HISTORY OF FORMAL EDUCATION IN TANZANIA

Beginning in the 1870s, a large number of Christian missionary schools were built across Tanzania, mainly by the Germans, British, and French (Topan

2008). At that time, approximately 125 indigenous languages were spoken in Tanzania but Swahili was already established as a trade language across the country, so it was the language most missionaries used in their schools (Topan 2008). During the German colonial period from 1890–1917, the Germans additionally established 60 secular, three-year Swahili-language primary schools, nine two-year middle schools and one high school, mostly along the coast of the Indian Ocean (Iliffe 1979; Topan 2008). From 1918–1961, British colonial powers built upon this system, expanding the number of schools, introducing English as a taught course in Years 3 and 4, and making it the language of instruction for Years 5 to 8 in secondary school (Topan 2008).

Under colonialism, small ethnic groups that were targeted by early and intense missionary efforts developed an educational lead over some larger ones (Iliffe 1979). Similarly, Christians generally gained advantages over Muslims and those without religious affiliations, and urban children received higher quality education than rural children partly because they were not preoccupied with agricultural responsibilities (Iliffe 1979). These patterns have had important, long-term repercussions, as Christians and certain small ethnic groups have continued to dominate political leadership in Tanzania, while larger ones like the Sukuma generally have been underrepresented relative to their size (Iliffe 1979; Omari 1987; Kessler 2006).

In the 1957 census, 16 percent of boys and 8 percent of girls aged 6–15 years in the Western Province (an area that overlapped with Sukumaland) were estimated to have had primary education (Abrahams 1967). A decade later, postindependence, half of Tanzanian children attended the first years of primary school (Varkevisser 1973). Most of the Tanzanian population did not speak Swahili as a first language, so their introduction to it in primary school was important in unifying the country (Topan 2008). The new socialist government soon made Swahili the language of instruction for the entire seven years of primary school. However, there was debate within the national leadership as to whether English should continue to be the language of secondary and tertiary education, since it might perpetuate the inaccessibility of higher education for the vast majority of the population (Topan 2008). In the end English did retain this role, reportedly because of a: "shortage of textbooks and resources in translation, shortage of trained teachers, [and] a general state of unpreparedness. . . . [In addition] English enables Tanzanians to have access to the outside world, to its knowledge, business, and global culture" (Topan 2008, 262).

In 1965, shortly after Tanzanian independence, only 10–15 percent of primary school children were admitted to secondary school (Topan 2008). Tanzania's first president, Julius Nyerere, soon implemented an "Education for

Self-reliance" policy which did not substantially increase secondary school participation but rather tried to ensure that primary education taught the skills needed for an agricultural society (Topan 2008). Active recruitment efforts also led to vast increases in the number of primary school pupils.

Working with a team of social scientists and educationalists in primary schools soon after national independence, Varkevisser (1973, 278) became concerned about what she referred to as the "stultifying" quality of education in rural Mwanza primary schools.

[An educationalist colleague] observed few occasions when teachers attempted to encourage children to pose questions; their responsibility was more to give answers, preferably in the wordings of their texts or of notes copied from the blackboard. Rote learning is perhaps inevitable in an educational system where test-scores derived from questions based on memory instead of insight determine whether a child will be one of the envied few with an opportunity to go on with his education.

Varkevisser (1973, 278–79) believed that Sukuma parents typically expected children to be obedient, but that children's experiences at home being responsible for younger siblings and engaging in imaginative and humorous discussion with grandparents and peers counterbalanced that submissive experience. She did not see a similar balance in schools:

It is startling to see how easily the same children who sit for hours on their school benches without discharging a flicker of initiative appear able, upon returning home, to shed their passivity when they shed their school uniforms and to emerge as active near-adults. Teachers seem ignorant of children's early capacity for independent action. They fail to harness the learning energy latent in their young students' proven self-reliance. Instead their authoritarian stance induces regression, battering students back into a state of dependence.

Varkevisser's critique reflected a much broader educational discussion that began in the 1960s and has continued internationally in the ensuing decades. Education specialists increasingly have promoted "competence-oriented" and "learner-centered" approaches to education, rather than traditional "performance-oriented" and "teacher-centered" approaches (Barrett 2007). Competence approaches are less authoritarian and more democratic, and focus on pupils understanding meaning rather than memorizing information (Barrett 2007). These teaching methods are also more tailored to the needs of individuals, which can require more complex teacher training and greater expense (Barrett 2007).

PRIMARY EDUCATION IN MWANZA REGION
AND TANZANIA AT THE TIME OF THE STUDY

National school systems within sub-Saharan Africa grew rapidly post-independence, despite having very limited resources. At the beginning of the twenty-first century they faced many challenges, including limited en-rollment and completion rates, and low levels of knowledge and skills even amongst those who did complete school (Johnson 2008; Lloyd and Hewett 2009). In several African countries, less than half of 15–24-year-old women could read a simple sentence after three years of primary school; even many of those who reached lower secondary school could hardly read or write (World Bank 2006). Within that context, the Tanzanian education system was considered to be particularly challenged—"a very late developer" (Cooksey and Riedmiller 1997, 123)—characterized by extreme underfunding, bureau-cratic inefficiency, corruption, and one of the smallest secondary and tertiary education sectors in the world.

When our study began in 1999, only 29 percent of men and 26 percent of women had completed primary school in Tanzania, and only 5 percent and 4 percent respectively had gone on to secondary school (National Bureau of Statistics and Macro International 2000). The older generations had the least experience of formal education; for example, 66 percent of men and 88 percent of women older than 64 years had never gone to school. In contrast, at that time over half of boys (51 percent) and girls (56 percent) of official primary school age (7–13 years) were registered as attending primary school. Notably, higher proportions of girls than boys attended school at the ages of 7–10 years, but by the age of 13 this shifted to higher proportions of boys than girls, and a large proportion of the primary school population was older than that. In 2003, for example, over half of Year 7 pupils were 15–17 years old, because many had only started school when they were nine or ten years old and many had repeated school years (Partnership for Child Development 1998; Bommier and Lambert 2000; United Republic of Tanzania 2003). At that time, only 19 percent of Year 7 pupils went on to secondary school (Palmer et al. 2007). Once in secondary school, students faced the great challenge of studying and taking exams in English, a language that the vast majority had been introduced to only at a very basic level in primary school.

At the time of our study, material conditions in Tanzanian primary schools were very poor, particularly in rural schools, which rarely had running water, electricity, or other basic facilities (Arthur 2001; O-saki and Agu 2002; Towse et al. 2002; Nilsson 2003; Renju and Nyalali 2008). Furthermore, teachers had received variable levels of training. Most of those trained in the 1970s and 1980s had only completed Year 7 of primary school themselves, and then had one additional year of teacher training college (Bennell and Mukyanuzi 2005). More recently, the national government set a goal for new teachers to have four years of secondary school and one to two years of teacher training college, but at the time of our study only 54 percent of Mwanza Region primary schoolteachers had that qualification (United Republic of Tanzania 1999). Many teachers perceived teaching as a "last resort," low-status, low-paid job, and they particularly wanted to avoid the isolation and hardship associated with rural settings (Towse et al. 2002). Rural Mwanza thus had some of the most underqualified and understaffed schools in the country, and only a minority of teachers were female (Bennell and Makyanuzi 2005). Despite limited training and a challenging work environment, however, many Mwanza teachers worked very hard and attempted to maximize the benefits of available resources, for example, trying to ensure that every child had a chance to use a book when possible (Renju and Nyalali 2008).

At the start of the twenty-first century, primary school teaching in Mwanza and elsewhere in Tanzania continued to be largely didactic, consisting almost entirely of lecturing, formal question-and-answer sessions, recitation, and having pupils copy sentences from the board (Cooksey and Riedmiller 1997; Arthur 2001; O-saki and Agu 2002). Emphasis was placed on memorizing information to pass national exams, rather than the development of critical thinking, knowledge application, or problem-solving skills. It was common for teachers and the children they appointed as prefects to practice corporal punishment, that is, to intentionally inflict pain to discipline a pupil, usually by hitting or caning them. Barrett (2007) noted that, in the absence of more progressive teacher training, some Tanzanian teachers nonetheless employed creative, interactive approaches which were rooted in local culture, such as games involving riddles and proverbs. In such a poor, performance-oriented setting, she further argued that it may be too much to expect teachers to have a learner-oriented approach, as they have very large class sizes and few resources, they are expected to follow a national curriculum, and they are evaluated specifically in terms of their students' achievements in national exams. At the time of our study, there were 931 primary schools and 40 secondary schools in Mwanza Region; the primary schools had an average of 675 registered pupils and nine teachers per school (United Republic of Tanzania 2003). Class sizes and teacher-to-pupil ratios have only worsened since our study, with class sizes of 100 to 200 pupils per teacher typical in the first two years of primary school in 2008 (Benson 2006; Barrett 2007).

In the next section we will draw on our study's findings to examine the topics raised above. Specifically, we will focus on children's relationships with their parents, peers, and teachers, as well as the general school conditions in study villages from 1999–2002.

FINDINGS

Parent-Child Relationships

In the first series of in-depth interviews, only 35 percent (22/63) of randomly selected respondents reported that their parents were in a monogamous marriage and that they lived with both of them. Forty-one percent (26/63) reported that their father was or had been polygynous at some point in their lives, but only 24 percent (15/63) reported that their parents continued to be in a polygnous marriage at the time of the interview. Most of those respondents lived with their mother full-time and their father when he visited on a daily, weekly, or yearly basis, but a few lived in a household with their father, mother, and one or move co-wives, or lived with their father and a co-wife because their mother had moved away for work or long-term medical care. Seven in-depth interview respondents reported that they lived with their mother alone (4) or with their mother and a step-father (3), and six said they lived with their father and a stepmother. The remaining 13 randomly selected respondents reported that they had not lived with a biological parent for many years, but instead with a grandparent, aunt, uncle, sibling, or, in one case, a husband. Eight of the 63 respondents said that their father (5) or mother (3) had died, and five said that they had never known their father.

In the study villages, relationships between parents and their prepubescent or adolescent children were typically formal. From a young age children were taught to be generally deferential towards adults and markedly so towards their parents, although older people sometimes commented that the younger generation was not as respectful as they themselves had been when they were younger. Researchers observed that children almost always initiated greetings by using the respectful term "*Shikamoo*" with their parents and other adults, the common practice when greeting someone of greater age or higher status in Tanzania. When giving this greeting in rural Mwanza, girls often curtsied and remained crouched or kneeling (figure 4.1), while boys stood still until

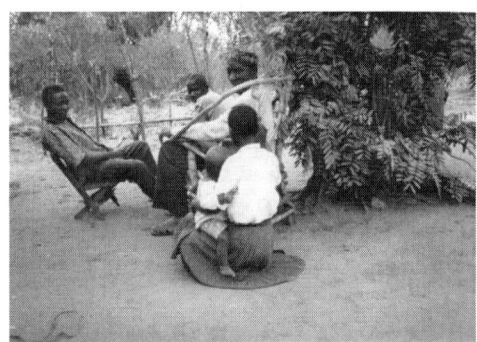

Figure 4.1. A girl holding a baby while greeting an elderly man and her brothers with a traditional curtsey.

the exchanges were completed. When talking with their parents, and especially their fathers, children usually did not look them in the eyes, behaved demurely, talked quietly, and rarely joked. Well into adulthood, people continued to demonstrate overt respect for their elders' decision-making.

Living within households, researchers developed the impression that most parents felt affection towards their children, but they were rarely demonstrative or direct in expressing this. Parental concern for their children's current and future welfare was often evident in the material support and practical training they provided, their general monitoring and regulation of their children's activities, and the primary care and advocacy they provided when their children were ill. Later in this book, for example, case study 3.1 describes how a father went to great lengths to ensure his ill child received good medical treatment, and how both he and the boy's mother closely cared for their son during that time.

Parents seldom worked alongside their children, apart from domestic work involving mothers and daughters or intensive periods of farm work. It was also rare to see parents spending their leisure time—something largely restricted to males—with their children, although parents sometimes ate their meals with their children. Women, girls, and small boys typically ate together near the cooking area, while men and older boys usually ate outside, elsewhere in the compound. A minority of households regularly had *shikome* fires where men and boys of about 6 years old and older sat in the late afternoon and evening, eating together and lingering afterwards as the men talked amongst themselves and the boys listened. However, this was reportedly less common than in the past, as explained by a 60-year-old man and two men in their 20s:

> They said that nowadays there are very few families in the village that sit around *shikome* fires. They said that young men prefer going for a walk in the village center and only return home briefly for dinner. They said that nowadays it is very rare to find a parent idly sitting with his children without any particular activity, for instance, eating. [PO-02-C-3-3m]

Parent-child relationships were also constrained by taboos in the study villages, for instance, adults rarely bathed in the presence of their children, although same-sex group bathing was common, and young men rarely drank beer in front of their parents' generation, even when they were old enough for beer drinking to be acceptable. Parents generally did not discuss sexual issues with their children, except sometimes indirectly, as when admiring or criticizing others' behavior. Unmarried children usually did not inform their parents of sex-related problems, because they believed their parents would not understand or would blame and punish them. For example, many girls told researchers they had been coerced to have sex but they tried to hide this from their parents. Similarly, adolescents who reported having had sexually transmitted infections said that they either had not told their parents, or they only told a same-sex parent after symptoms became severe.

Fathers were generally less approachable and stricter than mothers, so children feared their punishment more. It was considered acceptable for parents to use corporal punishment to train or discipline a child, including hitting or caning. However, in most families this seemed to be unusual and was rarely severe. A researcher recorded two examples one morning: "I heard a 3-year-old child crying. His mother was hitting him, telling him to greet his mother first and not wait to be greeted. Another neighbor called her 7–8-year-old child and asked him/her, 'Why haven't you swept the courtyard'? She also hit her child" [PO-01-C-2-5f]. Even when corporal punishment was infrequent, children were aware that it might occur and many told researchers that they hid forbidden activities specifically to avoid being hit or beaten by their parents.

Parents exercised considerable control over their children and strove to maintain this. As already discussed, much essential labor was performed by children from a young age (figures 4.2 and 4.3), particularly by girls, and this was seen as intrinsic to proper respect towards parents. The extent of young people's schooling was largely determined by parents, and parents generally tried to influence and restrict their children's sexual behavior and choice of marriage partners. Sons were usually dependent on their fathers for bridewealth. Children were expected to obey their parents closely until adulthood, and researchers rarely observed children openly disputing their parents' instructions. Disobedient or disrespectful children shamed their parents, and particularly their mothers, who usually were held responsible. Such children were perceived as a threat to the support parents expected in old age.

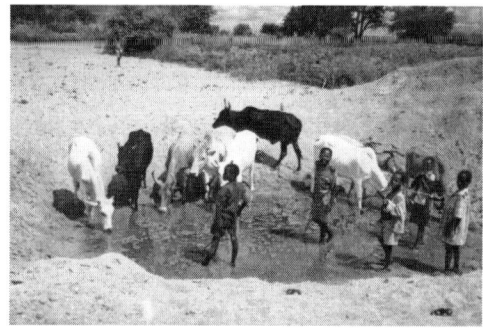

Figure 4.2. Boys herding cattle at a hand-dug water hole during the dry season.

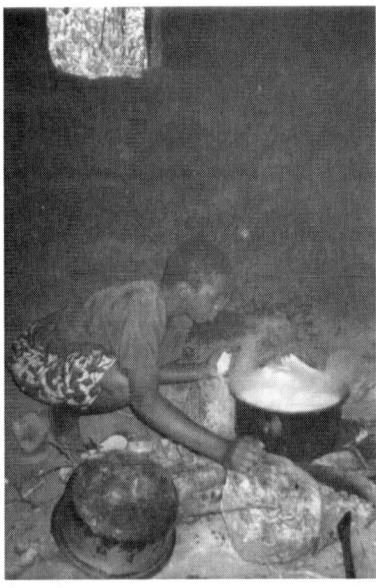

Figure 4.3. Girl cooking maize for a family meal. Cooking took place either outside of homes or within a room such as this, which might be used for sleeping or other purposes at other times of the day.

There were, however, some challenges to parental authority. The researchers occasionally heard young people openly argue with their elders, and older people sometimes bemoaned the passing of deferential practices, such as children only eating meat after the adults had had several helpings. Some older people also reported that the government was undermining parental control; for example, the possibility that authorities might restrict corporal punishment was resented by some older villagers. Covert resistance to parental power was also very common. The fieldworkers often recorded examples of children disobeying their parents when unsupervised, such as visiting a village center or attending a video show when this had been prohibited, which will be discussed more in the next chapter.

Peer Relationships

Our study found that, after their families, the two most important influences on young people's beliefs and behavior in rural Mwanza were their peers and schooling. Young boys and girls sometimes played together and shared tasks such as herding, but by the time they started school there was little opportunity for them to interact with the opposite sex publicly. Important exceptions were when young people were walking to or from school, on pathways when carrying out errand, and sometimes in the village center in the evenings when working or strolling there. Gender segregation was also relaxed when participating in church or political party choirs, mixed-sex cultivating groups, and holiday festivals or *ngoma* events, although even in such circumstances girls and boys generally stayed within their separate groups.

By school age, therefore, children in rural Mwanza mainly socialized with same-sex relatives, neighbors, and friends of roughly the same age. Most engagement with same-sex peers outside of school was in the course of domestic or agricultural work, such as fetching water or firewood, washing clothes, herding cattle, weeding or harvesting. Girls also regularly spent semi-leisure time together styling one another's hair. Boys had far less domestic work to do than girls, and their movements were much less restricted, so they spent more leisure time with their peers. They often hung out together at home or strolled together around the village. Many liked to play soccer, and some played cards or traditional board games.

One of the main ways in which young people interacted was through the *rika* laboring teams. *Rika* usually consisted of five to fifteen youths who cultivated each member's *shamba* in turn, but some of these groups instead hired themselves out to other farmers to cultivate their land. Parents accepted their children's *rika* participation as a way to ease farm work, and most youth were free to join a *rika* of their choice. During the cultivation season, young people might spend the whole day working with their *rika*, although groups that included school pupils usually worked after school hours and on weekends. Some *rika* dissolved at the end of the cultivation season, but some did other kinds of work together throughout the year, such as harvesting or felling trees for house building. The more established *rika* sometimes had formal leadership structures with an elected leader, a deputy leader, a secretary, and a treasurer.

Most *rika* were single-sex but some were mixed-sex, usually involving several girls and two to four times as many boys, as shown in figure 4.4. Within a mixed-sex *rika*, members tended to work alongside their own sex. Parents generally tolerated such *rika* more than other mixed-sex activities,

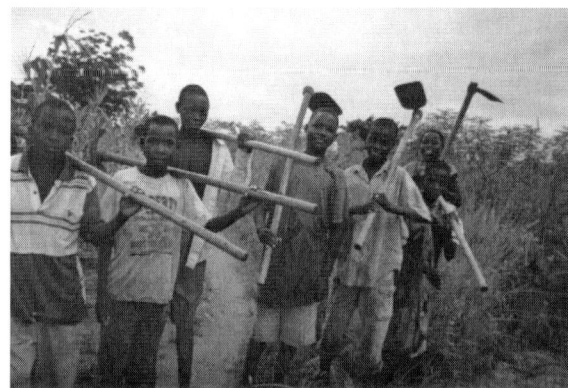

Figure 4.4.   A farming team (*rika*) made up of both boys and girls.

but some prohibited their daughters from working in them, fearing it would lead to sexual activity. Indeed, there were often reports of mixed-sex *rika* members being sexually involved, whether they had sexual liaisons during the working day, at an overnight assignment in a distant area, or at annual parties which *rika* threw to celebrate their achievements. Nonetheless, a few mixed-sex *rika* claimed to forbid such activity and their leaders reportedly fined young men suspected of having sex with female members. Once young women got married, they usually stopped *rika* participation, as it was considered less acceptable for married women and they had many other domestic and farming responsibilities within their husband's household.

At the start of the dry season following the main harvest, some *rika* became *ngoma* dance groups and performed at village centers on market days or holidays, as described in chapter 3. These groups predominantly were comprised of young men from their teens to their early 20s, but usually they included a few female teenagers as well. *Ngoma* dancers reported traveling from village to village performing *ngoma* throughout the dry season, making them absent from their village for weeks or months at a time. Such *ngoma* dancing usually was restricted to those who had left school.

General Primary School Conditions

Not all of the villages in our study had their own primary school, and some children had to walk as much as 6 kilometers each day to reach the nearest school. The material conditions of primary schools were very poor. Most consisted of two or three large buildings with several classrooms each, several houses for teachers, agricultural plots, and an earthen soccer field. Classrooms were constructed of earth or cement brick walls, iron-sheeted roofs, earth floors, and open doors and windows (figure 4.5). They usually were

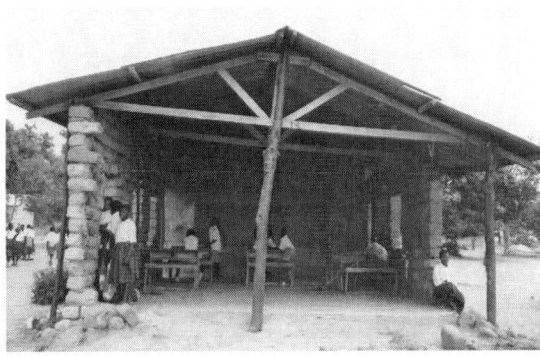

Figure 4.5. Primary school children in a classroom that is missing two walls. It was not unusual for classrooms to be in varying states of disrepair, with this being one extreme example.

equipped with a worn blackboard, chalk, and two-person desks, but there often were not enough desks, so some pupils sat on the floor, or several at one desk. Teachers sometimes had to manage with only one text book for the whole class, and sometimes with none at all. Schools did not have electricity or running water, and to relieve themselves teachers and pupils used pit latrines or, occasionally, nearby fields.

During the study period, annual school fees of Tshs 2,000 ($2.40) were abolished, but villagers still reported spending Tshs 6,000–8,000 ($9.60–12.00) per pupil per year for sports fees, running costs, paper and pencils, and school uniforms and shoes. In addition, school and village authorities sometimes raised school building and repair funds by requiring parents to contribute in cash or in kind. A few parents in our study said that they did not attend school meetings in order to avoid such demands. One head teacher reported he enlisted the **sungusungu** to ensure all parents made their contributions, and some parents specifically said they paid because they feared the **sungusungu**. Researchers often observed pupils carrying out chores around the school, tending school crops, or assisting in construction or repair work, and it was also not unusual for teachers to assign pupils to work in their homes. Some pupils said they did not mind this labor, but others said they felt exploited.

School Enrollment, Attendance, and Leaving

In the study villages, many children of primary school age attended school irregularly, and some not at all. In one school with 473 pupils, the head teacher said that recent census data showed an additional 113 village children aged 7–12 years had never started school. Researchers observed that such children tended to be very poor, from large families, and/or had year-round and day-long work, such as cattle herding. For example:

> [A 23-year-old man] said he never attended school because he was the only boy left at home to keep the cows after his brother had gone to school. . . . He said he could not ask his parents to take him to school, because . . . when you wake up in the morning, you find that the tasks you are supposed to do are already waiting for you. [PO-99-I-6-1m]

For those children who were enrolled in school, absenteeism was common because of family work responsibilities such as seasonal farming, casual labor, livestock herding, or market work. Sometimes a pupil was absent in order to raise funds to continue attending school. One boy, for example, told a researcher "he had gone to fish on Thursday, because he was accumulating money . . . for exam registration and the photographs required" [PO-99-C-

5-2f]. In several areas, particularly in the remote Sukuma villages, teachers attributed poor attendance to parents not valuing education.

Numerous young people told researchers how they had completely dropped out of primary school because of work obligations and/or an inability to pay school expenses. One head teacher estimated that only half of those starting Year 1 in his school would complete Year 7. In several villages some parents reported being particularly reluctant to use their scarce resources to pay for a girl's schooling, since they felt it would delay her marriage and their receipt of bridewealth, and it would be detrimental to both if she became pregnant out-of-wedlock. For example, when a pupil dropped out of Year 5 a teacher explained to a researcher: "Her father wants her to get married. He has stopped paying her school fees, and is waiting for a suitor to come by" [PO-01-C-2-1m]. Other reasons reported for dropping out of school included pregnancy, illiteracy, fear of punishment, frequent illness and/or ancestral disapproval of school. The last reason is illustrated by an encounter a researcher had with an out-of-school boy of about 10–12 years of age:

> I asked him if he goes to school, and he said he does not, asking me back, "Don't you see this?" and showing me a copper bangle he was wearing. Then he left. My companion told me that if someone, especially a youth, does anything against the liking of their ancestral spirits, like going to church or school, those spirits will make the person do something bad or strange, like cry loudly without reason. He told me that people who are believed to be connected to their ancestors in this way are made to wear a copper bangle. [PO-00-I-4-1m]

For those pupils who reached Year 7, the age range was often large because of variable ages at the start of schooling and the fact that many children repeated class years. For example, at the start of the *MEMA kwa Vijana* trial in 1998, the ages for Year 4–6 pupils recorded in school registers ranged from 9–22 years for boys, and 9–20 years for girls (Todd et al. 2004). Most Year 7 pupils, however, ranged from 14–18 years of age (Obasi et al. 2006).

The majority of pupils in our study who completed Year 7 failed their leaving examination and thus left school to take on adult work responsibilities. Of the minority of girls who did pass that exam, many did not attend secondary school because their parents said that they could not afford the fees. This was reported by several of the randomly selected girls who participated in the second in-depth interview series. In contrast, several of the boys in that interview series failed their examinations but then repeated Year 7 using an alias in order to re-sit the examination one to two years later. Although this was forbidden, it was not unusual for parents to pay teachers a bribe to allow a boy to assume the name of a registered pupil who had dropped out.

On leaving primary school, girls often married very soon; this process will be discussed in chapter 9. Completion of Year 7, or dropping out of school earlier, thus marked a transition to adulthood for most village youth, regardless of their age.

Teacher-Child Relationships

In our study villages, teachers' motivation seemed to vary considerably, ranging from those who were enthusiastic and strove to teach their pupils well, despite working with few resources and in difficult circumstances, to those who seemed poorly motivated and who frequently complained about pay, conditions, and pupils. One teacher observed: "Most pupils don't know the importance of school. . . . There comes a time when the teachers also get tired, so some pupils complete Year 7 without even knowing how to read and write" [PO-01-C-3-3m]. The researchers found that many teachers had a limited understanding of the subjects they taught, a view shared by some village authorities. One Village Chairman commented that, "Education currently is poor, because the teachers are unqualified, or rather, untrained," following this with the Swahili saying, "A blind man cannot easily lead another blind man" [PO-99-C-5-2f]. Teaching primarily focused on learning by rote, and there was little attempt to develop pupils' critical thinking skills. Teachers generally addressed pupils in an authoritarian way, and pupils would stand up to answer formally. There was rarely a mutual exchange of views and experiences, and teachers only occasionally engaged with their pupils casually.

In in-depth interviews, respondents were first asked to describe their general feelings towards school and teachers and then what they specifically liked about their school experience before they were asked if there was anything they specifically did not like. A minority of pupils hoped that school would be a means to build a better life. Some pupils reported liking certain subjects, sports, or spending time with their peers at school. When describing teachers they liked, pupils almost always mentioned a teacher's fairness and specifically that the teacher used little or no corporal punishment. For example, one recent school leaver said, "Many pupils like [a certain teacher] because he is polite and sympathetic. If you have made a mistake, you can defend yourself" [PO-01-C-2-5f].

When asked if there was anything about school that they disliked, almost every in-depth interview respondent immediately mentioned being hit or beaten by their teachers. Respondents particularly disliked what they perceived as certain teachers' excessive or unfair use of corporal punishment. Sometimes they also mentioned being hit inappropriately by a prefect. An example from an interview with a 15-year-old boy in Year 7:

R: [They hit us] if we do not bring things . . . such as a hoe, poles, grass, rope, or fertilizer for cultivating the school garden, or building fences and houses. . . . And they hit us sometimes when were are late to get to school, or we do not fulfill our duties. A teacher may not punish you on that day for that particular mistake, but he may choose to beat you another day for that same mistake. . . . They hit us on our buttocks and legs. And our palms and backs. I hate it. . . .

I: When we came to your school this morning, I saw a pupil hitting other pupils. Are pupils allowed to hit other pupils?

R: Yes, if they are prefects. . . . One can even cane you with five strokes. . . . There are some who hit any part of the body.

I: What would cause a prefect to hit a pupil?

R: When you are in the classroom, he may ask you for something, and you tell him that you don't have it, or that you can't give it to him. Then he waits for you during the time when you are doing manual work, and he gives you some tough work. And if you don't do that work, he beats you. He tells you to hold your ears and makes you bend over when he hits you.

I: Have you ever told a teacher that a prefect punished you for nothing?

R: No. They already know. . . . If you quarrel with a prefect and then go to the teacher, the teacher will also punish you. [II-99-I-47-m]

In all study schools, corporal punishment was used routinely for minor and major infractions, such as being late for school, perceived disrespect to teachers, or passing notes in class. Pupils feared the pain of such experiences, but they also strongly disliked the humiliation and shame involved in being verbally and physically degraded in front of their peers. This led some children to leave school and others to dread returning after the holidays. For example, a Year 6 girl in her early teens: " . . . said they were soon going to open the school and start beating [pupils] again . . . she longed for the next year to come, so that she will have completed school" [PO-02-I-4-5f]. Corporal punishment in schools usually involved beating with a slender, flexible stick, but it could include other forms of physical discomfort, pain, or humiliation, such as being made to kneel silently in front of a classroom for the entire class period. In one example, a researcher observed an entire class being forced to lie on the ground outside on their stomachs at the hottest time of the day. She recorded her observations:

Afterwards, a few were caned while holding their ears, while some dispersed. . . . [Later a pupil explained] that some were beaten because a pupil laughed and others responded. Another Year 7 girl complained that . . . lying on her stomach on the hot ground was torturous punishment. [PO-01-C-2-5f]

Corporal punishment was so established that no teachers and few parents questioned it. Pupils took it for granted and many considered it acceptable if used fairly and in moderation. However, there were generally one or two teachers per school who were widely resented by pupils for being particularly unfair and violent. A recent school leaver told a researcher, "I only like some of the teachers. I don't like [a certain teacher], because he hits so much. He can even hit you twenty times" [PO-01-C-2-5f]. There were only two participant observation reports of teachers being reprimanded for excessive use of force, both from the same village. One teacher was given a warning, and the other was transferred.

One reason pupils were beaten severely was if they were found to have had sex. Sometimes this was revealed when a girl became pregnant. In two participant observation schools and several of the schools where in-depth interviews were conducted, teachers took groups of school girls to a local health facility for mandatory pregnancy examinations. It is possible that some teachers and health workers did this practice out of genuine concern for the girls and their possible pregnancies, while others may have been financially motivated, as will be described below. Girls, however, universally reported strongly disliking these examinations, whether they were pregnant or not. For example, a Year 7 girl reported, "the mandatory pregnancy exam was embarrassing . . . as it was done by hand, they were told to remove all of their clothes, and the person doing the exam was a man" [PO-00-C-3-2f].

Teachers, pupils, and other villagers estimated that one to three girls per school became pregnant each year. Pregnancy was not legal grounds for expulsion, but in practice pregnant school girls did not expect, and were not allowed, to continue schooling in rural Mwanza. Sometimes, pregnant school girls were able to drop out without experiencing much stigma or punishment, but in each of the four study districts there were reports of a man, or his family, being forced to pay both the pregnant school girl's family and teachers. In exchange, teachers falsified the girl's school records, for example removing her name from the records or attributing her departure to another reason, and they did not report the pregnancy to the authorities so the man avoided legal punishment. In one village, the following incident was reported by several informants independently:

> The head teacher threatened that if he took the matter forward the boy would "die in jail." . . . After the young man and his guardian pleaded for the amount to be reduced, it was decided that . . . the daughter's father would get Tshs 100,000 ($120) and the head teacher would get Tshs 70,000 ($84). [PO-00-I-4-1m]

In two other villages, total fines paid to the girl's family and teachers were reported as Tshs 100,000–130,000 ($120–$156), with or without a cow. In a fourth village, a man whose son had impregnated a school girl explained that he only paid a relatively small amount to the girl's family and head teacher, because he had a good relationship with the teachers.

Finally, there were plausible first- and third-person reports of individual male teachers having sex with female pupils in eight of the nine participant observation villages and in one-third of in-depth interviews with randomly selected respondents. These reports involved recent cases of male teachers impregnating school girls, being caught having sex with pupils, and/or pressurizing girls to have sex. In participant observation villages, several of these accounts were known and discussed by the wider public because teachers were dismissed (one school), transferred (three schools), suspended (one school), fined (two schools), left the village voluntarily (one school), or married one of their pupil lovers soon after she finished school (two schools). Other reports were secret and were only reported to researchers confidentially. Teachers' sexual abuse of school girls will be described and discussed in depth in chapter 7.

Teacher-Parent Relationships

Adult villagers' views of teachers were ambivalent, reflecting their broader views on the value of formal education. A secondary school student explained why some villagers might not value schooling:

> *R:* Parents may forbid their children to go further in school, telling them, "You are grown up now, aren't you? Just go somewhere and find a wife. With the problem of unemployment, there is nothing you can do with school. Even children who study at the university level come back here and just become simple farmers. Education offers nothing." [II-02-I-315-m]

Teachers were considered by themselves and others to be distinct from most villagers, being from distant (sometimes urban) places, often not speaking a local language, and having higher education and a relatively secure income. They were therefore of higher status, which extended to their wives. For example, a farmer's wife recounted, "how the head teacher was told by other teachers to buy good things for his wife, so she can appear like a teacher's wife and not a villager. . . . [The farmer's wife] said that she is nothing compared to teacher's wives" [PO-01-I-1-2f].

Villagers generally respected teachers for their teaching role, but they sometimes also resented and even feared teachers, for a range of possible reasons, including their perceived arrogance and disdain towards local villagers, domination of village politics through their higher status, drunkenness or womanizing, and sexual abuse of pupils or exploitation of their labor. For example, while some parents supported or were at least resigned to their children working for the school or in the teachers' homes during school hours, others criticized it. A pupil's grandmother commented: "Do you think our school is a school? . . . The children are made to cultivate as if they were cattle" [PO-01-C-2-5f].

Parents rarely challenged teachers about their concerns and felt that they had little legal or bureaucratic recourse against them. Each school had a school committee, usually consisting of relatively educated parents and community leaders who were responsible for the daily running and improvement of the school. However, their authority seemed limited in some villages. During one participant observation visit, for example, a head teacher reportedly took a bribe of Tshs 40,000 ($48) to register a girl as transferred to another school, when in fact she had dropped out to marry. School committee members were angry that the money had not been shared with them, so the head teacher simply disbanded the committee until they dropped the issue.

In several villages, however, there were rumors about teachers being forced to move after they or their families fell ill because villagers bewitched them. For instance, a young shopkeeper

> said that if any teacher troubles the students . . . parents would fix them by using witchcraft. He gave an example of a certain teacher who . . . used to beat pupils frequently . . . the teacher was bewitched and started frequently getting boils until he decided to move to another village. [PO-99-I-6-1m]

Some teachers reported being bewitched themselves, and seemed frightened of the possibility of villagers taking revenge in that way. One teacher told a researcher that she was in the process of transferring to another school because of the "bad luck" she and other teachers had experienced in the village, including theft, fire, and her child's death, all of which she attributed to people's mischief, hatred, and/or witchcraft.

DISCUSSION

Research across sub-Saharan Africa suggests that parental authority, and more generally the authority of older generations over the young, has been dwindling for several decades (Caldwell et al. 1998). Large-scale factors which may contribute to this include the introduction of schooling, the extension of state administration, and increased involvement in the cash economy, urbanization, and labor migration (Caldwell et al. 1998). Children are no longer as economically dependent on their parents' generation, particularly with respect to land inheritance and bridewealth (Abrahams 1989). The widespread introduction of primary schooling also provides children with an alternative source of knowledge and authority to their parents. Parental control is sometimes further eroded by young people's mobility, and general social change can undermine the credibility of parents' advice, since children may see their parents' experiences as outdated (Bujra 2000).

In this and the last chapter we have seen that many of these large-scale changes had had an impact on life in rural Mwanza by the beginning of the twenty-first century. Nonetheless, many traditional aspects of village life and Sukuma childhood were remarkably resilient. Below we will discuss how childhood, adolescence, and adult authority have—or have not—changed in rural Mwanza over the last century. We will also consider the implications of our general findings on formal education for potential school-based adolescent sexual health interventions.

Childhood and Adolescence

In our study, we found that it was still common for girls of 8 years old or older to have many domestic responsibilities and to mainly socialize with same-sex peers. Older children continued to have typically submissive and formal relationships with their parents, and it was considered very inappropriate for parents and children to directly discuss sexual matters, as is typical of parent-child avoidance relationships. Like Varkevisser (1973), we also found ample evidence that prepubescent and adolescent children secretly engaged in activities which their parents discouraged or forbade, which will be discussed more in the next chapters.

However, one aspect of rural children's lives that *did* change markedly in the century prior to our study was experience of formal education. In the early 1900s, very few children in rural Mwanza had ever attended school (Cory 1953), but by the time of our study the majority did. Formal education altered childhood in rural Mwanza in many ways. It reduced the time children spent doing agricultural work, and it provided them with basic, new skills in Swahili language and literacy. Historically, young Sukumas married fairly soon after puberty but school pupils were not expected to marry, so schooling also led to a later age at first marriage, at least for girls (Żaba et al. 2009). This has contributed to the new phenomenon of "adolescence" amongst the Sukuma, that is, a stage of life when young people are biologically mature but not yet socially treated as adults. Caldwell and colleagues (1998, 149–50) discussed how schooling has contributed to the emergence of adolescence across sub-Saharan Africa:

Schooling removes teenagers from their houses and farms, provides them with information often at odds with parental instruction, and permits young people of both sexes to meet without family supervision. It prepares them for occupations different from their parents' and, inevitably, increases girls' age at marriage. . . . The result, especially as girls' age at first marriage rose and as more girls attended school, was an increase in premarital sexual activity, pregnancy, and childbearing.

In the coming chapters, we will describe how most adolescents in our study were sexually active by their mid-teens, a finding that is broadly similar to those of anthropologists working with the Sukuma in the early to mid twentieth century. Several early anthropologists described how unmarried teenage Sukuma girls were allowed a certain amount of sexual freedom as long as they were discreet, which typically involved sneaking out of their shared sleeping quarters or allowing a boy or man to sneak in for a sexual liaison after dark (Cory 1953; Abrahams 1967; Varkevisser 1973). In chapters 5 and 6 we will see how this basic practice was still common in rural Mwanza during our study, although the period of unmarried sexual activity was typically longer than in the past, specifically because of later ages at first marriage.

Schools and the Potential for Sexual Health Intervention

School systems offer an almost unparalleled opportunity to reach a large number of youth with low cost health interventions, particularly in sub-Saharan Africa. Given Mwanza's resource poor setting, the late age of most primary school leavers, and the low proportion that went on to secondary school, primary schools were in fact the only institution where an adolescent sexual health program could be implemented both on a large scale and at low cost at the start of the twenty-first century. A school-based intervention in that setting has the added benefit of being potentially sustainable long-term, as primary school teachers are often some of the most literate and educated individuals in rural areas, and once trained, they have the potential to deliver sexual health programs until they retire.

However, our study of the general school setting highlighted great obstacles to potential school-based sexual health interventions which go beyond the obvious constraint of severe material resource limitation. Many adolescents could not fully participate in such a program because they never enrolled in school, attended inconsistently, or dropped out. Many primary school teachers had little training beyond primary school themselves, and pupils were taught at a very basic level. Low baseline literacy, knowledge, critical thinking skills, and understanding of mathematical and biological concepts on the part of both pupils and teachers all have implications for the content and approach of any possible sexual health program.

Our study suggests that problematic teacher–pupil relationships also pose great challenges for potential adolescent sexual health interventions. At the time of our study, the basic approach to teaching had not changed since formal schooling was first introduced by missionaries, colonists, and the newly independent national government. Teaching continued to be highly authoritarian and performance oriented. The established teaching culture was characterized by recitation and corporal punishment and fundamentally contrasted with trust-building and participatory methods that are generally promoted in sexual health programs (Kuhn, Steinberg, and Mathews 1994; WHO 1997). For example, sexual health programs often seek to promote youth leadership and peer education, in the belief that they contribute to positive role modeling and skills development. However, pupils who are habituated to very subservient relationships with teachers may find it very difficult to take on effective leadership roles.

Sexual health intervention developers and evaluators elsewhere in Africa have found that substantive change to didactic and authoritarian school-teaching methodologies can be very difficult to achieve (Kuhn, Steinberg, and Mathews 1994; Shuey et al. 1999; Kinsman et al. 1999; Campbell 2003; Mukoma et al. 2009). While some success may be demonstrated in very intensive, small-scale interventions (Fawole 1999), it is much more challenging to take such efforts to scale without dilution of quality (Dusenbury 2005). Effective scaling-up may ultimately require much greater cost and fundamental changes in teacher training and supervision within the broader school system (WHO 2003; Barrett 2007).

In addition to teaching methods and general classroom dynamics, several official and unofficial school practices documented in our study had serious implications for teacher–pupil relationships, and thus potential teacher-led sexual health programs. Mandatory pregnancy examinations raise ethical concerns about pupil privacy and teachers' motivation, and sometimes led to pupils leaving school, being beaten and fined. Instead of reducing pupil sexual activity, forced pregnancy examinations and corporal punishment may have contributed to pupils' secretiveness about it.

Sexual abuse of school girls by teachers has been found in many countries in sub-Saharan Africa (WHO 1997; Mlemya, Justine, and Mgalla 1997; Kinsman et al. 1999; Jewkes et al. 2002; O-saki and Agu 2002; Panos Institute 2003; Andersson and Ho-Foster 2008). An abusive teacher might cause great harm to a sexual health program by modeling inappropriate behavior, by instilling fear and distrust of the program associated with the teacher, and even by exploiting sexual health classes as new opportunities to abuse pupils. Punishing such offences by transferring the guilty party simply moves the problem to another school. In such contexts, close supervision and appropriate responses are crucial within sexual health programs. In addition, there is a broader need for national policies and norms that better prevent, monitor, and correct such abuses (WHO 1997; Panos Institute 2003). A recent campaign in Kenya shows promise in this area, as authorities took advantage of the now widespread use of mobile telephones and sponsored a nationwide confidential helpline to identify teachers who sexually abused pupils. Their subsequent investigation led to the firing of over 1,000 teachers, mostly teachers working in rural areas (British Broadcasting Corporation 2010a).

Finally, while some teachers and villagers in our study seemed to have fairly positive and respectful relationships, in some villages substantial tensions existed between the two, which could affect the acceptability of teacher-led sexual health programs. Preexisting problems, such as teachers' alcohol abuse or sexual abuse of pupils, could create or reinforce controversy and stigma associated with a sexual health program in a community.

The Tanzanian primary school system was one of the most disadvantaged in the world at the time of our study. Some improvements have been made to it since then due to government efforts as well as nongovernmental programs working at a district level (United Republic of Tanzania 2003; World Bank 2004; Sedere, Mengele, and Kajela 2008). For example, the national Primary Education Development Plan dramatically increased primary school enrolment, refurbished and built new classrooms, and developed stronger local management and financial systems (Benson 2006). However, it has been far less successful in motivating teachers and improving teaching quality (Benson 2006). Substantial long-term improvements of infrastructure, resources, and teacher capacity and supervision remain critical. Such efforts may be important in improving adolescent sexual health even in the absence of specific sexual health programs.

Having described the main features of village life for young people in our study area, we will now address youth sexuality. In the next chapter we will begin by considering the predominant sexual norms that influenced young people, highlighting the contradictions between restrictive and permissive ideals and expectations, and describing how young people managed those contradictions.

NOTE

1. Some material in this chapter was adapted from: Plummer, M. L., D. Wight, J. Wamoyi, K. Nyalali, T. Ingall, G. Mshana, Z. S. Shigongo, A. I. N. Obasi, and D. A. Ross. 2007. Are schools a good setting for adolescent sexual health promotion in rural Africa? A qualitative assessment from Tanzania. *Health Education Research* 22(4):483–99.

Chapter Five

Contradictory Sexual Norms and Expectations[1]

The severity of the HIV epidemic in Africa has been attributed to a range of broad and interrelated factors, including poverty, inadequate health services, warfare, and the legacy of colonialism (Barnett and Whiteside 2002; Buvé et al. 2002; Kim and Watts 2005; Seeley, Dercon, and Barnett 2010). However, the overwhelming mechanism for HIV infection is sexual behavior, which is embedded in social relationships at a local level. This chapter focuses on the main features of sexual culture in rural Mwanza, highlighting its contradictory norms and expectations for young people. By "norms" we mean ideals of behavior shared by a social group which do not necessarily reflect actual behavior. Norms are not prescriptive in determining behavior, but rather people may draw on them to legitimate or criticize specific behaviors. If norms and other features of sexual culture are not understood, interventions that seek to reduce sexual risk behavior are unlikely to succeed.

Historically there has been substantial debate about whether sexuality in sub-Saharan Africa is essentially similar to that in the West or fundamentally different, and the HIV epidemic has given new salience to this discussion. Central to the debate is the question of whether sexual cultures in sub-Saharan Africa are fairly permissive compared with European cultures (e.g., Caldwell et al. 1989; Goody 1969), or whether they are mainly characterized by restrictive rules, ritual practices and self-restraint (e.g., Ahlberg 1994; Heald 1995). This debate has become highly polarized (Helle-Valle 2004). Protagonists have tended to mix findings from different historical periods and to generalize from one or two ethnic groups on different sides of the continent. Unfortunately this discussion has sometimes involved vague and value-laden terms such as "promiscuity" (e.g., Hrdy 1987; Miller and Rockwell 1988) and, occasionally, racist evolutionary theory (Rushton and Bogaert 1989). Social constructionist theory offers an alternate perspective that assumes sexual acts, orientations, and identities are constructed largely according to a society's culture at a given historical period, so they inevitably vary between societies (Vance 1991).

The debate described above has been highly polarized in part because data on sexual cultures are very limited. Most anthropological research in sub-Saharan Africa has focused on other topics and only incidentally thrown light on sexuality (Lindenbaum 1991). Early anthropology may have also relied too heavily on the accounts of elders who wished to present their society as respectable. In contrast, the social science research prompted by the HIV epidemic has primarily used surveys, which also have problems with data validity as discussed in chapters 1 and 2.

Most early anthropological research with the Sukuma suggested that there were fairly relaxed sexual mores for young people (Cory 1953; Tanner 1955a; Tanner 1955b; Varkevisser 1973). Based on his research in the early twentieth century, Tanner (1955a, 124) reported: "no attempt is made to chaperon young girls who are as yet unmarried, with the result that they have comparative freedom to sleep where they like and with whom they like." Varkevisser (1973) further suggested that, historically, grandmothers who shared sleeping rooms with unmarried young women were responsible for informally educating them about contraception and discouraging them from getting attached to particular young men, to reduce the chance that they might marry without bridewealth payment. *Ngoma* competitions and other events such as weddings and funerals provided an important opportunity for young people to find potential marriage partners, as Sukuma homesteads were often fairly self-sufficient and far apart (Varkevisser 1973). Virginity was not prized at marriage, but young people's unmarried sexual relationships were restricted in two ways: young women were expected to avoid conception and to be discreet, so as not to gain a bad reputation (Tanner 1955b). Both of these issues could affect a young woman's marriageability and reduce her potential bridewealth. A woman who lived independently of a father or a husband because of divorce or another reason was referred to as a ***shimbe*** (plural ***bashimbe***) (Varkevisser 1973) or an ***msimbe*** (plural ***wasimbe***) (Abrahams 1978) and expected relatively little or no bridewealth if she (re)married.

Much of the historical literature on East African societies inland from the coast of the Indian Ocean suggests that heterosexuality has been so much the norm in the last century that, for many people, same-sex sexual activity was unimaginable. Nevertheless, amongst the Sukuma in the mid-twentieth century, Tanner (1955b, 241) found that homosexuality was "a feature of a boy's life before puberty," and lesbianism "occurs between adolescent girls at a rather later age." Same-sex sexual activity has also been documented in the region during the last two decades, particularly amongst consenting men in urban areas and/or extremely marginalized boys and young men, such as street children, and the men who exploit them (Rajani and Kudrati 1996; Kajubi et al. 2008; Smith et al. 2009). Such same-sex activity has generally been well hidden. It has reportedly involved exploration, pleasure, assertion of power, and/or abuse, but until very recently it rarely seemed to be linked to personal identity.

In this chapter, we will describe and analyze sexual beliefs and values in rural Mwanza at the start of the twenty-first century. We will explore whether sexual norms were permissive or restrictive, the extent to which they conflicted, and how contradictions were managed by young people.

FINDINGS

Restrictive Sexual Norms

Heterosexuality

Heterosexuality was a widespread norm in rural Mwanza, and reports of homosexuality were very rare in our study. Villagers who were aware of the possibility of homosexual behavior had usually been exposed to it through Western media such as video shows. They generally found it repugnant and were deeply homophobic. To be the receptive partner in anal intercourse was considered particularly degrading. The rest of this chapter will focus exclusively on heterosexuality, but in chapter 8 we will present our findings on same-sex sexual activity.

School Pupil Abstinence

One of the most fundamental sexual norms in rural Mwanza, at least amongst adults, was that young people should not have sex until they have left school. As we saw in the last chapter, primary schooling often continued into the late teens and sometimes even the early 20s, especially for male pupils. In contrast, some children never went to school and approximately one-third to one-half of pupils dropped out before completing Year 7. For out-of-school youth in their teens, particularly boys, discreet sexual activity was tolerated and even expected, although like adults they were expected to avoid sexual relationships with pupils. Thus young people's sexual activity appeared to be judged by their school status and adult responsibilities rather than chronological age.

Pupil abstinence was the sexual norm that seemed to have the clearest generational differences in rural Mwanza. It was maintained by almost all adults, except those men who secretly exploited female pupils sexually. Parents tried to enforce the norm by prohibiting pupils from participating in unsupervised mixed-sex activities, particularly discos and video shows. This seemed to be effective with a small minority of adolescents, especially some who were extraordinarily ambitious and committed to further formal education, as they felt that sexual relationships would disrupt their progress in school.

Most pupils did not contest the ideal of school pupil abstinence in the presence of adults, but as they grew older the majority started to circumvent it and have secret sexual encounters at night, in remote spots, and/or when their parents were away. The main punishments for contravening the norm of pupil abstinence were beatings. For example, one school girl repeatedly received Tshs 500–1,000 ($0.60–1.20) from her 27-year-old sexual partner when they had sex, and then used the money to buy peanuts to eat as a midday meal at school. However, the researcher recorded, "One day the girl didn't share her peanuts with her younger sisters as usual, so they went home and told their father that the girl brings money to school these days. The girl's father beat her, for he suspected she has been given money by men [for sex], because he knows she is not given any money at home" [PO-01-C-2-5f]. Later that girl became pregnant and dropped out of school to have the child.

As noted in the last chapter, if a school girl became pregnant she invariably left school, and the boy or man usually had to pay a fine or bridewealth. The following example was provided by a five-month pregnant school girl:

> She said that, since her pregnancy became visible, some of her girlfriends don't visit and the boy who made her pregnant ran away. She said that she will not go to school again because of her pregnancy, although she greatly prefers to continue with education. When her parents discovered her condition they scolded her very much while telling her that she has lost a lot of their money. . . . They went to the boy's home, where they were compensated with two head of cattle and 30,000 Tsh [$36]. [PO-00-I-4-4f]

Several young men reported that they were wary of having sex with school pupils for fear of being prosecuted, fined, forced to marry the girls who they made pregnant, and/or bewitched by the girls' parents. The norm of pupil abstinence meant many adults were also opposed to the idea of a school-based adolescent sexual health intervention, and particularly instructions about condom use, because they believed it would encourage sexual activity.

Women's Sexual Respectability

In rural Mwanza, both men and women frequently used sexual respectability to categorize each other, but it was particularly important for women. The main categories of adult women, in order of sexual respectability, were as follows:

(a) monogamous married women;

(b) unmarried young women living with their parents who were not known to have ever been sexually active, although it was difficult to maintain this reputation for more than one to two years after leaving school;

(c) *wasimbe*, a term which in our study villages meant almost all other never married, divorced, or widowed women of reproductive age, most of whom were mothers; and

(d) women who were perceived to be very promiscuous, known variously as *wahuni* (badly behaved people, implying sexually "loose" in this context), *daladala* (bicycle taxis or minibuses, from the English "dollar, dollar") or, most derogatory, *malaya* (prostitutes).

We found that women who were considered to be *wasimbe* included some who lived in their parental homestead and some who lived independent of a parent or a husband. The diverse types of women who were commonly categorized as *wasimbe* in rural Mwanza are illustrated by comments made by young men in group discussions and participant observation:

P: An *msimbe* is woman who has delivered a baby.

F: Even a Year 5 pupil?

P: Yes. If she delivers a baby her breasts will definitely fall. You think by looking at her, "This one is married." But she may say that she isn't, so you think, "Aha, so she is an *msimbe*."

F: How does someone feel when she is called an *msimbe*?

P: Those women feel bad to be called an *msimbe*. [GDII-00-C-12-4m]

An informant said there is a type of *msimbe* who became an adult without getting married, while her younger sisters got married and left her at home. I asked what makes a girl not get married, and they said it is just an *mkosi* [jinx]. . . . Another informant said that not only does a jinx make a girl not get married, it makes her not be cheerful or charming towards people, she doesn't work with effort, she doesn't greet people, and she may even have a habit of standing on paths talking to boys. They said that, "A man is never overtaken by events, and never gets old. If a man has property, even if he is 90 years old he can still marry a young girl who has just completed Year 7. But a girl loses 'marketability' early." [PO-02-I-4-5f]

Wasimbe constituted about one-quarter to one-third of women in most villages. Many villagers differentiated between two kinds of *wasimbe*. Those who were believed to have had few sexual partners, who had been abandoned when pregnant, and/or who had previously been married were generally given more respect, and they often eventually (re)married. Most junior wives in polygynous marriages had once been perceived as this type of *msimbe*. In contrast, there were women who had never married and who were perceived to "love carelessly"—that is, to have multiple, indiscreet partnerships—and they were accorded less understanding and respect. A young divorced mother of two explained, "There are two types of *wasimbe*, those who are uncontrollable and those who can reform themselves. The uncontrollables are those who won't even listen to their parents" [PO-00-I-4-4f].

One of the main criteria of a woman's eligibility for marriage, and thus the bridewealth that could be demanded for her, was sexual respectability. A Village Executive Officer observed that

> when a boy elopes with a girl, it means he reduces the cost of bridewealth . . . because he has already had sex with the girl and it is already known by the people. If the girl's parent refuses to accept that small bridewealth payment, he leaves the girl, who has a slim chance of getting married as she is already an *msimbe*. [PO-01-I-4-5f]

Women primarily maintained their respectability by hiding any out-of-wedlock sexual relationships they had. If a woman was known to have been sexually active, she could still promote her respectability by not openly initiating sexual encounters, not agreeing to sex too quickly, and not being known to have had several sexual partners. Other threats to a girl or woman's respectability were accepting a low amount of money for sex, wearing immodest clothing, attending video shows, having a sexually transmitted infection, aborting a pregnancy, living alone, and having previously resided in large towns.

Having a child outside of wedlock was often referred to as "giving birth at home" (*kuzalia nyumbani*), that is, while living in one's parents' household rather than one's husband's. Such children took the formal name of their maternal uncle or grandfather, and sometimes were financially supported by them. Older villagers said that in recent decades such births had lost much of their previous stigma. However, some villagers regarded never married mothers as *wahuni*. Single mothers typically were less eligible for marriage than other young women, had greater material needs, and were more reliant on sexual partners for income.

Female jobs in the cash economy that primarily involved contact with men were generally done by *wasimbe*, such as selling food at kiosks or brewing and selling beer. Like virtually all sexually active unmarried women, *wasimbe* received money or gifts in exchange for sexual encounters. This linking of sex with money or gifts was not regarded as inherently immoral, and most of the transactional sex discussed in this book was not regarded by villagers as prostitution, which generally *was* considered immoral. Within each village only a small number of women were perceived to be *malaya*. They typically had this reputation because they were believed to openly solicit sex, to have a relatively high number of sexual partners, to change partners frequently, to not be selective of them, and to be indiscreet.

Importantly, the categories above could be permeable and transient, particularly a woman's identity as either **msimbe** or wife. Women were not expected to remain virgins until marriage, although they preferred to maintain this impression. Marriage could take several different forms, and divorce and remarriage were fairly common, as will be discussed in chapter 9.

Men's Sexual Respectability

In contrast to women, high numbers of sexual partners and greater sexual activity often enhanced men's reputations amongst other men, and this will be discussed more later in this chapter. Women generally did not admire this, but appeared resigned to it, and might blame and disparage the mistress rather than the husband in extramarital sexual relationships. However, researchers occasionally witnessed both married and unmarried women's heated condemnations of particular men's sexual irresponsibility or faithlessness, particularly when men did not support their offspring. For instance, when a man boldly stated that he had no intention to marry, an older woman interrupted: "What about the two girls who you made pregnant? Aren't they your wives?" [PO-00-I-4-4f]

Taboos against Discussion of Sex

Sexual issues were rarely discussed publicly, and explicit discussion was regarded by some as obscene. Numerous euphemisms were used for sexual intercourse, such as "act of marriage" (*kitendo cha ndoa*). Parents rarely provided sexual information to their children, and sometimes said a school-based sexual health intervention was unacceptable because it involved discussing sexual issues across generations and between sexes. For example, a Village Executive Officer said, "The way they teach at public meetings is a shame, as some people have their mothers and their in-laws with them, making it difficult for people to see that what they are being taught has merit" [PO-01-I-4-5f].

There were, however, some notable exceptions to the cross-generational taboo on discussing sex. Older women sometimes discreetly advised young unmarried women within a household on pregnancy prevention and young married women on fertility enhancement. Occasionally parents advised their children on the treatment of sexually transmitted infections, particularly children of the same sex. Furthermore, in many homes small children shared sleeping rooms with their parents, where they probably witnessed their parents' sexual activity. Prepubescent children typically shared rooms with older, same-sex siblings and cousins, and also in that context many children observed their older relatives' sexual activity, when their partners snuck into the room.

Religious Beliefs about Abstinence and Fidelity

The role of religion in shaping sexual norms did not emerge prominently from the participant observation research. In the few very devout Christian or Muslim families, parents were unusually restrictive of their children and especially their daughters, preventing attendance of *ngoma* events, videos, and discos, which were regarded as sinful. These parents were probably the most careful to prevent their children's sexual activity, and a small minority of informants attributed their celibacy to such restrictions and/or their own religious beliefs. However, formal religions were probably more influential in shaping ideals of sexual conduct and women's sexual respectability than in substantially reducing young people's actual sexual activity. Some youths in strictly religious households said that close parental monitoring simply made them even more secretive than other youth. For example, in some strict households young women reported meeting their partners for hurried sex in the evening, leaving the house for only a few minutes under the pretence of going to the latrine.

Permissive Sexual Expectations and Norms

The restrictive ideals described above coexisted with other norms which encouraged sexual activity. These were mainly maintained by males and young women.

Sexual Pleasure, Biological Need, and Masculine Identity

In rural Mwanza, sexual desire and satisfaction were the overwhelming motivations for boys and men to have sex. For example, a 20-year-old man explained: "The reason I first decided to have sex . . . is simply as the Sukuma say, 'the old man rises' [the penis becomes erect]" [II-00-C-83-m]. Similarly, a 19-year-old man in Year 6 "said that there are many pleasures in the world, but the pleasure of sex tops all others" [PO-01-C-3-3m].

Both sexes, but particularly men, talked about male sexual activity as an essential biological drive. As a young man in a group discussion explained:

P: If you are really normal, if you are not impotent, you must have sex with a girl. Because if not, you might sleep at night and dream that you are with a girl, and you'll find your genitals really disturb you. So once you wake up you are compelled to immediately go have sex [with a girl]. [GD-02-I-1-1m]

Men were proud to be sexually "strong," particularly to ejaculate multiple times in the course of one sexual encounter. Impotence was considered humiliating and the subject of much gossip. It was attributed to witchcraft or transgressing taboos and was generally treated by traditional healers. Many young men were pleased to make their partners pregnant because it demonstrated their potency and fertility. Similarly some parents were reported to "inwardly rejoice" when they learned that a son has made an unmarried woman pregnant, as it publicly proved his manhood [PO-99-C-5-2f]. A female primary school teacher explained:

> Their joy is due to the knowledge that their [male] children are now mature, that they are not defective. She said that fathers can't tell their children or others about their joy, except when they meet at a pub or in other places where they boast that their children are perfect men. [PO-02-C-3-3m]

For almost all men, but particularly those not yet married or with children, sexual experience was prestigious and intertwined with their masculine identity. Fieldworkers frequently observed boys and young men hanging out together talking about their sexual conquests at the village center or elsewhere. In the following example a female researcher witnessed an exchange between a 25-year-old house builder (Mashaka), his 20-year-old unmarried female cousin (Fatuma), and a male guest:

> Mashaka told his guest that he has the ability to seduce any woman. Fatuma, who was listening, told the guest that Mashaka was a liar as he gives most of his property to one *msimbe*. Mashaka said he also had another lover who is not an *msimbe* and who wanted to marry him, but he broke up with her. Fatuma objected, saying that it was the woman who left him, because he had planned to elope with her, but she ran away with another man. Fatuma said that when Mashaka found out he became so angry that he threatened to make formal charges against the woman for taking his property, and to strip her clothes off her when he saw her on a path. Mashaka then said that it does not matter who broke up with whom, because when that woman eloped with the other man Mashaka had already made her pregnant. [PO-02-I-4-5f]

This exchange also highlights how men may have sometimes embellished their sexual experience for their peers, and possibly downplayed their emotional involvement in a relationship once it ended.

Sex was also discussed amongst men around the evening *kikome* fire at home, sometimes even between fathers and their older sons, legitimating sexual activity and in contravention of cross-generational taboos. For example, one evening at a participant observation household:

> My host started telling the older youth that they should use condoms when having sex. He said that he has heard stories that his younger brother is having a sexual affair with a certain girl. The young men strongly argued that they usually use condoms when having sex and that they have them in their rooms. My host went out for a short time and his younger brother told a visiting young man, "He is telling us to use condoms while he himself is a great womanizer and does not use them." These comments were made while the older sons of my host were present and listening. [PO-99-C-2-1m]

The participant observation data suggest that peer pressure might have been as important a motive as sexual pleasure for adolescent boys to start sexual activity. Boys older than 14 who had not yet engaged in sexual activity were likely to be ridiculed by their more sexually experienced peers. One 21-year-old informant who chose to be celibate while he was still in school described how peer pressure led him to sometimes fabricate sexual experience:

> He said those youths who have never had sex are laughed at or jeered at by those who already have started having sex, saying they are silly, they don't know how to seduce. When such incidents happened to him he pretended he had had sex. [PO-00-C-3-3m]

Boys known to be sexually inexperienced were subjected to insults such as "impotent," "cowardly," or "woman," and a few were even shunned by their peers. To avoid being scorned, most boys strove to gain sexual experience. Pressure from friends could make it very difficult for even the most resolute to maintain their abstinence. For example, a 19-year-old man recalled why he first began having intercourse at the age of 11:

> He decided to have sex due to the pressure he was getting from youth who already had begun having sex. He said that his friends laughed at him, saying that he was afraid to seduce girls, or that he was impotent. He decided to begin sexual relations in order to rid himself of the shame that confronted him every time he met his friends. [PO-01-C-3-3m]

For boys in their early to mid teens, their own sexual pleasure and satisfaction could be of less importance than their reputation with their male peers. For example, a 27-year-old man recounting his first sexual experience when he was in Year 5:

> The informant said that when he had sex with that girl, he did not enjoy it much. He said that he was very afraid and he did it quickly. He said that at that time he

had not even begun to ejaculate. He said that the next day when his friends asked him if he managed to have sex with the girl, he told them that he had managed to do so. He said that he felt very good telling his friends about having sex with the girl. [PO-02-C-2-1m]

The prestige of male sexual experience related to sexual conquest and the ability to seduce many partners. A 25-year-old farmer explained, "The people who are most respected in the village are those who own many head of cattle, the prominent farmers, those who are known to be rich, the men with many wives, and the young men who have many lovers" [PO-00-C-9-3m]. Male sexual prestige was entwined with economic status because of the money or gifts required in exchange for sexual encounters. The interlinking of the prestige of wealth and masculinity was illustrated by the practice of *kubenchiana* at discos which was described in chapter 3. By paying to dominate the dance floor with a desirable partner, young men demonstrated their affluence publicly and this translated directly into access to women, enhancing their sexual activity and reputations.

However, young men had to balance the esteem of perceived sexual experience against the risk of jealousy and suspicion of unfaithfulness from sexual partners, and punishment from adult authorities. Rather than publicize the details of their sexual relationships, they thus often preferred a reputation of sexual experience based on rumor. In the first series of in-depth interviews, for example, sixteen of the twenty-nine randomly selected male pupils reported that they had had sex, and almost all said that their close friends knew this, but seven said they had never told anyone specific information about their first sexual experience.

Sex as a Female Resource and the Principle of Reciprocity

For young women, sex was regarded primarily as a resource that they could exploit, and virtually all sexual encounters outside of marriage involved material exchange, unless they were physically forced, which was rare. Material exchange for sex was so established that almost any gift from a young man to a young woman, such as a snack, soap, payment of video show entrance, or a "loan" of money, was seen by both parties as a contract to have sex. Wives particularly resented husbands' extramarital relationships, because they required the husband to give other women money that could otherwise have been used for their household.

The size of the gift given for each sexual encounter varied according to the man's affluence, the woman's prestige, and their relative experience and negotiation skills. School boys with the least money typically gave sugar cane, soap, or Tshs 100–500 ($0.12–0.60) per sexual encounter, while older men typically gave Tshs 500–2,000 ($0.60–2.40). Young women were given more if they were believed to have had few sexual partners, to be difficult to seduce, or to have urban sophistication. At one *ngoma* event, for example, a boy tried to give a female researcher a piece of sugar cane, and when she declined his friends laughed, saying, "Such [young women] are for beer, they are not like those here in the village, who are bought sugar canes [for sex]" [PO-00-I-4-4f].

Young women often showed each other what they received from their sexual partners, and there was an element of peer pressure to acquire commodities. For example, a 20-year-old woman who lived in extreme poverty with her widowed mother reported:

> Her boyfriends used to give her Tshs 2,000 ($2.40) while she was still in school, and she spent it all on food, like fried rice cakes. She said that, if a girl is not given money [by her boyfriend], other girls laugh at her at school [because she cannot] buy food at break time. [PO-01-I-1-2f]

Many young women used their earnings for essentials, such as soap and clothes, especially as parents expected girls to procure such items independently by the time they reached their mid-teens. Some young women supported other members of their family with gifts and money that they received for sex, although this was hidden from male heads of household. Some impoverished mothers encouraged their daughters to have sex specifically to help support the family, but it was not necessary to be very poor for a daughter to contribute in this way. For example, a 21-year-old woman whose family was supported by her father's boat transport business:

> *R:* One of my [recent] boyfriends was a businessman, he buys fish wholesale. We had sex at his home around 10 pm, and he gave me Tshs 4,500 ($5.40). I gave it to my mother and she went to buy herself clothes. I just told her that so-and-so had given it to me. She asked me, "Who is he to you?" I told her, "He is my lover."
>
> *I:* And when you told her that he was your lover, what did she say?
>
> *R:* She didn't say anything. [II-02-I-288-m]

Gifts were generally concealed in order to hide relationships, but no one considered material exchange for sex problematic in itself. To the contrary, a girl or young woman who received a small gift, or nothing, was generally scorned and considered to lack self-respect, while women prepared to have sex for free might be condemned as sexually loose and a *mhuni*. The underlying logic of many comments about transactional sex was the principle of reciprocity, or mutual give and take.

The continued provision of money or gifts for sexual encounters within a relationship was assumed to ensure a woman's fidelity, except with women reputed to be *daladala*. If gift giving was not maintained or substantially diminished, relationships often ended quickly, or the young woman secretly found another boyfriend. The amount exchanged for sex generally fell during a relationship, giving young women an incentive to change partners. Only a few informants of both sexes belittled the importance of the money or gifts men provided before or after sexual encounters, implying that such exchange reflected affection and did not motivate young women to have sex. Given its importance in the sexual relationships of unmarried youth, material exchange for sex will be described in depth in chapter 7.

The Inevitability of Sexual Activity Unless Prevented

One of the dominant features of sexual culture in Mwanza was the assumed inevitability of sexual activity. There was a widespread expectation that social contact between the opposite sexes would lead to sex unless it was prevented, so long as those involved were not related, young children, or old. Sexual activity was thus believed to be constrained primarily by externally imposed restrictions, particularly sexual segregation, rather than self-imposed discipline. This belief stemmed from several factors already discussed: the notion of sex as biologically driven, the central role of sex in masculine identity, and the important economic opportunity sex provided for young women. It was also linked to a general belief that sex is not only natural but health-giving. Most thought that anyone who was physically fit—particularly males—must have had sex, and that once experienced it was very difficult to abstain and maintain one's mental well-being. A young man stated that: "Sex helps people calm their minds; if someone does not have sex, his mind is restless" [PO-01-C-2-1m].

Young men and women assumed that nearly all of their peers had experienced sexual intercourse by the age of 15. Similarly, a Village Executive Officer estimated that only 5 percent of girls refrained from sex before leaving primary school. The expectation that social contact led to sex made it difficult for young people to maintain nonsexual friendships with the opposite sex. Public contact between young men and women was rare, but when it occurred, young men assumed they should take the opportunity to start sexual negotiations and young women anticipated this.

Sexual License at Festivals and Social Gatherings

Another widely held expectation was that normal restrictions on sexual activity were relaxed at festivals and special social gatherings. This primarily was maintained by young people, but apparently was also condoned by many older people. Four main factors seemed to underlie this: the usual social controls were not as effective given the crowds, movement, and/or darkness after nightfall; the sexual license had a symbolic or ritual function; adults felt a celebratory, permissive mood which led them to indulge their children; and/ or young men had more money than normal at these events, which facilitated greater alcohol use for some and sexual activity for many. Many different kinds of special events were associated with greater youth sexual activity, some of which primarily involved school pupils, while others involved village youth more widely or villagers of all ages.

Special events primarily involving school children included inter-village sports competitions which might require overnight stays, and "LY" ("Last Year") Day, a celebration that marked pupils' final school day with games, food, videos, and a disco. Having sex on "LY day" was significant for many youth because it symbolized the social transition of leaving school. Many young men described how this day was, "very important to many youth—especially those very restricted at home by their parents—to achieve their plans to have sex" [PO-00-C-3-3m]. For some this involved having sex for the first time, but for others it was having sex at home for the first time, or having sex with two girls in one day.

Festivities involving young people both in and out of school included annual *rika* parties and traditional Sukuma *bukwilima* marriage ceremonies. As noted earlier, some *rika* hosted parties to celebrate their achievements at the end of the year. Sometimes adults chaperoned these events but then left after a couple of hours, possibly drunk themselves, and the youth then focused on sexual liaisons. *Bukwilima* weddings were the most widely admired form of marriage celebration, although they had become infrequent by the time of our study. In this form of wedding, the bride and groom each selected the same number of same-sex friends to help prepare for the main ceremony, a process that involved several overnight stays. *Bukwilima* weddings offered the clearest example of ritualized sexual license, because the bride's friends were paired with the groom's friends and the young women were expected to provide their male counterparts with food and bathing water, which often led to sex. An example provided by a 26-year-old man:

> He said that he greatly enjoys attending *bukwilima* events because he manages to have sex with new girls at them. For example, although young adolescent girls made up the last *bukwilima* party, he was nonetheless able to get one as a lover. He said that it is very hard for a young man or a girl attending *bukwilima* activities to return home later without having had sex. [PO-01-C-9-3m]

During the *bukwilima* celebration parents seemed to tolerate this increased sexual license, and it also seemed common at other kinds of wedding celebrations in rural Mwanza.

Events involving all age groups at which young people tended to be more sexually active included weekly markets, weddings, funerals (which were often large gatherings over several days), *ngoma* events, and holidays such as Christmas, Easter, **Bulabo**, *Saba saba*, and *Nane nane* (August 8th, the Tanzanian Peasant's Day holiday). In the following field notes, a researcher described young people's semi-open sexual negotiation at a *Saba saba ngoma* event:

> While still watching the *ngoma,* one boy with a bicycle continuously rang his bicycle bell. People who were watching the *ngoma* turned their heads to look at him. A young woman who was standing near me said that when he rings his bell he is indicating that he is looking for his partner. She said when some girls are at a big gathering, they check to see if their lover is looking for them whenever they hear the jingle of a bell. Arrangements to have sex were done outside of the *Saba saba* grounds before and after the *ngoma*, and inside the grounds while the *ngoma* was underway. I saw one girl standing with a boy and holding his radio while they talked, others being bought sugar cane, and others talking in kiosks inside the *Saba saba* grounds. Some boys followed me and said that they wanted me. Some bought sugar canes and brought them to me. Others called out to me, "You must use your youth before you die." [PO-00-I-4-4f]

On several Christian and some other national holidays, it was accepted that young women greeted men with the expression, "*Halleluya*," which literally meant "praise and thanks to God," but in this context was a request for a gift or money, as noted in chapter 2. When a man gave a *Halleluya* gift to a girl or woman who was not his relative, it was widely understood that this would be reciprocated with sex. A female researcher described *Halleluya* exchanges she witnessed during Christmas celebrations in one village center:

> At the beginning I stood with seven other young women who were all smartly dressed, but they dispersed and went in different directions. One joined me again and told me that if girls stood together then their chances of getting "*Halleluya*" were minimal and that is why they had preferred to disperse. I noticed most of those girls talked to two or more men, sometimes holding hands with them and receiving money, sweets, sugar cane, or peanuts. Some disappeared completely. . . . It was a bit chaotic as it was dark and people moved up and down with no one seeming to pay particular attention to the others. Those who were standing were mostly male-female pairs. I noticed young girls in Year 2 being seduced. For example, an early adolescent girl was greeted with a "*Halleluya*" by an older man. The man started caressing her and speaking to her seductively. He told her to pick up her "*Halleluya*" from him later, on the way home. Even the married women said "*Halleluya*" and were given money by men. [PO-99-I-1-2f]

DISCUSSION

Norms, Expectations, and Behavior

In rural Mwanza, young people's heterosexual activity was constrained by norms shared by most villagers that school pupils should be abstinent, women should maintain their sexual respectability, and sex should only be discussed in particular social contexts. These norms were of far greater importance in restricting or modifying sexual behavior than the threat of HIV infection, which was only rarely mentioned by young people as a personal concern, as was found elsewhere in Tanzania during the same time period (Dilger 2003); perceived susceptibility to HIV will be discussed further in chapter 11. Despite the influence of restrictive norms, expectations of how people behaved in practice encouraged sexual activity, and these expectations may have had normative elements, for instance, the belief that heterosexual sex is natural and healthy, or that sex without compensation demeans a woman. These expectations meant that sexual relationships were not as restricted as suggested in research literature that has highlighted rules, ritual practices, and self-restraint in sexual cultures in sub-Saharan Africa (e.g., Ahlberg 1994; Heald 1995).

In our study population, some norms or ideals were clearly espoused, such as feminine and masculine sexual respectability, pupil abstinence, the naturalness of sex, women's right to receive something for sex, and its role in masculine identity. However, only the first of these norms was universally endorsed, while different social groups supported or contested the others to varying degrees. Other norms were discerned from patterns of behavior and the occasional expression of values, including taboos against the discussion of sex, and special sexual license at festivals. Again, different social groups support these to varying degrees. The fundamental reason why the restrictive norms did not neatly predict behavior was that they were contradicted by the permissive norms. Consequently, individuals had to manage conflicting expectations.

Generational and Gender Conflict

Generational differences in the endorsement of sexual norms reflected broader generational conflicts. Young people's esteem amongst their peers was raised through consumption, which young women largely achieved through, and for men largely consisted of, transactional sex. Conversely, parents expected children to respect and obey them, and to delay sex until they left school: it was shameful to have children who flouted these norms. Parents' attempts to control their children's sexuality can also be interpreted in economic terms, as bridewealth involved a significant transfer of wealth between families and it was affected by a woman's sexual reputation. This will be discussed more in chapter 7.

In the early twentieth century, anthropologists characterized young Sukumas' sexual culture as fairly permissive as long as discretion was maintained (Cory 1953; Tanner 1955a; Tanner 1955b), but in the last half century a new restrictive norm was established. The ideal of strict abstinence for school pupils was probably introduced by Christian colonialists and missionaries (Van Eeuwijk and Mlangwa 1997). However, as discussed in chapter 3, it was only after national independence in the early 1960s that a large proportion of rural children started attending school. This norm thus only became a core part of Sukuma culture after independence, and it exemplifies a fundamental tension with the new social category of "adolescence" (Murcott 1980; Caldwell et al. 1998).

In our study, differential endorsement of norms and expectations also reflected differing interests by gender. At the heart of these was the sexual double standard, whereby men openly expected monogamy of their partners but not of themselves, and the related division of women into sexually respectable and disreputable. Unmarried men and women's expectation and practice of monogamy will be discussed in depth in the next chapter.

Contradictions Managed through Concealment

While several norms seemed to inhibit sexual activity, others seemed to condone or encourage it. Young people managed these contradictory norms and expectations primarily by concealing their sexual relationships, in particular from their parents but to some extent also from their peers. This avoided punishments and reduced the risk, for men, of being forced into marriage if they impregnated their partner, and, for women, of jeopardizing their sexual reputation and eligibility for marriage. For both sexes it avoided accusations of being unfaithful to another sexual partner and the jealousies that might involve.

Unwillingness to acknowledge sexual activity has long existed amongst the Sukuma. As Varkevisser (1973, 268) noted: "It is traditionally acceptable for Sukuma girls to enjoy their freedom at night, so long as they avoid shaming their parents. . . . The mere glimpse of a daughter talking on the road to a possible lover is sufficient provocation for a parent to beat the girl." Secrecy has also been found to be central to sexual cultures elsewhere in sub-Saharan Africa, with discretion sometimes also perceived as more important than following restrictive sexual mores (Setel 1999b; Nzioka 2001; Arnfred 2004; Helle-Valle 2004; Leclerc-Madlala 2009). Such discretion is a prerequisite for managing different sexual identities in different social contexts, as discussed in chapter 1 (Helle-Valle 2004).

In rural Mwanza, concealment of young people's sexual relationships almost certainly contributed to short relationship duration, overlapping or concurrent partnerships, and high levels of partner change. There was little scope for peers to strengthen a couple's relationship through social recognition and, conversely, less risk of sanctions if one had other sexual partners. Furthermore, hiding relationships gave little opportunity for a couple to develop intimacy through nonsexual contact. Indeed, even if a couple wanted a nonsexual companionate relationship, it was very difficult to have given general segregation of men and women. Another factor discouraging longterm relationships was that men usually gave less for second and subsequent sexual encounters with a partner, giving the partner a dwindling incentive to stay in the relationship.

A further consequence of clandestine relationships was that many adult villagers and broader authorities did not recognize or acknowledge the prevalence of young people's sexual activity. Lack of awareness or acknowledgement of youth sexual activity can hamper the development of national policies addressing adolescent sexual health and also reduce the legitimacy of programs that promote premarital partner reduction, monogamy, or condom use (Van Eeuwijk and Mlangwa 1997; Baylies and Bujra 2000). Finally, the deep-seated habit of concealing sexual experiences, particularly from adults, helps explain the limited validity of young people's survey and interview reports of sexual behavior, as described in chapter 1 and 2.

CONCLUSION

In this chapter we have considered how sexual beliefs were socially constructed and subject to social change in rural Mwanza, including shifting power between generations, integration into the cash economy, and the spread of schooling. In our study we found that sexuality was more complex than suggested by either side in the debate about whether sexual cultures in sub-Saharan Africa are permissive or restrictive. The case study series in the next section of the book will describe typical unmarried young people's lives and particularly their experiences managing the contradictory sexual norms and expectations described in this chapter. The following chapters will then examine unmarried young people's sexual behavior in depth, moving from the macro-social level of relationships in chapter 6 to the interpersonal, microsocial level of negotiation and specific sexual activities in chapters 7 and 8, respectively.

NOTE

1. Some material in this chapter was adapted from: Wight, Daniel, Mary L. Plummer, Gerry Mshana, Joyce Wamoyi, Zachayo S. Shigongo, and David A. Ross. 2006. Contradictory sexual norms and expectations for young people in rural northern Tanzania. *Social Science and Medicine* 62:987–97.

Case Study Series 1

"We'll Have Sex Again When the Opportunity Arises"

Typical Young People's Lives and Premarital Sexual Relationships

The case studies in this series describe five individuals' family and school backgrounds, socioeconomic activities, and sexual relationship histories in detail, to illustrate typical experiences of unmarried young people in rural Mwanza during the study period. These case studies describe how youth tried to manage complex and sometimes contradictory social norms and expectations, particularly as related to their sexual behavior and risk.

For example, Ndila's case study (1.1) demonstrates how male pupils in early adolescence tended to have rare, opportunistic sexual encounters with girls of the same age or younger, but that the frequency of their encounters increased as they became older, gained experience, and had more income to use for material exchange. Saidi's case study (1.2) in turn illustrates how many out-of-school young men devoted a great deal of time to secretive, open-ended, and sometimes overlapping sexual relationships. Bulugu's case study (1.3) demonstrates how a young man engaged in a traveling occupation had sexual partners in both his village and a nearby town, effectively bridging different populations of women.

In contrast to the male examples above, Flora's case study (1.4) demonstrates how early adolescent school girls frequently experienced intense sexual pressure from boys and men, particularly girls who were perceived as hard-to-get. Typically, as in Flora's case, any intentions such girls had to delay sexual debut were worn down over time. Kabula's case study (1.5) illustrates how girls in rural Mwanza had very little access to the cash economy and this strongly influenced their sexual behavior. Initially, Kabula's main motivation to have sex was a desire for snacks at school and small luxuries, but she eventually had a child out-of-wedlock and then depended on material exchange for basic necessities for herself and her child.

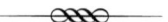

1.1. NDILA: A YOUNG MAN'S TRANSITION FROM EARLY CHILDHOOD, THROUGH SCHOOL, TO YOUNG ADULTHOOD

Ndila was 16 years old and in Year 6 of a *MEMA kwa Vijana* control community school when he participated in his first in-depth interview. He was reinterviewed by the same interviewer two years later, when he was an out-of-school farmer still living within his mother's household.

Ndila was born in a district town where his father worked as a health inspector. His parents were Christian and Sukuma. They separated when Ndila was a few years old, and he did not see his father again. Ndila then moved to a village where he lived with his maternal grandfather until he was 8–9 years old. At that time, Ndila became chronically ill with stomachaches and headaches, and his family eventually sent him to another village where he received treatment from a traditional healer. Ndila explained: "I could not be cured at a hospital. I was suffering a lot—my head was in terrible pain due to a witch. The traditional healer told me who the witch was" [II-00-C-84-m].

When Ndila was believed to have been cured, his family was unable to pay the Tshs 20,000 ($24) fee, so Ndila continued living with and working for the traditional healer until the bill was paid. At 11 years of age, Ndila then moved to his mother's village and began Year 1 of school. He lived with his mother and a half-sister in a two-roomed house made of poles and grass. His mother farmed potatoes, cassava, and other crops, and she also had a sardine-selling business.

Ndila helped with the family farm during the rainy season, but during the dry season his after-school hours were free, as was the case during his first interview. He explained: "Yesterday I went to school, and after that I went to play soccer. Then I just came home and waited for food, and had supper before bed. . . . During the dry season, you just roam about, as there is nothing to do" [II-00-C-84-m]. Ndila sometimes went to the video shows or discos, where he stood outside with other boys dancing to music if he could not pay entry. Ndila also participated in a same-sexed *rika* of youth who helped farm one another's farms, but they did not hire themselves out for a fee. He raised his own chickens and pigeons, selling the pigeons for Tshs 500 ($0.60) each. He used his earnings to pay for exercise books, clothing, and entertainment. Ndila's mother paid for his school fees, uniforms, and shoes.

Ndila prided himself on never having missed a day of school between Year 1 and Year 5. Like almost every in-depth interview respondent, when asked if there was anything he disliked about school, Ndila mentioned being beaten by teachers:

N: I like all of the teachers, except one. He/she was very much against me, and used to beat me. Yes, that one I didn't like very much.

I: Does it mean that he beat you even if you did not do anything wrong?

N: Yes. He might perhaps find you wearing a watch, and he would tell you to take it off. You just oblige.

I: And if you refuse?

N: He is a teacher. How could you refuse? [II-00-C-84-m]

Ndila estimated that he was 8 or 9 years old when he had his first sexual experiences with girls he met while herding cattle in his grandfather's village. This activity almost always involved an element of play, such as pretend wrestling, joking, or imitating a mother and a father at home. Ndila said such play almost always led to vaginal intercourse, although he did not yet ejaculate at that age.

Ndila said that the first time he had sex was with a girl in Year 1: "You got hold of each other and began wrestling. Then if she threw me down, she had sex with me while she was on top. If I threw her down, I had sex with her while I was on top" [II-00-C-84-m]. He reported that he and this girl did this almost every day for many months. Around the same time, Ndila said that he also had sex two times with a second girl. He followed her to where she was collecting firewood, and their relationship also began playfully: "She would make jokes like, 'You are still a child.' I would tell her, 'I like/love you,' and she then would [pretend to] insult me or hit me. When she did, I simply laughed. I just slowly continued with her like that, until she finally agreed" [II-00-C-84-m]. Ndila reported that he only had sex once with his third partner, because she was a girl in Year 2 who only herded cattle briefly, while on a school vacation. He explained: "We pretended to cook food made out of mud. We then made small straw houses out of poles, and got inside and [had sex] while we pretended to sleep there" [II-00-C-84-m]. Ndila said that he did not give money or a gift to any of these partners. He explained, "They were still young. Perhaps a girl does not ask for money until she grows up and realizes she can, when she is 10 or 13 years old. Then she becomes aware that that is what is done" [II-00-C-84-m].

After Ndila stopped herding cattle he did not have sex again for a number of years, including the years he lived with the traditional healer and his first years of primary school in his mother's village. As a school boy in early to mid adolescence, Ndila was also typical in that he frequently approached girls for sex, but he had little money and he rarely succeeded in convincing them. During that period, he described his own motivation for sex as purely physical, while he believed girls were only motivated by money.

Ndila did not have sex again until he was 13 years old and in Year 3, when he seduced a classmate on their way home from school:

N: I told her, "You know my problem." After some discussion, then she knew. She told me that I should come the following day and bring Tshs 100 ($0.12). I had the money, because sometimes you just do casual labor and you get wages. The next day I gave her the money while at school. She agreed and said, "Maybe during the break." During the break we left the school and went to the hill [for sex]. We returned to the school when the bell rang. [II-00-C-84-m]

When asked why he picked that girl and not another as a sexual partner, Ndila said that he had approached many girls, and she was simply the first one who consented. Ndila reported that they did not have sex again, because other boys influenced her: "They told her, 'Just reject him. That one does not have money. You should just take us instead.'" [II-00-C-84-m]

Ndila got his next sexual partner at the beginning of Year 4. She was an out-of-school girl who he met while strolling in the village one evening. He pursued her for several months, and ultimately convinced her to have sex outdoors during the Easter celebrations. He said that he only gave her Tshs 50 ($0.06) for each sexual encounter, but she did not have any money at all so that was enough for her. They had sex outdoors three times over several weeks. At the time of the interview, 1–2 years had passed since he had last seen her, but Ndila still considered himself to have a sexual relationship with her. He explained: "We are still continuing, but it is just that her elder sister came to take her away for work elsewhere." [II-00-C-84-m] He said that he had not had any other sexual relationships since being with her.

During the first in-depth interview, Ndila did not believe that there was any way to prevent pregnancy while having sex. At Ndila's request, the interview was conducted in Sukuma, but he could not correctly explain the Sukuma term for sexually transmitted infections (**bunyolo**). He said: "**Bunyolo** are only transmitted through the air . . . if a person with **bunyolo** passed here, and there was someone with his mouth open, then the illnesses would get in his mouth." [II-00-C-84-m] Ndila had heard of AIDS, and described it as an illness that made people very thin. He did not believe that anyone in his village had ever had AIDS, or that he could ever get it. He knew that AIDS was sexually transmitted, but he also believed that it might be caused by witchcraft:

> *N:* When a man has sex with a woman, he gets it. And then when he goes to have sex with another one, she gets it.
>
> *I:* And how else might they get AIDS?
>
> *N:* Maybe by being bewitched. Maybe he annoyed a witch sometime . . . maybe by frequently insulting him/her. [II-00-C-84-m]

Ndila knew that condoms could be used to prevent transmission of AIDS by sexual intercourse. He described a condom fairly well:

> *N:* A condom is white. It feels the same as when you touch a plastic bag. It is made the same as a man's penis looks. You put it on a penis so that it protects . . . then you go to have sex with her. . . . Afterwards you remove it and throw it in the latrine. We saw condoms at school, a teacher had brought them. We blew them up. Of course, he just gave them to the boys. [II-00-C-84-m]

When the researcher interviewed Ndila again two years later, Ndila had finished Year 7 but he had not passed his Primary School Leaving Examination, so his mother had arranged for him to return to school using the name of a student who had dropped out. At the time of the interview, Ndila was still waiting to resume school while living in his mother's compound, where he had built himself a one-roomed *maji*. He attended African Inland Church services on Sundays and performed in the choir, including taking overnight trips to other villages to perform on religious holidays. Ndila also sometimes attended weekly or monthly video shows and discos.

During his second interview, Ndila said he occasionally treated himself for health problems at home. For example: "When I had a fever I bought some tablets from the shops and swallow them to be cured. But when I cut my leg, I bought two-colored pills [tetracycline capsules] and opened them to pour the powder on the wound" [II-00-C-284-m]. Ndila continued to occasionally have severe headaches. He explained: "You know there is something like a worm in my head. It wriggles there and starts dancing. Then my head starts aching" [II-00-C-284-m]. He still believed in witchcraft and traditional medicine, but he had come to believe that Western medicine could effectively treat this condition. Eight months earlier he had travelled to a large hospital where he had been treated with aspirin, an antimalarial drug, and other medications. However, Ndila did not trust the capacity of his local health facility: "Hospitals are excellent because people get treated and whoever is treated gets cured. But not [the local facility]. Medicine is not available there. You just know that there is nothing here. Absolutely nothing" [II-00-C-284-m].

At the time of the second interview, Ndila had a small plot of land where he grew cotton. He had earned Tshs 10,000 ($12) from his cotton crop the year before, which he used for clothing and household expenses. Ndila also worked in two farming *rika*. The first *rika* was a church group of eight men and twelve women, both married and single, who were saving their combined earnings to buy guitars for the choir. Ndila's second *rika* was composed of ten out-of-school young men who planned to host an all-night disco at one of their houses at the end of the season. Ndila said they planned buy a cow and a goat to serve guests during the day, as well as hire a disk jockey who came with tape cassettes of Congolese dance music and female dancers for night-time entertainment. Ndila only expected male villagers to come to this event, and they all expected to earn money from their investment in it.

During his second interview, Ndila's description of his earlier sexual history was consistent with what he reported in his first interview. He said that he had had three more sexual partners since his first interview. He met the first one at a market in a neighboring village, when he was still in Year 6. He said that they had sex three times, but she then married another man so their relationship ended. He then met a different girl at the market, who he had sex with outdoors about seven times. Ndila said that they never quarreled, but they broke up because they "ceased communicating with each other" [II-00-C-284-m]. Five months later, when Ndila was 17 years old and in Year 7, he began a sexual relationship with a 15-year-old out-of-school girl who he met on her way to a well. They had had sex every two to three weeks in the ten months since then, when she was on an errand in remote areas or in her room at night. She shared a two-room house with her brothers, and Ndila had to pass through her brothers' room to enter her room. He explained: "I knock. They invite me inside, saying, 'Come in.' You just greet them, then you walk straight past, there is no conversing" [II-00-C-284-m]. He usually gave this girl lotion, body oil, soap, and/or Tshs 200–500 ($0.24–0.60) for each sexual encounter.

As an older school pupil and recent school leaver, Ndila had more income, sexual experience, and frequent encounters than he had had in early adolescence. There was nonetheless often a gap of many months between his relationships, and he said that he had never had concurrent partners. During both interviews Ndila said that he selected his partners for their physical attractiveness, but at the second interview he also mentioned other attributes that he valued, such as faithfulness. Also, although all of his relationships continued to involve material exchange, he had come to believe that some women were additionally motivated by sexual desire: "What attracts a man to a woman is his [penis], when it starts swelling and becomes erect and he just longs to seduce a girl. . . . And it is the same thing for a girl. A certain part of her genitals becomes erect, something pointed called a clitoris" [II-00-C-284-m].

During the same month as his second in-depth interview, Ndila participated in the 2001–2002 *MEMA kwa Vijana* trial survey. Like 86 percent of the male participants who were tested for five sexually transmitted infections at that time, Ndila tested negative for all five (Ross et al. 2007). During the second interview, Ndila reported that he had never used condoms or other contraception. When asked whether he would use a condom if a sexual partner requested it, he immediately replied: "I would think that that girl has diseases, and reject her" [II-00-C-284-m]. Later, when asked whether he might ever be able to get AIDS, Ndila again said, "No, not at all. Only people in towns have AIDS" [II-00-C-284-m].

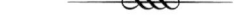

1.2. SAIDI: A MALE FARMER

During the first round of participant observation in a *MEMA kwa Vijana* control community, Saidi was a 22 years old and had completed primary school two years earlier, so he was not a trial member. His parents had had fifteen children together before his father died eleven years earlier. Saidi lived in his mother's compound with a 20-year-old sister and a 15-year-old brother, both of whom were trial members, as well as three of Saidi's nieces by another sister, all of whom were also in primary school. The household was very poor, and the family subsisted by cultivating a small agricultural plot. The seven family members lived in three rooms without even the most basic amenities, such as doors or a pit latrine.

Saidi said he first learned about sex by observing an older brother when he snuck girlfriends into their shared home at night. He said that he himself first had sex when he was 17 years old and in Year 5 of primary school. At that time an older, more sexually experienced friend made all of the arrangements for him to have sex. After that first sexual encounter, Saidi arranged his own relationships directly or through letters delivered by intermediaries. Saidi said that his sexual liaisons with younger adolescent girls usually took place in isolated places out-of-doors during the day or in empty classrooms in the early evening, when a girl had gone on an errand, such as to chop firewood. If the girl was older and slept in her own room, he instead snuck into her room after 11:00 p.m. and left very early in the morning. He said that on two such occasions he had almost been caught by a girl's parents, but that both times he managed to get away without them discovering his identity.

Saidi also took advantage of special celebrations to have sex with partners who had strict parents. For example, in his village the Catholic church held a vigil on Christmas Eve that could be attended by people of different denominations. At midnight children and youths left the church and held a singing procession that went from house to house, stopping and singing at each home until they were given a small amount of money, such as Tshs 50 ($0.06). Saidi, who belonged to the Protestant African Inland Church, explained why he joined the procession:

> He said that he joined the procession to meet a sexual partner who he ordinarily has difficulty meeting for sex at night, because she shares a sleeping house with her parents. He said that usually they remain behind while letting the others proceed. Once the others are a good distance away, they go have sex in a house or in the maize fields, and re-join the group in the morning. [PO-02-I-1-3m]

Saidi estimated that he had had more than ten sexual partners, most of them in the prior three years. Many of his partners were school girls, because he had very limited income and they typically expected less in exchange for sex than other young women. All of Saidi's sexual relationships were secret and opportunistic, and some overlapped with other sexual partnerships in an open-ended way. In those relationships, if sexual activity with one partner ended—and this was attributed to circumstances rather than bad feelings between them—then Saidi believed that they might reengage in sex if the opportunity arose again. During the first participant observation visit, he perceived his two most recent partners in that way. One of them had recently married a man in a nearby village, but Saidi had never quarreled with her so he believed that they still "could have sex again any day they happen to meet" [PO-01-I-1-3m].

Saidi was emotionally attached to his other recent partner, a secondary school student. They had first become sexual partners three years earlier, when he was in Year 7 and she was in Year 6. While in school together, they had had fairly regular sexual contact:

> Saidi said that they had always had sex in the bushes or in the classrooms, and that very often they had sex on festivals like Christmas, New Year, Easter or *Saba saba*, when most of the girls are free to walk about until night fall, which Saidi called a "time for sin." Saidi said he used to give her Tshs 200 ($0.24) if he had it, and sometimes even Tshs 500–1,000 ($0.60–1.20). [PO-01-I-1-3m]

Once this girl went away to secondary school in the district capital, Saidi did not see her often. Nonetheless, he continued to perceive her as one of his girlfriends:

> He said that he had sex with her twice last year when she was on holiday in the village [her first year of secondary school]. He said he has not yet had sex with her this year. However, he said, "We have a good relationship and we'll have sex again when the opportunity arises." Saidi said that he likes/loves her very much, because she discusses topics in a mature way. [PO-01-I-1-3m]

When the researcher returned for another participant observation visit one year later, Saidi was working as a casual laborer in a cotton plantation in a neighboring village, where he earned Tshs 800 ($0.96) per day. He had also built his own *maji*, where he slept alone within his mother's compound. At that time Saidi reported that he continued to miss his girlfriend in secondary school, and wished he could see her more. He was thus disappointed to learn that she had visited the village over the Christmas holiday but she had not tried to see him before leaving again: "He said that he was feeling very bad to have missed his partner that he likes/loves so much" [PO-02-I-1-3m].

Saidi's emotional attachment to this young woman did not discourage him from taking advantage of increased sexual activity during the holiday period. For example, on New Year's Day the researcher observed a 23-year-old friend of Saidi trying to arrange a new sexual relationship for Saidi:

> We were standing on the roadside when three girls passed who Saidi's friend knew. Saidi's friend asked Saidi which one he liked/loved amongst them . . . Saidi showed him one who was taller than the rest, and his friend went to call her. His friend talked to all of the girls for two minutes, and then he took the one Saidi chose by the hand and pulled her aside. After talking with her for about three minutes, he left her and returned to where we were standing. He told Saidi that the girl was in a hurry, so they would meet another day when she had ample time to talk. [PO-02-I-1-3m]

During that participant observation visit, Saidi said that he had had one new sex partner during the prior year. While that woman had been interested in continuing the relationship, Saidi had decided to end it after one sexual encounter for reasons he did not specify. More generally, Saidi explained that what attracted him and other young men most to a young woman was appearance, but if a man also considered marrying her, she should be monogamous, respectful, and work hard at cultivation, cooking, and other domestic chores.

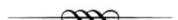

1.3. BULUGU: A MALE BICYCLE TAXI DRIVER

When a participant observation researcher met Bulugu, he was a 19-year-old bicycle taxi driver in a *MEMA kwa Vijana* intervention community. Bulugu had finished primary school two years earlier so he was not a trial member. He regularly went to a nearby town for his work, where he had a girlfriend who worked in a restaurant. Sometimes they met for sexual liaisons at his house, and sometimes he spent the night with her at her house in town. Early in the participant observation visit Bulugu told a researcher that his girlfriend had had a previous sexual relationship with a truck driver, but that that relationship had ended and now she wanted to marry Bulugu.

Several days later the researcher met Bulugu again, and Bulugu told him that he had ended the relationship because he discovered his girlfriend had other sexual partners. He had gone to visit her one evening at her work place, and after sharing sodas together she went to serve male customers behind a closed door in the back. He felt suspicious, so he went to look for her, and he found her outside having sex with a customer near the toilets. He was furious but decided not to confront her, as the researcher recorded in his field notes:

> The girl later came back and asked him if he had seen any person who came with a flashlight to the back. He told her that he did not see anyone. He told me that he later spent the night with the girl in the hotel having sex. He told me that he has now decided to leave her, since if he becomes ill with a sexually transmitted infection he will trouble his family and he will also trouble himself. [PO-99-I-6-1m]

Bulugu told the researcher that he did not want to use condoms to prevent sexually transmitted infections, because they reduced his sexual pleasure. Instead, he said that in the future he would only have partners who were not *wahuni* like his former girlfriend. Bulugu hoped to begin a new sexual relationship immediately, and he had already negotiated a sexual liaison with a village girl he had just met:

> Bulugu told me that in the past two days he and another bicycle taxi driver have been going after some girls who live in a nearby village. The girls hired their bicycles and when they were taking them to their destination, the men approached them about sex. The girls told the men to fetch them today to bring them to the village to sleep with them. Bulugu said that they would use his place. [PO-99-I-6-1m]

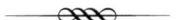

1.4. FLORA: A FEMALE PUPIL IN EARLY TO MID-ADOLESCENCE

During the first participant observation visit in Flora's village, she was 13 years old and had just completed Year 5. Flora was in a *MEMA kwa Vijana* intervention school and had participated in the intervention, but she was too young to be eligible for the biological survey, so no biological data were collected for her. Flora's parents were monogamously married farmers, and she herself was a member of a *rika* made up of neighborhood children of 10 to 13 years of age. She sometimes also sold fried rice cakes in the market place on evenings and weekends. She and her family were Catholic and regularly attended church.

Flora told the researcher that she frequently was accosted by men and boys who wanted to have sex with her. The researcher noted:

> Flora said that both married and single men disturb her at the market by asking to have sex with her. She said some even wait for her by the path on her way home, taking advantage of the darkness. Flora said she ignores them and starts running home. She said it has also occurred when she goes to the shallow pond [5 km away] to fetch water. Young men stop her and say, "I like/love you." Flora said that she has never seen some of those men before. [PO-99-I-1-2f]

On numerous occasions when the researcher accompanied Flora to the market or elsewhere in the village, the researcher's observations confirmed these reports. Flora almost always firmly rejected her suitors and tried to ignore them, and she made a point of not taking substantial gifts that were offered to her. During the Christmas Day festivities, for example:

> Flora said if she asked for *Hallelluya* gifts from the opposite sex [mostly relatives], they gave her about Tshs 50 ($0.06), but if it was from fellow girls it was Tshs 10 ($0.01). Flora said that there was a young married man who gave her Tshs 5,000 ($6). She said she returned it because most men give a lot of money to girls who they have always admired but have been unable to get, and if she had taken such a huge amount of money the man would have followed her later [for sex]. She prefers taking a little money, less than Tshs 100 ($0.12), so that if a man demands it back one day she can easily find it and give it back. [PO-99-I-1-2f]

Despite Flora's stated practice of only taking small *Hallelluya* gifts, the researcher observed how one persistent secondary school student pursued her after having given her a gift the day before:

> The young man bought a bottle of soda for Flora, but Flora refused to take it. Flora's girlfriend told her to take it, but Flora said she was already drinking a soda. The man tried to talk to Flora, but she totally refused to respond and instead talked to me alone. I noted that when men tried to seduce Flora's friend, her friend laughed shyly with them, but Flora openly resisted by frowning and going away. When we left for home at 8:30 pm the young man tried to follow us. Flora refused to even turn around, and when we parted she ran to her home nearby. I saw the man turn and go back towards the market place. [PO-99-I-1-2f]

During the first participant observation visit Flora's resistance to such frequent and persistent sexual requests probably contributed to common perceptions of her as a virtuous girl who was highly desired both as a sexual partner and a potential wife. For example, the researcher's female host, a beer brewer in her early 30s and a mother of six, described how she wanted Flora to marry her cousin's son:

> My host said that her cousin has many cows and plans to go straight to Flora's parents to propose this to them. She said that they can't refuse ten cows or more, given that marriage proposals are rare these days. She said that they have looked at Flora's character and see it is worthy of a marriage proposal, and moreover, she

is beautiful and young. Flora is not aware of this plan, nor are her parents. My host said they also have plans to sweet talk the teachers into removing Flora's name from the school register [so she could marry before completing school]. [PO-99-I-1-2f]

When the researcher returned to the village the next year, Flora was 15 years old and had just begun Year 7. She and her family had converted from Catholicism to Seventh Day Adventism, but they continued to attend church regularly within their new religion. In the past year, two men from the district capital and one from elsewhere in the village had approached Flora's parents with marriage proposals, but her father had told them that she needed to finish primary school before marrying.

During the second participant observation visit, Flora told the researcher that she had had sex for the first time some months earlier when she was 14 years old, as described below:

> Flora said she had had sex in the bushes in the evening. She said she received Tshs 2,000 ($2.40) before she had sex and later used the money to take her dress to the tailor. She said she felt very bad after having sex. Flora said that the man with whom she had sex had been pestering her for a long time until she finally agreed to it. Flora said that she also decided to have sex because different men had told her that, if she has not had sex at her age, she would have problems later when she gets married. Also she heard other girls discuss their boyfriends, and thus decided to "taste" it. [PO-01-I-1-2f]

Flora's first two sexual relationships had been negotiated by a young woman who was four years older than her but in the same class. This classmate first facilitated a one-month sexual relationship between Flora and the classmate's uncle. When that ended, she arranged a relationship between Flora and the classmate's cousin, a kiosk owner. This was Flora's sexual relationship during the second participant observation visit. Her intermediary explained that she delivered letters between the two partners, and provided Flora with an excuse to visit a partner for sex during her morning break or after school, under the guise that Flora was visiting the intermediary. Her intermediary reported that whenever Flora visited her boyfriend the kiosk owner she was allowed to unlock a drawer where he kept money and take out Tshs 1,000 ($1.20).

During that participant observation visit the researcher observed that Flora continued to be approached at the market and elsewhere by men seeking to negotiate sex with her, and Flora largely continued to ignore them. Flora also told the researcher of a married teacher who repeatedly had tried to pressure her to have sex with him. As noted in chapter 4, there were plausible reports of sexual relationships between male teachers and female pupils in almost all of the participant observation villages, but Flora lived in a village where such reports were extraordinarily numerous, and almost every male teacher was implicated. An exchange between Flora and her teacher was typical:

> Her teacher called her into the office when other teachers were away. He asked her whether she had handed in the exam [and] pretended to argue with her . . . He then said he had just misplaced it. He told her she was the best girl in class with

45 percent, but he wanted to give her another 15 percent. She agreed to the free marks, and the teacher started caressing her breasts, buttocks, and hands . . . [and] asked her for sex. . . . She told the teacher to wait until when she completes Year 7, and the teacher agreed. Flora said that whenever she meets this teacher when she is alone, he tells her that he is still waiting for her promise. . . . Flora said that this is one of the reasons that she may leave the village immediately after she completes her Year 7 examination. [PO-01-I-1-2f]

In addition to the sexual experiences above, during the second participant observation visit Flora told the researcher that recently a man who had a repu-tation as a "girl spoiler" had tried to rape her. Flora said that the man had long sought to have a sexual relationship with her, and his sister ultimately facilitated the assault:

On a Sunday morning around 10 am the man's sister came to where Flora was sell-ing fried rice cakes and told her to take some to her house to leave on the table. The house is next to the market. When Flora took the fried rice cakes there the man's sister followed her and locked the door behind her. Flora said that she did not know that the man was in the house, but he immediately woke up and started touching her. Flora said that he tried to give her money, but she would not touch it. She said that they struggled with each other and finally she removed one of her shoes, hit him on the face, and threatened to make noise if he continued. Flora said that the man's sister heard the struggles and eventually opened the door from outside. . . . Flora said that she hates that man, and when she sees him she feels bad, because she remembers that experience. She did not tell her parents for fear of being rebuked and blamed for having gone to the man's house. [PO-01-I-1-2f]

During the second participant observation visit, Flora said this man did not succeed in having intercourse with her, but when recounting the experience again one year later, she said that he in fact had. During that third participant observation visit, Flora was 16 years old and had just completed Year 7. She had passed her Primary School Leaving Examination and won a place at secondary school, but her parents said that secondary school was too expensive, so they planned to send her on a one-year tailoring course instead.

At that time, Flora told the researcher that she had recently been in a sexual relationship with the acting Village Executive Officer. Flora had learned about condoms from the *MEMA kwa Vijana* Intervention, and she said she insisted that this partner use them because she feared becoming pregnant. He did not bring a condom the first time they arranged to have sex, so she refused to have intercourse. He then brought and used a condom the next time they met for sex. The relationship did not go beyond these two sexual encounters, however, because the man's wife found out:

The man's wife followed Flora to the shallow pond where she was drawing water, and wanted to beat her. Flora said that it was the man's fault that his wife knew about it, because after having sex with her he started following her and openly de-manded more encounters. [PO-02-I-1-2f]

During that third participant observation visit the researcher observed that other men continued to approach Flora for sexual relationships. She also saw that Flora curtailed her movements in the village center specifically to avoid the teacher who continued to pressure her for sex. It was clear that Flora's reputation within the village had changed, in part because of the public accusations made by the Village Executive Officer's wife. Flora was no longer perceived as a highly respectable school girl, and one informant referred to her as a *mhuni*. For example, the researcher's host, who previously had praised Flora's virtuosity:

> My host mentioned that Flora and another girl have had sexual relationships with the acting Village Executive Officer. She said that she learned about this from the man's wife. My host said she wonders why young girls like having sex with married men, some of whom are older than them by far. [PO-02-I-1-2f]

During the third participant observation visit Flora confided to the researcher that she had had symptoms of a sexually transmitted infection for over a year, namely a genital rash, sores, itchiness, and unusual discharge. She said that she did not feel she could go to a health facility for diagnosis and treatment, because she feared her visit would not be confidential. The researcher commented in her field notes:

> Flora said that since the local health inspector came from within this village he was bound to tell others about it, and that the health inspector's wife could gossip about it with other women at the market place. I tended to believe this, as I had spent one evening with Flora, the health inspector's wife and another woman selling fish at the market. I heard them gossip about other women and girls, mainly about *uhuni* [bad behavior] and sexual partners. . . . Flora said, "If I start to tell the doctor that I have this and that pain, he/she will ask me a lot of questions. Really, I just can't do it." [PO-02-I-1-2f]

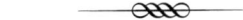

1.5. KABULA: A YOUNG WOMAN'S TRANSITION FROM SCHOOL TO SINGLE MOTHERHOOD

Kabula was 18 years old and in Year 6 in a *MEMA kwa Vijana* control community school when she participated in an in-depth interview. The same interviewer then interviewed her again two and one half years later, when Kabula was a single mother living with her son within her parents' household.

Kabula's parents were monogamously married farmers. She was the oldest of her parent's five surviving children; another four of their children had died. Her family was Sukuma and Catholic. Their household of seven people lived in two houses built of mud bricks and thatched roofs. Kabula slept with her sisters in the same two-room house as her parents. Kabula's father set a strict curfew for her, and he hit her if she returned home late.

Kabula helped farm her parents' fields and participated in the daily domestic chores typically shared amongst women within households, including fetching firewood, hauling water, cleaning, and cooking. As a school pupil, she earned money by cultivating a small portion of her parents' farm for her own personal use. She earned Tshs 1,500–3,000 ($1.80–3.60) annually from her cotton crop, and Tshs 2,000 ($2.40) from her rice crop, which she had used to buy a dress and a pair of shoes, and to pay part of her school fees.

Kabula was enthusiastic about school, and especially enjoyed learning to read and write. The only thing she disliked about school was sometimes being beaten, for example, once when she did not bring Tshs 200 ($0.24) in school fees:

K: The teacher asked for school fees. He/she beat me here, there, I don't know where all. I bled. I went home crying, hiih! My parents looked for money. They went around searching until they got it. I went home at 8 am and they got it by 11 am, so I went back to school then.

I: Have you been hit by any other teacher while you were at school?

K: Yes, by many. If you have no money, they hit you. If you have not washed, they hit you. Even if you forget something, they hit you. [II-99-C-69-f]

During the first interview, Kabula said that her first sexual relationship began when she was 16 years old and in Year 4, and that it continued until she was in Year 5. Her partner was an older villager who came to her room for sex at night. The first time he gave her Tshs 1,500 ($1.80), but later he gave her about Tshs 600 ($0.72) for each encounter. When asked what she did with the money, she laughed, and said, "I was still young, I used to bring it to school for food, and the rest I gave to other people." She ended the relationship when the man repeatedly promised to give her money after sex, but then did not do so.

In Year 5, Kabula said that she began a sexual relationship with an out-of-school farmer of about the same age. Two to three nights per week he knocked on her window and snuck into the room she shared with her sisters, where they had sex from about 10 pm until midnight. She believed that her sisters were not awake and aware when this happened. This partner gave her Tshs 500–600 ($0.60–0.72) for every sexual encounter, which she used to buy peanuts or gum at school. That relationship lasted one year, but Kabula said she had broken up with that boyfriend just days before the interview because he had another sexual partner:

K: We have separated. I told him, "Get out and go!" He got another girl in another village. We went to the market there. We met that girl, and people began to joke with her. She was annoyed. They left her there crying. They began telling him, "Iih, let us go to so-and-so, your lover." They were telling him this, and he became angry then. He told me [later] that it was lies. I told him to go away. [II-99-C-69-f]

In addition to the two sexual relationships described above, Kabula reported that she had had sex with another man in her room for Tshs 500 ($0.60) one month before the interview. This man knew that she already had a regular partner. She did not yet know whether he wanted to continue having sex with her beyond that one encounter, but she seemed open to the idea.

At the time of the first interview, Kabula said that her parents had never told her anything about sex. She said that she feared getting pregnant, but she did not know of any contraceptive methods. If she became pregnant she said she would "just have the baby" and continue living with her parents. Kabula had heard of sexually transmitted infections, but she had never thought about whether she might get one. She did not know how HIV/AIDS was transmitted, or what could be done to prevent its transmission. She had never been to a health facility, but she had once been treated in a traditional healer's compound for several days with something the healer diagnosed as meningitis.

During her second interview, Kabula explained that she had finished Year 7 but she had not passed her Primary School Leaving Examination. In her first year out of school, she sometimes earned money as a casual laborer farming cotton, maize, cassava, or rice on other people's farms during the rainy season. After she had her baby, her parents gave her land to farm rice and cotton for herself, from which she had earned Tshs 11,500 ($13.80) the year prior to the interview, which she used to buy gunny sacks. She also began a home business making *gongo* to pay for her and her son's needs. She learned that business from her parents.

During the second interview, the interviewer asked Kabula how many sexual partners she had ever had. At first, Kabula said that she had only had two partners. The researcher then reminded her that she had reported three partners during her first interview, and Kabula corrected herself to say that she had had four partners in total. While Kabula's description of those four partners were detailed and plausible, all but one were quite different from what she had reported in her first interview. For example, she again reported that she first had sex when she was in Year 4, but in the second interview she said her first partner had been a school boy in Year 3 with whom she had sex 2–4 times per week for six months, not an older villager who she saw regularly for a year, as she reported in the first interview. In the two interviews combined Kabula described six distinct sexual relationships in detail, suggesting she had had at least that many, rather than the four total she reported in the second interview. Such inconsistencies were not unusual in in-depth interviews. This methodological problem is described and discussed in more detail in the next chapter.

During the second interview, Kabula said that she had had two sexual partners in the two and one half years since her first interview. The first was a young man from a neighboring village who worked at a cotton ginnery. She said he was about the same age as her and they first had sex when she was staying in her grandfather's house in the other village. When she returned to her parents' household, he continued to meet her for sex at night one to three times per week, each time bringing her Tshs 500 ($0.60) or a gift, such as kerosene or body oil. When describing her different sexual partners, Kabula said that this young man was the one who she most liked/loved. She also said that he was the one who made her pregnant.

Kabula's pregnancy within a couple of year's of leaving primary school was not unusual. Four months earlier, she had participated in the *MEMA kwa Vijana* 2001–2002 survey, where 19 percent of female participants tested positive for pregnancy (Ross et al. 2007). In addition, of those who reported that they had never been pregnant during the first survey in 1998, 46 percent reported that they had been pregnant by the time they were interviewed three years later.

Kabula told the interviewer what happened after she became pregnant:

K: Two months elapsed and I did not get my period, so then I knew. I just kept quiet. I was afraid.

I: How did others know that you were pregnant?

K: They saw me. They saw my womb was just bulging [laughter], it was just forging ahead.

I: Was there any person who asked you whether you were pregnant?

K: Yes. My [24-year-old] paternal aunt. She told me, "I think you are pregnant." I used to deny it. But she would say, "But really, you are pregnant." When I was about six months pregnant my father asked me one day. I agreed that I was pregnant. He asked me, "Where did you get that pregnancy from?" [laughter] I just kept quiet. He persisted in asking me: "Whose?" I told him. My parents then kept quiet. Then they said that they should look for people to take me to inform the man and his family. So they took me there. [The man] denied that child, so I decided to leave him. . . .

I: And did your partner later tell you that he wanted to continue having sex with you?

K: Yes. Later he said, "I denied [paternity] because I was afraid of your father."

I: What was he afraid of?

K: I don't know, maybe of being beaten. Later he told me, "I shall come [to have sex] today," and I said, "You are coming today—why? You denied the child. You are coming again so that we do what?" I did not want it. I left him and went home. [II-02-C-269-f]

After having her son, Kabula said she started a new sexual relationship with an out-of-school youth who was three years younger than her. It was unusual for a young woman to have a partner so much younger than her, and she said even he was surprised when she approached him with interest: "He said, 'But you—you are really old, you have a child!'" [II-02-C-269-f] Nonetheless, he quickly became interested in her and they began meeting for sex outside of her house about twice per week. She explained that she no longer let her sexual partners enter her room at night: "He doesn't come in, he just stays outside. We have sex in the shrubs there. I leave my child sleeping inside. By the time he wakes up, I have already come back" [II-02-C-269-f].

At the time of the second interview, Kabula said that this young man wanted to marry her, but he had not yet convinced her. She said that his mother and siblings knew of their relationship, and that they liked her:

K: Even now when I see his mother and siblings they insist that I go there. They want me to marry him. . . .

I: Why do you refuse?

K: [laughter] There isn't even a reason.

I: Do you ever think of getting married?

K: I will get married. [II-02-C-269-f]

Despite the open nature of Kabula's relationship within her partner's family, she continued to hide her sexual activity from her own parents:

K: When my boyfriend gives me money, my mother doesn't ask where it comes from. She just thinks, "Perhaps she got that money from selling *gongo.*"

I: And have you ever told your mother that you have a sexual partner?

K: I never have.

I: Why haven't you told your parents?

K: They can beat me. [II-02-C-269-f]

In summary, over a period of five years, Kabula seemed to have at least six long-term (6–24-month) sexual relationships involving one to three sexual encounters per week. She hid all of these relationships from her parents, even after she became a parent herself. Each of Kabula's new relationships seemed to start a few weeks before or after an old one ended, so she rarely went without a steady sexual partner, and two relationships sometimes overlapped.

Kabula said that she had never been taught any information about sexually transmitted infections, and that she had never experienced symptoms of one. This may have been an honest response, as many people have no overt symptoms when they have such infections. However, during the 2001–2002 *MEMA kwa Vijana* survey, Kabula was one of the 27 percent of female participants who tested positive for Trichomonas, which was one of the six sexually transmitted infections measured for females (Ross et al. 2007).

Kabula said that she did not know how sexually transmitted infections could be prevented during sex, although she had vaguely heard of condoms: "I just hear about condoms, but I don't know what they are. At the hospital, there are those posters pasted up, you see 'Condoms' written on them and then you ask yourself, 'What is a condom?' But I don't know" [II-02-C-269-f].

Kabula had delivered her son in a health facility in a neighboring village, and spoke favorably about it. At the time of the second interview, she said that she still had never used a contraceptive and did not know how to prevent pregnancy, although it is likely that she received some kind of family planning information at the health facility after delivering her son. Kabula said that she herself had not been to a traditional healer in recent years, and she had never taken her son to one. However, her son wore a **lupigi** (a protective charm) that her father had made for him after obtaining herbs from his own father. She explained: "My child was suffering. A lot of saliva was coming out of his mouth and he would cry. Then the **lupigi** was put on him and he became well" [II-02-C-269-f].

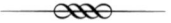

CONCLUSION

The case studies in this series illustrate how unmarried youth in rural Mwanza managed some of the contradictory sexual norms and expectations described in chapter 5, including restrictive norms of pupil abstinence or female sexual respectability, and permissive expectations of male sexual need, or sex as a female resource. In the next chapter we will examine common sexual relationship patterns for unmarried young people both in and out of school. Within that broad topic we will address some of the issues raised here, including limited emotional intimacy within relationships and experience of concurrent partnerships. Later chapters will address other topics illustrated by these case studies, such as sexual coercion and violence (chapter 7), contraception (chapter 10), and illness causation beliefs and treatment-seeking practices (chapter 11).

Chapter Six

Unmarried Young People's Sexual Relationships

In any cultural context, sexual relationships can be unique, complex, and dynamic. The term "relationship" itself is difficult to define, because it can encompass anything from a one-off encounter with a stranger to a long-term partnership involving occasional or frequent sexual encounters. In both low and high income countries, researchers trying to understand sexual relationships and their implications for sexual health have struggled to accurately assess variables such as the emotional nature of relationships, their overall timing, duration, and overlap, and the frequency of sexual encounters within them (Gersovitz et al. 1998; Gorbach et al. 2002; Kraut-Becher and Aral 2003; Ferguson et al. 2004; Nnko et al. 2004; Helleringer and Kohler 2007; Nelson et al. 2007; Thomas and Cole 2009; Harrison and O'Sullivan 2010). Each of these can be difficult to measure at one point in time for one partnership, and even more challenging to assess over time in fluid relationships. The diversity of relationships and their complex interconnection make them even more challenging to examine at a population level.

To date, research on sexual relationships in sub-Saharan Africa has generally taken one of two forms: survey research on key variables, such as age at first sex, number of partners, or type of partner, or anthropological study which generally considers the social nature of partnerships, such as kinship structures, lineages, and marriage alliances (Gersowitz et al. 1998; Kaaya et al. 2002; Thomas and Cole 2009).

Surveys can offer valuable insights into different kinds of low and high risk sexual relationships at a population level. For example, survey research in sub-Saharan Africa has found that men and women who report multiple sexual partners are consistently more likely to be HIV-infected than people who report fewer partners (Chen et al. 2007). However, as discussed in chapters 1 and 2, survey questionnaires are usually structured and short, so researchers have little time to build trust with respondents and little flexibility to tease out the complexities of sexual relationships (Nelson et al. 2007). Even variables which might seem straightforward to measure—like age at first sex, or lifetime number of partners—can be fraught with problems, particularly if respondents have limited knowledge of their own age, poor math skills, difficulty with recall, or concerns that their behavior might be socially undesirable, none of which are unusual in sub-Saharan Africa (Gersowitz et al. 1998; Brewer, Garrett and Kulasingam 1999; Stycos 2000; Gersovitz 2007; Beguy et al. 2009).

These problems are compounded when collecting more complex data, such as the timings and durations of multiple sexual relationships. Concurrent relationships—those in which one or both partners have other sexual partners while continuing to have sexual encounters with their original partner—warrant close examination for their potential importance in HIV transmission. However, given the challenge of collecting data on them, few studies have directly focused on them in sub-Saharan Africa to date (Research to Prevention 2009; Lurie and Rosenthal 2010; Harrison and O'Sullivan 2010).

Similarly, little research in sub-Saharan Africa has focused on the role that emotions, and particularly love, play in initiating, maintaining, and ending sexual relationships, especially for unmarried youth (Thomas and Cole 2009). "Love" can involve a variety of powerful emotions related to kinship or personal ties, including strong affection, attachment, tenderness, devotion, loyalty, and concern. In some high income countries, researchers have attempted to distinguish lust from love, and particularly from romantic love. "Romantic love" has been defined as an intense attraction that involves idealization of a partner, with an erotic component and an expectation of a shared future (Jankowiak and Fischer 1992; Giddens 1992). In romantic love, a person believes a partner's character uniquely complements his or her own, "making one's life complete." This has been described as a quasi-religious, transformative, and sublime experience that overshadows physical attraction and other relationships and obligations in a couple's lives (Vaughan 2009). Romantic love is generally perceived as a precursor to "companionate love," in which love, sexual satisfaction, and intimacy come together when a couple lives together long-term, often in marriage.

Giddens (1992) hypothesized that romantic love was not common in pre-industrial Europe but became prevalent there as a result of industrialization, increased individualism, and the growing trend to see one's life as a narrative. Historically, anthropological research with different ethnic groups across sub-Saharan Africa has rarely mentioned romantic love, and has sometimes specifically stated that it does not exist (Jankowiak and Fischer 1992). Some have argued that romantic love became more important in sub-Saharan Africa during the twentieth century due to influences of Christianity, colonialism, modernization, and globalization (Little 1973; Caldwell et al. 1998). During that period greater individualism, economic freedom and exposure to Western media amongst young men are believed to have resulted in more young people choosing their own spouse, including sometimes marrying out of love rather than obedience to parents or economic obligation. Romantic love reportedly became an ideal for some educated urban African women by the 1950s (Little 1973) and was adopted by some urban African men more recently (Samuelsen 2006). "Love" was also perceived as an acceptable explanation for first pre-marital sex in a survey of urban young women in Mali in the late 1990s (Gueye, Castle, and Konate 2001), although it is unclear whether young women meant an idealized, romantic love, or love of a different form.

Other recent studies have suggested that love and particularly romantic love are rare in young people's sexual relationships (Vos 1994; Balmer et al. 1997; Nzioka 2004; Silberschmidt and Rasch 2001; Undie, Crichton, and Zulu 2007). Instead, it has been reported that, for young men, desire, peer pressure, or boosting of masculine prowess are the main motivations to have sexual relationships, while for young women the main incentive is material exchange, similar to the findings we described in the last chapter (Meekers and Calvès 1997; Gueye, Castle, and Konate 2001; Nzioka 2004).

This chapter will examine the nature of unmarried young people's sexual relationships in rural Mwanza. We will mainly focus on social factors that influence sexual relationships, although we recognize that relationships are influenced by many psychological and physiological factors as well (VanWesenbeeck et al. 1999). In order to assess typical behavior and to reduce bias from third-person rumor or scandal (Neighbors et al. 2006), the analysis in this chapter draws almost entirely on first-person accounts and strong observational evidence.

The description of our findings will begin with definition of sexual terms, followed by estimations of the proportion of young people who had had sex and typical ages at first sex. We will then describe three common, overarching sexual relationship patterns, as well as the specific characteristics of pre-adolescent, school pupil, and unmarried young adult relationships. Finally, we will describe our findings related to broader relationship issues such as emotional intimacy, lifetime numbers of partners, concurrency, and sexual mixing patterns.

FINDINGS

Definition of Sexual Terms

In all methods researchers were careful to clarify sexual terminology with respondents, to reduce the chance of ambiguity and misunderstanding (Sanders et al. 2010). Throughout survey questionnaires and at the onset of in-depth interviews, researchers used the terms *kufanya mapenzi* (to make love) and **kwilala** (to have vaginal intercourse). The Swahili term was a euphemism because pilot studies found that some more explicit terms were offensive to the general public, while others were inoffensive and technically accurate but unfamiliar to most people. To insure that respondents did not misunderstand these terms to mean a different activity (such as non-penetrative sex), researchers initially gave a standardized definition: "when a penis is inside of a vagina (or a man or boy's private parts are inside a woman or girl's private parts)," and also provided several widely used synonyms.

During in-depth interviews and participant observation, if respondents preferred to use other terms, researchers tried to confirm that those terms indeed meant vaginal intercourse and sometimes adopted them themselves in subsequent conversations with that respondent. Terms that both sexes used included "cooperating with him/her" or "pounding each other." Young men sometimes instead used terms like "banging a woman," "doing a woman," and "business," while young women used expressions like "working," "getting used to a man," and "pounding and winnowing"; the latter was also the name of a famous dance. Terminology used for other sexual activities will be described in chapter 8. If not otherwise specified, "sex" as used here refers to activity that included vaginal intercourse.

Informants also used a range of terms to describe their sexual partners, and many of these words could describe both casual and more committed partners of either sex, such as *rafiki* (friend), **mung'hya** (girlfriend), **nsumba** (boyfriend), *mpenzi* (lover), *hawara* (lover or mistress, depending on context), and *mchumba* (lover or fiancé/fiancée, depending on context). If a young man believed his partner had other partners he might refer to her as a *daladala* or **nyembe go ha nzila** (a mango tree that grows along a public path, with fruit that anyone can pick). Some young women who maintained a partner primarily for material support referred to him as a goat, particularly when using the phrase *kuchuna buzi* (to skin a goat, or to receive ample money for sex).

Words commonly used to describe sexual negotiation included *kutongoza* (to seduce) and *kuhonga* (literally "to bribe," but in this context meaning material exchange for sex); both terms described the man taking the active role and the woman the passive one. The most common words used to describe emotions and affection within sexual relationships were *kupenda* and **kutogwa**, both of which can be translated as either "to like" or "to love" in English. To better understand the specific emotions involved when those terms were used, researchers often asked respondents for further explanation and tried to interpret the terms in the context of broader remarks and observations.

Age at First Sex

In both *MEMA kwa Vijana* surveys and HALIRA research it was challenging to collect accurate data on whether young people had begun to have sex, and if they had, what their age was at sexual debut. In the 1998 assisted self-completion questionnaire survey, 55 percent of boys (average age 16) and 21 percent of girls (average age 15) reported having had sex (Plummer, Wight et al. 2004). Reports were similar for randomly selected boys in the 1999-2000 in-depth interview series conducted 9–18 months later (55 percent, average age 17), but were substantially higher for randomly selected girls (67 percent, average age 16). The higher reporting for girls in in-depth interviews might have been attributed to the smaller number of respondents or their greater age, except that many of those who reported sex in in-depth interviews again denied it in concurrent or later surveys (table 6.1) (Plummer, Ross et al. 2004). Close examination of the survey reports at an individual level also revealed that many respondents' reported experience of sex was inconsistent within and between surveys. On the same day as the 1998 survey mentioned above, for example, a subsample of young people also participated in a face-to-face questionnaire survey. The overall proportions reporting sexual experience were similar in the two surveys, but 38 percent of males and 59 percent of females who reported sex only did so in one of the two questionnaires (Plummer, Wight et al. 2004).

During the second series of in-depth interviews in 2002, 72 percent of randomly selected men (average age 19) and 82 percent of women (average age 18) reported that they had already had sex. Even in that interview series, however, there was strong evidence that some respondents falsely reported abstinence. For example, a few months before their interview, one of the eight men and two of the six women who reported never having had sex tested positive for one to two sexually transmitted infections and/or pregnancy in a trial survey.

It was also difficult to estimate the typical age at first sex in our study population. Table 6.2 shows survey and in-depth interview data on age at first sex for young people who reported that they had had sex. Within both the *MEMA kwa Vijana* trial and the HALIRA qualitative study, many young people—especially boys—reported very early ages at first vaginal intercourse, such as 8, 9, or 10 years of age. In the 1998 assisted self-completion questionnaire, for example, 35 percent of boys and 12 percent of girls who reported sex said that they were 11 years old or younger the first time they had vaginal intercourse (Plummer, Wight et al. 2004). In that survey, the median age at first sex for those who reported it was 13 for boys and 14 for

Table 6.1. In-Depth Interview Respondents' Reported Experience of Sex

Data are compared for the 1998 and 2000 MEMA kwa Vijana assisted self-completion questionnaire (ASCQ) and face-to-face questionnaire (FFQ) surveys, as well as 1999–2000 HALIRA in-depth interviews (IDI).

IDI Respondents	N	Number (Percent) Reporting Sex					
		1998 ASCQ N = 43	1998 FFQ N = 73	1999–2000 IDI N = 73	2000 ASCQ N = 56	2000 FFQ N = 62
Males	31	11/20 (55)	14/31 (45)	18/31 (58)	13/23 (57)	19/27 (70)
HIV-positive	2	1/2 (50)	1/2 (50)	2/2 (100)	2/2 (100)	2/2 (100)
No sexually transmitted infection	29	10/18 (56)	13/29 (45)	16/29 (55)	11/21 (52)	17/25 (68)
Females	42	3/23 (13)	5/42 (12)	30/42 (71)	17/33 (52)	20/35 (57)
Specific positive biological test:						
HIV	5	0/2 (0)	0/5 (0)	4/5 (83)	0/3 (0)	1/3 (33)
Gonorrhea*	1	0/1 (0)	0/1 (0)	1/1 (100)	0/0 (na)	0/0 (na)
Pregnancy	3	0/2 (0)	2/3 (67)	3/3 (100)	2/2 (100)	2/2 (100)
Sub-total positive biological test	9	0/5 (0)	2/9 (22)	8/9 (89)	2/6 (33)	3/6 (50)
No sexually transmitted infection or pregnancy	33	3/18 (17)	3/33 (9)	22/33 (67)	15/27 (56)	17/29 (59)
Total	73	14/43 (33)	19/73 (26)	48/73 (66)	30/56 (54)	39/62 (63)

N = number
na = not applicable
*One randomly selected female in-depth interview respondent tested positive for gonorrhea during the 1998 MEMA kwa Vijana trial survey.
Adapted from Plummer, Ross et al. 2004.

Table 6.2.   Age at First Sex for Youth who Reported having had Sex

Data are compared for the 1998 *MEMA kwa Vijana* assisted self-completion questionnaire (ASCQ) survey and 1999-2000 HALIRA in-depth interviews with randomly selected respondents.

	Number (Percent) Reporting Sex					
	Males		Females		Total	
Age at First Sex (Years)	ASCQ N = 1603	In-Depth Interview N = 16	ASCQ N = 508	In-Depth Interview N = 22	ASCQ N = 2111	In-Depth Interview N = 38
≤ 11	567 (35)	4 (25)	62 (12)	1 (5)	629 (30)	5 (13)
12	163 (10)	1 (6)	54 (11)	1 (5)	217 (10)	2 (5)
13	174 (11)	2 (13)	65 (13)	1 (5)	239 (11)	3 (8)
14	241 (15)	5 (31)	112 (22)	5 (23)	353 (17)	10 (26)
15	197 (12)	3 (19)	115 (23)	8 (36)	312 (15)	11 (29)
16	134 (8)	0 (0)	65 (13)	4 (18)	199 (9)	4 (11)
17	70 (4)	1 (6)	23 (5)	0 (0)	93 (4)	1 (3)
≥ 18	57 (4)	0 (0)	12 (2)	2 (9)	69 (3)	2 (5)

N = number

girls. However, individual-level reporting was again highly inconsistent: in surveys held on the same day in 1998, only 64 percent of those who reported sex also reported the same age at first sex in both surveys (Plummer, Wight et al. 2004).

When data from all of the *MEMA kwa Vijana* and HALIRA research methods are considered together—including participant observation, in-depth interviews, and surveys—they broadly suggest that over half of boys and girls in our study population had had vaginal intercourse by the age of 15 years. Those methods also suggest that, at that age, a larger majority of girls than boys were sexually active, and many—if not most—sexually active girls had sex frequently (e.g., weekly), while sexually active boys typically went for many weeks or months between sexual encounters. By their late teens, a large majority of both unmarried young men and women were sexually active and typically had sex on a weekly basis.

Relationship Types

The study identified three types of sexual relationship which school pupils and out-of-school youth commonly experienced. These were relationships which involved one-time encounters; those which involved occasional opportunistic encounters within an open-ended timeframe; and those which were steady, sometimes semipublic partnerships, which involved more frequent encounters. The first two types of relationship often involved encounters with a partner who was a visitor to the village, or alternatively, encounters which took place when a villager travelled elsewhere. For each of these three types of relationships, sexual encounters increased around special events, as described in the last chapter. By the time they reached their late teens, it was not unusual for a young man or woman to have experienced each of these three types of relationships once or multiple times.

In the second series of in-depth interviews, over half of randomly selected males (71 percent) and females (56 percent) who reported sex also said that they had had one or more one-time sexual encounters. As noted above, such relationships frequently involved sex with a stranger around a special event, but they could also be preplanned or spontaneous with someone else in the course of daily life. They generally did not continue beyond one encounter, because one of the two did not enjoy the experience, the young man was unable to provide money or a gift for a second encounter, or the couple simply did not see one another again. Notably, several in-depth interview respondents did not report onetime encounters when first asked about their lifetime number of sexual partners, and only mentioned them when asked about them directly.

The second common type of sexual relationship was open-ended and involved occasional, opportunistic sexual encounters over weeks, months or years. These relationships were usually, but not always, casual. If the couple did not actively end the relationship—as might occur if bad feelings developed between them—they might resume sexual activity if the opportunity arose again. Such a couple might not have sex for an extended period because they were geographically separated, busy with other activities, unable to arrange private encounters, or (in the case of boys) unable to raise sufficient money or gifts. However, if the right circumstances occurred, such as if they met at a festival when neither had a partner that night and the young man offered an appropriate gift, then they might readily have sex again. In such circumstances, mutual attraction and familiarity could make sexual negotiation with a previous partner much easier than with a new partner.

The third type of relationship involved sexual encounters at fairly regular intervals, typically once per week but ranging from several times per week to once per month, for a finite period ranging from a few weeks to a couple of years. This last type of relationship was unusual for early teenagers, particularly boys, but gradually became more common and involved more frequent sexual contact by the late teen years. This category included semi-public, "main" sexual relationships, but it also included some more secretive, overlapping sexual relationships, as when a young man or woman regularly met different partners on different nights of the week. For instance, a 20-year-old man who had recently completed Year 7 described having two concurrent steady sexual relationships: "With one I am just continuing having sex every two days. That one is for the night. The other one is for the day, maybe . . . maybe once per week, as she lives far away." [II-00-C-83-m]

Each of these three types of relationships were commonly reported by sexually active adolescents and young adults, although their typical extent and nature varied depending on gender and school status, as will be described below.

Preadolescents

When in-depth interview respondents were asked to describe their earliest sexual experiences, about one-quarter of boys and a smaller proportion of girls mentioned "playing" at sex in their pre-adolescent years, particularly while herding livestock. Case study 1.1 provides one example. Such experiences also were reported frequently in participant observation research. Tending goats or cattle took young boys to isolated areas for many hours of the day, but the work did not require much active attention. There they might engage in sexual play with the few girls who also tended cattle, or girls who went to remote areas to fetch firewood or water.

Prepubescent sexual activity was often described as exploratory, game-like imitation, in which children pretended to be their fathers and mothers, or other relatives who they might have seen having sex in a shared bedroom. For example, an 18-year-old boy in Year 6 and a 15-year-old boy in Year 7 said:

> Many young people, even they themselves, had learned about sex through different play/games, including imitating their fathers and mothers and hide-and-seek. During the latter, they used to hide with girls and then had sex with them before they returned to continue the game. [PO-01-I-7-3m]

Most boys who talked about this play said it involved vaginal intercourse, typically describing how the boy or the girl placed the erect penis inside of the vagina, and then they actively engaged in intercourse for 10–15 minutes before they removed the penis again, because the boys did not yet ejaculate at that age. Three other aspects of prepubescent sexual activity distinguished it from later typical sexual partnerships. First, boys did not give girls money or gifts in exchange for sexual encounters. Second, boys sometimes reported not experiencing pleasure in their first attempts at intercourse, and sometimes experiencing pain. Third, it was not unusual for the girl to be one to two years older than the boy, and to directly initiate the sexual activity. For example:

> He said those girls with whom he was herding cattle used to call him, they would embrace him and begin caressing him. After seeing that he had an erection, they undressed themselves and lay on their backs and placed him on top of them, and then he inserted his penis into their vaginas. [PO-00-C-3-3m]

Most boys who described such experiences reported that, once they began school, three to six years passed before they again had sex in their early to middle teen years.

Male Pupils

Many early adolescent school boys reported frequently approaching girls to try to negotiate sex, but rarely succeeding, as illustrated in case study 1.1. School boys had little money or gifts to offer a girl in exchange for sex, so they typically invested a lot of effort in wooing and declaring their liking or love for a girl during prolonged periods of negotiation, using peer interme-diaries, letters, and a direct approach. One 16-year-old in Year 7 explained:

> *R:* The relationship between a boy and a girl begins at school, when a boy and a girl do school work together. If the boy has a desire to have sex with her, then he will let the girl know. If she refuses he would have no alternative but to fol-low her. Yes, and in the long run, he gets her, because he will use all means to succeed. [II-99-I-42-m]

In their early teen years, school boys had the greatest chance of having a sexual relationship with girls who were the same age or younger than them, because such girls typically were inexperienced and expected relatively little in exchange for a sexual encounter. These sexual relationships usually involved one or a few brief, rushed, and opportunistic sexual encounters, for example, in bushes, an empty building, or a latrine. Half of male in-depth interview respon-dents who reported sex said that they only had sex with their first partner one time, but occasionally early adolescent relationships lasted as long as a year. A boy may have known a girl for years before becoming sexually involved with her, but they typically had little opportunity to talk together one-to-one both before and during their sexual relationship. There were only rare reports of school boys having an emotionally intimate sexual relationship.

The frequency of sexual encounters in pupil sexual relationships usually depended on the couple's freedom of movement and the boy's resources. In their early to mid-teens, it was not unusual for sexually active school boys to only have sex once or twice per year, but by their mid-teens they might have sex about once per month, and by their late teens about once per week. By their mid to late teens, most sexually active school boys reported having had several sexual relationships.

One boy, for example, reported he began his first sexual relationship when he was 14 years old and in Year 5 after meeting his partner where she sold porridge in the village center in the evening. She was about the same age and he gave her Tshs 200 [$0.24] for their first encounter. They continued to meet off-and-on for out-of-door sexual encounters until he was in Year 6, when a male friend convinced him to find a new partner:

I: What were the reasons that lead to your break-up?

R: My friend told me to drop her. He told me to look for another one. He told me, "Why only one girl, every day? Find another one."

I: But did you still like/love her?

R: I still liked/loved her.

I: Did you tell her that you were leaving her, or did you just leave her?

R: I just left her. [II-99-C-41-f]

Soon afterwards, this boy began a new sexual relationship with a girl in Year 7 from another school. He met and first had sex with her at a soccer match, after he gave her Tshs 500 [$0.60]. They continued meeting for sex about once per week for six months.

As school boys grew older, their experience, confidence, and access to cash usually also grew, as did their pool of potential partners, because the number of sexually active girls of the same age or younger increased as they aged. As a result older school boys were more successful both in directly negotiating longer term sexual relationships which involved regular sexual encounters and also in finding new partners soon after a break-up.

Sexually active school boys rarely were concerned about preventing pregnancy, although if one of their partners became pregnant they usually greatly feared being held responsible for it. In several villages, individual school boys reported that they had made a school girl pregnant, but they kept it a secret by convincing the girl to name an out-of-school sexual partner as the father.

Female Pupils

In their early teen years, school girls often had their first sexual relationships with same aged or slightly older school boys, as described in the section above. As they grew older, however, adolescent girls learned from other girls and out-of-school youths and men that more could be obtained from a relationship with someone out of school, and they began to pursue such relationships instead or as well as those with school boys.

For example, one 14-year-old girl in Year 6 first had sex with a classmate in Year 4 in exchange for a very small amount, but she subsequently decided to only take lovers who had more to offer. She explained:

R: One boy right here in Year 6 asked me for sex and I refused. I asked him for money and he refused. I asked for body oil and he refused. So I rejected him.

Another one in Year 7 has just begun seducing me. He gives me money. I buy body oil, exercise books, and pencils with it. I have never had sex with him, but I plan to do so soon. If it is a matter of having sex in the bush, we will just do it. There is yet another man at that kiosk. He wants me right now. I used to go inside his kiosk and he gave me exercise books, pencils, and sweets.

I: If he asks you to have sex with him, will you accept or refuse?

R: I will accept, because I have consumed his property. [II-99-C-51-f]

Sometimes a girl developed a particular liking for a school boy so she continued to have a sexual relationship with him even if he gave her relatively little. Rarely, however, did school girls describe having an idealized, romantic attachment to a particular sexual partner in or out of school.

In addition to offering a school girl more in exchange for a particular sexual encounter, an older and/or out-of-school partner could usually provide her with money and gifts on a regular basis, contributing to longer-term relationships with more frequent sexual encounters than school girls had with their male classmates. These out-of-school men were typically a couple of years to a decade older than their school girl partners. In addition to the longer-term sexual relationships described above, school girls, like school boys, occasionally had one-time or casual sexual encounters, particularly around special events. Primary school girls sometimes used traditional pregnancy prevention methods such as drinking an ash solution or wearing a protective charm, but they only very rarely reported use of modern contraception.

School pupil couples tended to have sex out-of-doors. Older, out-of-school youths instead often had sex with school girls in their private rooms or rooms they shared with other boys in their household. However, if a school girl's partner was married then the couple typically had sex in an isolated field, a friend's house or a guesthouse. In some villages there were also specific locations which many couples used for illicit sexual encounters, such as fishermen's huts, *ngoma* huts, caves amongst boulder outcrops, or certain unoccupied buildings. There were also numerous accounts of a girl allowing a boy or man to sneak into her sleeping room for a sexual encounter at night, whether her younger female relatives were present or not.

Sexual relationships between school girls and older partners were very secretive, especially if the man was married. School boys and out-of-school youth might discreetly approach a school girl in a public setting, such as a market or a festival, but older men were more likely to approach them in isolated settings, such as when meeting them on an errand. In many cases, school girls seemed to have some choice and agency in their relationships with older partners. However, in almost all study villages there was evidence that some men in positions of authority—such as teachers, health workers, and government officials—abused their power to force school girls into sexual relationships.

Case studies 1.4, 1.5, 2.1, and 2.3 provide more detailed descriptions of school girl sexual relationships.

Unmarried Out-Of-School Young Men

As discussed in chapters 4 and 5, once young people left primary school they quickly took on most responsibilities of adulthood, regardless of their absolute age—whether they were, for example, 15 or 21 years old. However, if they stayed in their village most unmarried out-of-school youth continued to live in their parents' households and to abide by their rules. It was assumed that a son would eventually bring a wife into the household, while a daughter would eventually move into her husband's parents' household. Young men tended to remain unmarried longer than young women after leaving school. For example, of the randomly selected pupils who participated in in-depth interviews in 1999–2000, 93 percent of the men who were reinterviewed 2–2½ years later reported that they were unmarried, compared to only 48 percent of the women.

In the first years after leaving school, many young men wanted to delay marriage until they were more financially secure. A 16-year-old farmer who had completed Year 7 explained:

> *R:* My friends and I discuss how to raise the standards of our lives. One might say, "This year, I will do my best to cultivate, so that I can buy a bicycle." Another might say, "This year, I want to do my best to do what? To get married." Now when someone says something like that you give him advice. You tell him, "Postpone marriage. First get property or money. When you have enough, that is when you should get married." We advise each other like that. [II-00-I-98-m]

Many young men also seemed to enjoy being single in their first years out of school, for they were earning more money than ever before and they wanted to explore the greater sexual freedom this facilitated. After leaving school they typically began to have sex more often and with more partners than they had before. Some said they did not want to commit to one sexual partner because they found it exciting to seduce new ones. Seduction went hand in hand with young men's main forms of entertainment and relaxation, such as hanging out in the village center in the evening, or attending videos, discos, *ngoma*, or holiday events. As discussed in chapter 5, there was often an unspoken expectation that unmarried young men were sexually active, and young men often felt entitled to pursue sexual liaisons. For example, during a village-wide meeting held to discuss security issues, young men did not hide their displeasure when someone suggested punishing young women who were caught walking with a lover after dark:

> The Village Chairman talked about girls who are taken by men for the night. He said they should go early, before the security patrol starts, otherwise they will be arrested. . . . One man got up and said that a by-law should be passed so that if a girl is arrested going to a man's place at night, she will be whipped by the *sungusungu* because of her bad behavior. I heard some of the boys sitting near me mutter, "Now you have proposed a bad idea. Should we stop taking girls for the night?" One of the boys said, "I don't care what they do, but should we stop having a good time just because of security patrols? That is not possible." [PO-01-C-2-6f]

Young men were widely reported to be attracted to female newcomers to a village "like bees to honey" [PO-01-I-4-5f]. A 22-year-old shoe shiner recounted how he had had sexual relationships with a primary school pupil and others locally, but he considered village girls to be "backwards" and unattractive. He instead sought to seduce visitors to the village:

> He said that his latest [sexual partner] was a visitor, and he was happy because he had got her before any other local man. He said that his relationships with girls end when they leave the village. He told me he has specialized in sexual relationships with visitors because they have not been polluted by men in the village. He said he knows no girl in the village who has less than two boyfriends, and hence he fears them. [PO-99-C-5-2f]

When young villagers themselves travelled to other villages to visit relatives or attend a wedding or funeral, they were sometimes sought after in similar ways and had sex with new partners on such trips.

Many out-of-school young men had sexual partners who were also out-of-school, but some pursued relationships with school girls despite the norms against this because they found school girl youthfulness or relative inexperience attractive, and/or they did not have enough money to support a relationship with an out-of-school woman. Out-of-school men went to great lengths to hide such relationships, including sometimes denying a pregnancy, as reported earlier for school boys. For example, in one participant observation village a 22-year-old man (Nicolaus) tried to ensure that his school girl sexual partner (Anjelina) attributed her pregnancy to another partner (Peter), a 21-year-old man. Adults in all three families were aware of the likely cover up. The researcher's field notes:

> Nicolaus said that last night he went to Anjelina's home to plead with her not to identify him as the baby's father, but he found she had already identified Peter

instead. Peter has now run away from home to avoid being arrested for that offence. Nicolaus's mother said that when she heard that Anjelina was pregnant, she was extremely frightened, because she had seen Nicolaus standing privately with Anjelina so she knew they were lovers. Nicolaus's mother said that it is common to have a pregnancy attributed to you that is not yours, especially for school girl pregnancies. . . . [Two weeks later] Peter's father went to the school today to pay the pregnancy fine for Peter. He said many times he warned his sons not to have sex with pupils, but Peter didn't take heed so now he has to carry his own burden. He said that Peter was not as sharp as other village men, as some make pupils pregnant but convince them to name other men as the fathers. He said that doing this is just an ordinary thing in the village, but for it to work the man held responsible must also have had sex with that girl. . . . [Later] Nicolaus told me he convinced Anjelina not to name him by being close to her after she became pregnant and promising to give her Tshs 10,000 [$12] later, if she does not reveal he is the father. Now that everything is over he said he might not give her any money at all. He said that Anjelina's aunt even helped him convince Anjelina not to name him as the father. [PO-01-C-3-3m]

Some young women in such circumstances were strategic in identifying the man they most wanted to marry as their baby's father, whether he was the likely biological father or not, so Anjelina may have preferred that Nicolaus did not assume responsibility for her pregnancy. This practice was common enough that it will be discussed more in chapter 9.

Although most single young men did not want to have children soon after they finished school, they usually were not concerned about pregnancy prevention, and condom use was rare. It was not unusual for unmarried young men to have a series of partners in close succession or to maintain open-ended, concurrent relationships. The duration of their sexual relationships were highly variable, as were the frequency of encounters within them. When asked how long a couple's sexual relationship normally lasted, a 20-year-old man explained:

R: Well, it depends on their understanding. It can be one week. Let us say one week goes by, and then you separate. You see, someone else might take over as a new lover, just like that. Sometimes a relationship can be as long as a month or a year. You may perhaps make her pregnant, and then she becomes yours. [II-99-I-24-m]

Sometimes a young man had an out-of-school partner with whom he had a discreet but semipublic relationship, so that the two were recognised as a couple within a broader group of peers (figure 6.1). As most young men got older they became more interested in having such a relationship with a young woman they might want to marry later, that is, one who was hardworking, respectful, and monogamous. A partner's faithfulness was highly valued by

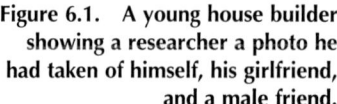
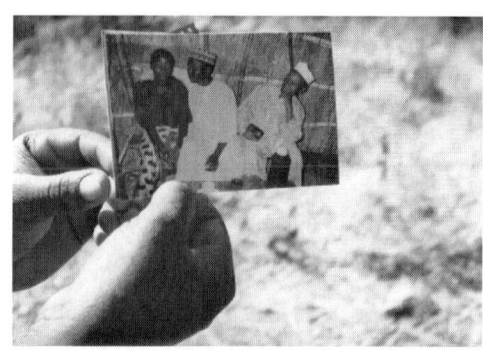

Figure 6.1.   A young house builder
showing a researcher a photo he
had taken of himself, his girlfriend,
and a male friend.

young men, and many reported ending a main sexual relationship after discovering that their partner had other partners. When asked to describe their
feelings for steady partners, young men often used the words *kupenda* or
kutogwa. Rarely, however, did they seem to idealize their partner as someone
uniquely suited to them.

Case studies 1.2 and 1.3 also provide examples of unmarried young men's
sexual relationships.

Unmarried Out-Of-School Young Women

The vast majority of young women were sexually active by the time they left
school, and it was common for those who were not married to have a steady
sexual partner who they met for sex once or twice per week. If such a relationship ended, there was usually only a short gap (such as one week) before
a new one began. In addition, like unmarried young men, unmarried young
women engaged in one-time encounters or casual relationships involving occasional encounters.

Unmarried young women considered wealthy men to be particularly desirable partners, such as those with a good income from the government or
fishing, or those who owned a kiosk or mill. Male newcomers to a village—
especially those from urban areas—were often perceived to have more money
and style than local males, so they were considered very desirable. In a group
discussion one young male villager explained, "If a young man comes to this
village from Mwanza City and wants ten women, he could even get twenty"
[GD-00-C-10-1m].

Unmarried young women typically worked long days in their farms and
homes, and sexual relationships could provide a welcome contrast to that, as
they might enjoy the attention and flattery of sexual negotiation, the excite-
ment of rule-breaking, and the experience of new gifts or activities paid for
by a sexual partner. A small minority of unmarried young women also men-

tioned physical pleasure as a motivation for some sexual relationships. For example, a group discussion participant:

> *P:* You can go to one partner, and when you arrive he touches you nicely. You see, he just caresses you, you both satisfy each other's sexual drive. You can leave there feeling good. And there is another one, you say, "Let me go and take money from this one, then I will buy a dress tomorrow. When I wear it for my other man, I will have a good time." This one gives you money and the other one is just for having a good time. [GD-00-C-10-1f]

Many unmarried young women also reported being attracted to a particular sexual partner because of his good behavior, such as being polite, respectful, hardworking, and monogamous. Young women often reported having greater affection for one partner than for other prior or current partners, and hoping that a favorite partner eventually would marry them. However, they were usually also pragmatic and prepared to marry a different partner if their favorite relationship did not work out. For example, a 21-year-old woman who was pregnant with her second child and still living with her parents:

> She said her child's father is a farmer and provides for the child's needs. She said that he still comes to her home at night to have sex with her, and early in the morning he leaves before people wake up. She said that if he asks her to marry him she will accept, and if he doesn't then she will get married to someone else. She said that she has never taken her child to her partner's home, because her father does not allow her to do so. [PO-00-C-3-2f]

It was not unusual for single mothers and other young women who were perceived to be **wasimbe** to have relationships that were commonly known but not publicly acknowledged. Couples in such relationships could be somewhat open and develop a kind of routine, for example, spending time together when mingling in a group of mixed sex peers at *ngoma* celebrations or the village center in the evening. However, such activity could negatively affect a woman's reputation. As one 20-year-old woman explained, "Some girls, especially **wasimbe**, disrespect their parents and even openly go to their boyfriends' home before their parents have gone to sleep" [PO-00-C-3-2f].

Young women in steady relationships, like young men, usually expected their regular partners to be monogamous, and might end the relationship if they learned that this was not the case. There were reports, however, of individual young women continuing a relationship with a steady partner despite his infidelity, because the partner provided for the woman well and she still hoped to marry him. Occasionally single mothers also reported wanting to conceive again even if they were not married, especially if they thought this would prompt a partner to marry.

Other examples of out-of-school young women's premarital sexual relationships are described in case studies 1.4, 1.5, and 2.3.

The Emotional Nature of Relationships

Adolescence and young adulthood were times of great discovery, exploration, and transition for young people in rural Mwanza, as elsewhere in the world. Often sexual relationships began in an opportunistic and exploratory way with neither partner having a clear expectation that it would end or continue beyond their first sexual encounter. The mutual attraction that led a couple to have an initial sexual encounter could evolve into a longer term sexual relationship. Whether such a relationship involved occasional or frequent sexual encounters depended on how strongly the couple liked one another and their specific circumstances, such as how convenient it was for them to meet, whether either partner already had a steady partner, and whether the young man could offer money or gifts on a frequent basis.

References to *kupenda* and **kutogwa** came up repeatedly in our study. Possibly the most common statement made by boys and young men trying to persuade a girl or woman to have sex was, "*Nakupenda*" or "**Nakutogagwa**"—"I like/love you"—whether they had just met or had known one another for years. Similarly, when young people were asked to describe their emotions or attraction for a partner, they often simply said, "I liked/loved him/her." Sometimes it seemed clear in the context of a statement whether someone meant "like" or "love," but sometimes this was quite ambiguous.

The emotional nature and intensity of unmarried young people's sexual relationships varied. In almost all relationships, however, young people liked a partner when they first became sexually involved, even if they had very little knowledge of one another. It was rare for a young woman to report voluntarily having sex with a man who she disliked, and in fact, a lack of such selectivity was considered one of the most important characteristics distinguishing prostitutes from other women having sex in exchange for money or gifts. Sometimes unmarried girls or women seemed to be neutral or indifferent towards particular partners—maintaining a sexual relationship for the sole purpose of material support—but they did not actively dislike the man. The extent to which a woman liked a man was often the deciding factor in her choice between suitors who offered the same amount of money, or in her choice to have sex with a particular suitor even if he had little to offer her in exchange. Sometimes, a young woman's liking seemed to have a passionate quality to it, although the degree to which this was emotional, sexual, or both was usually unclear. In one village, for example, young women were observed testing their response to their sexual partners through the flutter of their heart beats when they looked at them.

The very limited nature of one-to-one contact beyond sexual encounters meant that unmarried couples usually had limited knowledge of one another and little opportunity to become emotionally close. This was particularly true for school pupils whose occasional rushed sexual encounters were likely to take place outdoors during the day. Encounters which took place at night around public events and entertainment sometimes provided couples more time both to talk and to have sex. The greatest potential for an unmarried couple to develop physical and emotional intimacy seemed to occur if they met at night on multiple occasions over weeks or months, particularly young adults who spent many hours together after dark. However, unmarried young people rarely expressed a wish to share activities with, or to get to know, someone of the opposite sex other than to arrange and to have sex. Sexual intercourse also rarely seemed to have symbolic significance as an expression of a couple's emotional intimacy.

There were exceptions to this general pattern. For example, one young man disclosed that he had had a long relationship with a young woman, involving only talking, playing, and caressing, until his male friends goaded him into having intercourse with her. Evidence of emotional attachment seemed greatest in some steady, semipublic relationships involving young people in their late teens or early twenties. Occasionally, couples demonstrated their commitment and caring by being extraordinarily generous in the material exchange for sex that took place within their relationship, the young woman either asking relatively little or the young man offering relatively more than typically expected. One 16-year-old boy in Year 6 described such a pattern in his two-year sexual relationship with an out-of-school girl:

> He has had intercourse with her more than ten times. He said that he enjoyed all those times, and he thinks his partner also enjoys it, because she has never rejected him, nor has she asked for money, and he has never given her anything for sex. He feels that they like/love each other very much. [PO-00-C-9-3m]

Premarital sexual relationships varied in their expectation of monogamy. However, there was considerable evidence of possessiveness and jealousy in some premarital relationships, particularly in steady, semipublic ones. For example, in most study villages, there were first and third-person accounts of young men who demanded gifts back after learning of a lover's infidelity, even ripping a partner's clothing off of her in public. In another example, an 18-year-old mother described how her boyfriend, the father of her child, attempted to test her fidelity by sending two male friends to try to have sex with her. She rejected the two suitors, but when she learned what her boyfriend had done she was angry with him and they broke up.

Our study found that young men and women in steady relationships usually felt strongly about being their partner's sole sexual partner. However, it was much less common for a young person to perceive a certain partner as his or her "one and only," even in steady relationships. As already noted, many young people were emotionally attached to a particular partner and hoped to eventually marry him or her, but they did not seem to romantically idealize that partner as the *only* person with whom they could perceive having a sexual relationship and a shared future. Even in such relatively committed sexual relationships, young people might still have other, less serious relationships which fulfilled a particular desire for sex or money, or which served as a kind of marital "backup" in case the main relationship did not work out.

Having emotional intimacy and an in-depth knowledge of a partner was also not usually seen as critical to marry. For example, in the second series of in-depth interviews most of the married randomly selected respondents reported that they had met their spouse for the first time one to two months before marrying, regardless of whether they married by engagement, elopement, or simply moving in together. Typically the critical issue in deciding to marry was not emotional intimacy but whether both partners were at a stage in their lives when they wanted to marry, which usually was soon after leaving school for young women and about five years later for young men.

While accounts of idealized, romantic love were rare, in most villages there were reports that traditional medicine could be used to make a particular person irresistibly and exclusively attracted and devoted to someone else. Descriptions of such "love medicines" were widespread and diverse but few people were believed to actually employ them. The most widely reported medicine was said to treat a condition called *damu nzito* (heavy/thick blood), which was believed to make people—mostly women—unattractive. The treatment was believed to improve a person's general attractiveness so that he or she might find a sexual partner or spouse. A different medicine was believed to make an individual passionately desirable to a particular person only. This medicine was most often blamed if a woman's husband became extraordinarily devoted to a mistress or co-wife, in which case the other woman might be accused of having used a medicine to bewitch him. Alternatively, men were sometimes reported to use such medicine to seduce a hard-to-get woman. A 59-year-old man and his 32-year-old wife gave the following explanation:

> They said that after a man has used those medicines to get a woman to have sex, he can alter the medicine if he then wants to break-up with her. The male informant said that he once used such a medicine to help a friend get a girl whose par-

ents had refused his proposal of marriage. He said that the medicine worked and that girl decided to run away from home and marry his friend. [PO-01-I-7-3m]

In these accounts the bewitched person was perceived to lose control over his or her feelings and actions and to become exceptionally devoted to a particular sexual partner at the expense of other social obligations and relationships. However, those individuals were not held responsible because traditional medicine, and perhaps a witch, were believed to be at fault.

Total Number of Partners

In both *MEMA kwa Vijana* surveys and the HALIRA qualitative study obtaining accurate estimates for an individual's lifetime number of sexual partners was sometimes quite challenging. For example, of the pupils who participated in both face-to-face and assisted self-completion questionnaire surveys on the same day in 1998, only 47 percent of those who reported sexual experience reported the same lifetime number of partners in both surveys (Plummer, Wight et al. 2004).

During the first in-depth interview series with randomly selected pupils, boys who reported sex (average age 17) said they had three partners on average, compared to two on average for girls who reported sex (average age 16). Participant observation data suggest that these estimates may have been valid, although it also seems possible that girls underestimated their total number of partners for fear of stigma. In addition, for both males and females reports may have sometimes been underestimated because of the constraints of the interview format. In the first in-depth interview series it was not unusual for a respondent to first deny ever having had sex and then only to describe their first sexual relationship slowly, after repeated assurances and follow-up questions by the interviewer. Typically respondents were only briefly asked about other sexual relationships towards the end of the interview, and their responses were fairly superficial.

In the first in-depth interview series, the estimation of lifetime number of sexual partners was further complicated by a possibility that some boys may have overreported their total number of partners. In their second interviews a few male respondents reported fewer total partners than they had in the earlier interviews. Some boys may have exaggerated their total number of partners in the first interview, in order to appear more masculine. Others seemed to have changed their personal definition of "sex" or "sexual relationships" as they grew older. For example, during his first interview one respondent listed prepubescent sexual partners when asked to count all of the partners he had ever had, but he did not initially list them in response to the same question in his second interview. When reminded of those earlier reports he acknowledged them but explained that he no longer considered those girls to have been sexual partners, even though their sexual play had included vaginal intercourse.

In the second series of in-depth interviews, the average number of sexual partners reported by randomly selected sexually active respondents was the same as reported earlier, that is, three for males (average age 19), and two for females (average age 18). Participant observation research again suggests this may have been a valid average of lifetime partners for young men. With greater sexual experience and confidence and less stigma associated with their sexual activity, some young men may have felt more able to report their sexual activity honestly and accurately in the second interviews without trying to either hide or embellish it. However, these interviews were also constrained by time limitations, which may have contributed to underreporting of sexual partners. Most respondents had more complex sexual relationship histories as they had grown older, and this seemed to make it more difficult for some to accurately recall all partners.

Participant observation and the in-depth interviews themselves strongly suggest that some female respondents underreported their number of partners in the second in-depth interview series, although not necessarily for the same reasons as they might have during the first series. Having left school and grown older, some young single women in the second series seemed more comfortable acknowledging their sexual activity. However, out-of-wedlock sexual activity was still stigmatized for women, particularly for the half of female respondents who had already married by their second interview. In those interviews, most young wives initially claimed that their husbands were the only sexual partners they had ever had. Many of these women had reported different partners in their first interview. When reminded of this, most of these respondents acknowledged the validity of their earlier reports but denied that they had had any other partner than their husband since then. A few young wives adamantly denied their earlier reports throughout the entire second interview, particularly those who had a different interviewer than they had had the first time.

For example, in her first interview a 16-year-old school girl described her first sexual experience at the age of 15, including the man's enthusiastic pursuit of her, his sister's involvement in the negotiations, and their subsequent sexual encounter at his sister's house, when he gave her Tshs 2,000 [$2.40]. However, in her second interview this young woman reported that the first time she had sex was with her husband, who was clearly not the same man she had described earlier. She denied her earlier report but then said that she had only told the first interviewer about one other sexual encounter, when she was held down by two men and had been forced to have sex in a cemetery. Her detailed description of this incident made it also seem plausible, but in fact she had not reported it in the first interview.

In another example of inconsistent reporting by married women, during her first interview a 21-year-old woman provided detailed and plausible descriptions of sexual relationships with four shopkeepers and two pupils, but she consistently denied all of those relationships in her second interview. In that interview, she initially said that her husband was the only sexual partner she had ever had, and she had only met and married him three months earlier. By the end of the interview, however, she also acknowledged having had a one-time sexual encounter with a different man during the same month when she met her husband. However, she still denied her earlier reports. Such evidence of bias raises questions about the validity of married women's responses to questions about either premarital or extramarital relationships.

When the different *MEMA kwa Vijana* and HALIRA data sources are considered together, they broadly suggest that most adolescents had had several sexual partners by their mid to late teens. These estimates do not include prepubescent sexual experience, whether such activity involved vaginal intercourse or not. As already noted, adolescent girls typically had more frequent sexual activity than boys of the same age, and they may have also had more partners on average. In addition, by their early twenties most unmarried young men and women had had several more partners.

Concurrency

In our study, villagers often criticized people—particularly women—who were believed to have multiple sexual partners out-of-wedlock. Some unmarried, sexually active youth generally tried to be monogamous due to personal belief, religious teachings, concern about their sexual health, or simply because they were satisfied with the sexual activity or material exchange they received within their main relationship. Others were monogamous due to external factors, such as young men who were not able to financially support multiple relationships, young women who wanted to protect their reputations, or any young person who feared losing a sexual partner because of infidelity. Nonetheless, our study found that experience of secretive, overlapping sexual relationships was not uncommon amongst young people, especially by their late teen years.

Certain types of concurrency were socially acceptable and even admired in rural Mwanza, particularly formally within polygynous marriage or informally amongst men in general. For example, a young man in a group discussion:

P: We youths usually tempt one another. You'll find that perhaps you have a principle to have one partner only. Now, when you first started seducing girls, if you say that you only have one, your peers definitely won't understand you. Your friend will say, "I have had so many, I can't even count them." Now, you get tempted, thinking "Even I should add a second one, and then later maybe get another one." [GD-02-I-1-36m]

Young adolescent males in our study did not often have overlapping partners, since they usually only had sufficient income to support occasional sexual encounters. When they did have concurrent relationships it typically involved a onetime encounter at a special event overlapping with an open-ended relationship. For example, one 16-year-old described having had four sexual relationships with same-aged school girls: the first was a onetime encounter when he was 13 years old, followed by a two-month relationship and then a one-year relationship, as well as a one-off encounter that took place with a fourth girl while the third relationship was still ongoing.

Sometimes young people did not recognize such relationships were concurrent. For example, some adolescents initially reported never having had overlapping relationships but then acknowledged having had one or more one-time sexual partners while still in the midst of a longer-term, open-ended relationship. There were many other instances, however, when youth knowingly had concurrent relationships, as when young adults with one "main" relationship occasionally or regularly had more secretive sexual relationships. A young man explained this in a group discussion:

> *P:* You can even have alternating girlfriends. You can plan: "Today I should go to her, tomorrow to another, and the day after tomorrow to another. You might have several but the liking/love differs. There is one you will like/love most, so you give more to her. [GD-02-I-1-36m]

Often concurrent relationships were less planned than suggested by the young man above. In most villages, for example, incidents were reported in which two young men arrived at a house on the same night expecting to have sex with the same young woman; such incidents usually ended in some kind of confrontation and/or break-up. The open-ended nature of many young people's sexual relationships also helped foster spontaneous concurrency. For example, after three participant observation visits to an inland village, a male researcher noted:

> It was very rare to find young people who had a steady relationship with only one partner. I found that young men who are sexually active have several girls who they have sex with. For example, at an *ngoma* gathering or market day they would look for a girl who had had sex with them before. If they saw such a girl they would approach her for sex. If the girl refused they would look for another girl with whom they had a similar relationship, or they would look for any girl who was around and willing to have sex with them on that particular day. [PO-02-I-4-1m]

Some unmarried young women also maintained more than one sexual relationship at a time. For example, during one participant observation visit a researcher shared a room with a 21-year-old woman (Esther) who, unusually for a woman, was still in Year 7. During the research, Esther had a regular, semipublic relationship with Nyanda, the 28-year-old leader of her *rika*, who she one day hoped to marry. She described what drew her to him:

> Esther said she likes/loves Nyanda more than her other partners because he is kind, he buys her exercise books, pens/pencils, and sweets, and he gives her a lot of money. She said that he recently gave her Tshs 800 [$0.96], with which she bought three second-hand blouses. Also, he doesn't drink beer, he busies himself, and he is hardworking. She said she also likes/loves Nyanda because he is handsome: as brown as she is, and somewhat fat [healthy/attractive]. She said she becomes very happy whenever she sees him. [PO-00-I-4-4f]

Esther's father had discovered Esther and Nyanda having sex two years earlier, and the matter was resolved when Nyanda's parents agreed to pay a fine, because Esther was a school girl and Nyanda was believed to have taken her virginity. However, Esther confided to the researcher that she had had three other sexual partners before Nyanda. Esther and her parents expected her to marry Nyanda once she left school, so her mother did not confront Esther when she sometimes returned home late the morning after a nighttime sexual encounter with Nyanda.

Despite Esther's hopes of eventually marrying Nyanda, she sometimes still had sex with her very first sexual partner, and possibly others. The researcher recorded the following interactions after one *ngoma* event:

> [Esther's second sexual partner] bought her sugar cane for Tshs 10 [$0.01] and, when he gave it to her, told her something in a seductive voice, and then Esther broke out with sharp laughter. [Later, her first sexual partner] called her, but Esther did not respond. He told her, "Esther, you pretend not to hear me because you have a visitor [the researcher]. If you don't want my money, then give it back to me." Esther then slowed her pace and talked with him, and he looked pleased after talking with her. When Esther went home to sleep tonight, she told me that she would wait until the children were asleep, and then she would carefully get up and go to [her first partner's] house in order to satisfy him with sex. [PO-00-I-4-4f]

Male and female informants involved in concurrent relationships rarely seemed to view the overlapping nature of their relationships as inherently wrong or immoral. However, they usually strove to hide them to avoid possible jealousies, breakups, and (especially for girls and women) stigma they might experience if they became public knowledge. As discussed in chapter

5, the discretion that young people practiced to hide sexual relationships from parents and older villagers often also effectively hid them from other young people, which was important in maintaining concurrency. For example, a young man in his early 20s

> said that girls have many boyfriends and that is why they would not like being seen with any one of them in public, because the other ones may start fighting him. There are no interactions between boyfriend and girlfriend in public, because even the boys can have more then three girlfriends. [PO-99-C-5-2f]

In each village, mill workers, shopkeepers, bicycle taxi drivers, and other young men who provided needed goods or services, earned an above average income, and had high contact with girls and women tended to report more sexual activity—and more partners—than other young men. These accounts were supported by the disproportionate number of girls and women who reported having such men—particularly shopkeepers—as sexual partners. It was more difficult to identify groups of unmarried young women who were particularly likely to engage in concurrent sexual partnerships. Generally, however, material exchange was an important motivation for young women who reported concurrency, whether as a means to access entertainment and gifts or to meet subsistence needs.

Unmarried young villagers who travelled for school or work were more likely than other villagers to maintain concurrent partnerships in different locations, as will be discussed in the next section. In addition, it was not unusual for young people whose main partner travelled to have a different partner in the village during their absence. Young women usually did this to supplement their income, but attraction and other factors could also play a role. Men who travelled might commonly have one-time encounters with strangers, but our findings suggest that women who remained behind in the village were more likely to have open-ended relationships with someone known to them, possibly resulting in long-term concurrent relationships when the traveling partner returned and/or travelled again.

In one inland village, for example, a 27-year-old man described how he had a long-term sexual relationship with a young woman whose official fiancé only visited once per week:

> He told me that they started their sexual relationship [three years earlier] and that the girl likes/loves him very much. That same year he made her pregnant, but after the pregnancy reached five months she had a miscarriage. He told me that last year she ran away from home and went to live with a young man from another village. Later she returned home and the young man came to introduce himself to her parents, to say that he wants to marry her. He said that the young

man is now her official fiancé and openly stays overnight with her when he visits the village on weekends. Nonetheless my informant still goes to her home to have sex with her on other nights of the week. She sleeps with small children in her room, and usually they are already asleep when he sneaks in. Some days she instead comes to sleep with him at his home. The girl is now pregnant again. She told my informant that the pregnancy belongs to him but not to worry, because she will make sure that her fiancé believes the pregnancy belongs to him. [PO-99-C-2-1m]

Concurrency seemed to be most widely and openly practiced in fishing villages where a sizeable proportion of the male population travelled regularly for work and had partners in different locations. Numerous young women in fishing villages also reported having concurrent partnerships. These women generally made an effort to be discreet about their more casual relationships, but their main, fishermen partners were sometimes aware of them and tolerated them. In contrast to these first-person accounts, however, in fishing villages there were also third-person reports that, if a woman was found to be unfaithful to a fisherman, he and his friends might gang rape her to punish her.

Case studies, 1.2, 1.3 and 2.3 provide additional examples of concurrent sexual relationships prior to marriage.

Sexual Mixing Patterns

In rural Mwanza, we found several distinct networks or populations that were "bridged" by individuals who had sexual partners in different groups. Important examples already described above are older men and younger women who bridged predominantly same-aged sexual networks about five to ten years apart.

Most young people had sexual partners who resided in the same village but another important bridging group already mentioned is individuals—usually young men—who travelled for work or school and had sexual partners both in and outside of a village. Such mobility took different forms. In all villages, there were people who routinely travelled to larger villages and towns for a few days or a week of work, often to sell agricultural products or to purchase manufactured items. Some villagers also moved between a study village and nearby villages or towns on a daily basis, such as those who provided a bicycle taxi service, peddling while the passenger sat on the bicycle seat behind them. In most villages, there were also young people—mainly men—who moved to towns or Mwanza City for one or more years of employment, men usually working as casual laborers and women in domestic service or food services. As previously noted, in some villages a large proportion of men travelled for extended periods to work in fishing or mining. Finally, there were a small number of men with homes in urban areas who traveled to villages on a onetime, occasional, or frequent basis, such as bus drivers, video show hosts, *ngoma* dancers, or carpenters who built school furniture.

Our study suggests that all of these forms of travel contributed to partner change and concurrency. Young men who travelled for work usually earned sufficient money and had ample opportunity to have sex frequently, because many young women who worked in guesthouses, food kiosks, and bars supplemented their income through sex with customers. In addition, some men had sex with prostitutes while traveling, particularly in male-dominated locations such as mines or fishing camps. There were also reports of men having sex with other men or boys in isolated fishing camps, which will be discussed more in chapter 8. Men who travelled to the same place on a regular basis (such as bicycle taxi drivers), or for extended periods of time (such as miners), often had a steady partner both in their village and in the other location, as illustrated by case study 1.3.

When young men and women returned to their home villages after an extended period away, they were often seen as newly desirable because their experiences beyond the village were considered exciting and interesting, and the men often had more cash than locals while the women had more modern or urban hairstyles and clothing. For example, when a domestic worker (Ligwa) in her 20s visited her village after an extended stay in Mwanza City, the researcher accompanied her as she walked around the village reestablishing contact with prior sexual partners:

> At one place she left instructions that they should tell a certain man that Ligwa wants to be bought some sandals. That woman told her, "As soon as he returns, he will definitely follow you." They all laughed together. At the next place a woman began asking Ligwa why she hasn't come there for a while, saying maybe Ligwa has procured another lover who has taken over from the woman's brother-in-law. Ligwa told the woman that when her brother-in-law returns she should tell him Ligwa wants him to buy her a pair of sandals. The woman said that was not a problem, except that she shouldn't "skin" her brother-in-law and take all his money. When a friend of Ligwa came by, she passed on greetings from a third man. After hearing this Ligwa said, "So he still likes/loves me. One day we quarrelled so much that I thought our relationship had completely ended." While on our way home, Ligwa said that the young men are her lovers. She said that she doesn't like/love the second one very much, but that that woman is their intermediary and really helps her to get a lot of money from him. [PO-01-I-7-5f]

Finally, visitors to villages were known to have sex with local women during their stay. This could take place within steady, occasional, or one-time relationships. For example, a male video attendee said "The young men who brought video shows usually have sex with village girls after they allow the girls to watch the video free of charge. Girls see those men as having money and thus being potential long-term providers." [PO-99-I-1-2f]

Case studies 1.3 and 2.3 provide more detailed descriptions of people who travelled outside of their village and sexually linked town and village populations.

DISCUSSION

Relationship Types

It was not possible to assess the exact prevalence of different kinds of sexual relationships in this study, but the unusually large scale of the research helped to broadly identify several common types of sexual relationship. Our finding that prepubescent Sukuma children sometimes "played" at sex as part of larger games mimicking adult life are in keeping with the historical literature, as anthropologists documented similar practices during the twentieth century (Tanner 1955b; Varkevisser 1973). Prepubescent sexual play might not typically be considered part of a sexual relationship history. However, we consider it such here because in rural Mwanza it usually involved vaginal intercourse, or at least an attempt at it, and even if the boy did not ejaculate it might still have implications for sexual health. Such play often involved older girls than boys, and older girls might have been exposed to sexually transmitted infections from other, older partners. In addition, even before the advent of antiretroviral therapy in sub-Saharan Africa a small minority of HIV-infected infants survived into late childhood and adolescence, and a larger proportion receiving therapy do so today (Birungi et al. 2009; Ferrand et al. 2009). Such children might engage in typical prepubescent sexual activity, as will be seen later in this book in the example of case study 3.1, an adolescent boy who probably was HIV-positive since infancy.

By the time school boys and girls in our study population reached their mid to late teens it was not unusual for them to have had several sexual partners, but the nature of their relationships typically differed. First, school girls were sometimes substantially younger (e.g., five to ten years) than their partners, and second, their relationships tended to involve more frequent and numerous sexual encounters. It also is possible that, by their mid-teen years, school girls had more lifetime sexual partners on average than school boys of the same age. Probably all of these factors contributed to young women having higher rates of sexually transmitted infections than young men. For example, in the *MEMA kwa Vijana* 2001–2002 survey, 14 percent of males (average age 19) and 28 percent of females (average age 18) tested positive for one or more of the five sexually transmitted infections that were tested in both men and women (HIV, herpes, gonorrhea, Chlamydia, and/or syphilis) (Helen Weiss, personal communication).

Most sexually active adolescents reported having had one and often more onetime partners; such sexual encounters were common for pupils and out-of-school youth of both sexes. Often these encounters involved sex between strangers who did not meet again. Respondents frequently did not consider such partners when asked about their total number of partners or their experience of concurrent relationships, which highlights the importance of specifically asking about onetime encounters in establishing sexual histories.

A study in Uganda found that the risk of contracting HIV in one sexual encounter ranged from one in one hundred to one in one thousand, depending on how long the HIV-positive partner had been infected (Wawer et al. 2005). Unprotected, onetime sexual encounters thus do not necessarily place an individual at high risk of HIV infection. However, some sexually transmitted infections are much more infectious (Fishbein and Pequegnat 2000; Pinkerton 2003). In addition, when onetime encounters are fairly common, as seemed to be the case in this young population, the possibility of individuals eventually being exposed to a partner with HIV or another sexually transmitted infection increases.

Many young people in our study also had open-ended relationships which involved occasional, secretive sexual encounters. Typically such couples knew very little about one another and did not make a specific commitment to continue the relationship. However, after each encounter they parted amicably and in the absence of a clear ending to the relationship—as sometimes, but not always, happened when one of the two got married—it was fairly easy to have further sexual encounters weeks or months later if the opportunity arose. Some other research in southern Africa has documented young people's casual, short-term sexual relationships (e.g., Jana, Nkambule, and Tumbo 2008). However, we have seen little documentation of the kind of casual, open-ended, and sometimes long-term sexual relationships we found in this study (e.g., Harrison and O'Sullivan 2010).

In rural Mwanza young people's openness to spontaneous and opportunistic sexual encounters such as those described above possibly resulted from an experimental and exploratory stage of life as they transitioned from childhood to adulthood (Dehne and Riedner 2001; Gorbach et al. 2002). However, these relationship patterns may also reflect a broader cultural openness to chance amongst the Sukuma and other local ethnic groups, similar to what Johnson-Hanks (2005, 363) described in Cameroon as "based not on the fulfillment of prior intentions but on a judicious opportunism: the actor seizes promising chances."

The third common type of sexual partnership identified in our study usually began by the middle to late teen years, when most young people experienced one or more "main" premarital sexual relationships that were recognized by peers and involved frequent sexual contact. Like other premarital sexual relationships, these ones almost never involved condom use and often were not mutually monogamous, so even if they were long-term they were not necessarily protective of sexual health, as has also been found elsewhere in sub-Saharan Africa (Meekers and Calvès 1997; Halperin and Epstein 2004; Moyo et al. 2008).

Emotional Intimacy

The emotional nature of young people's sexual relationships was a topic of interest from the onset of this study. Participant observation researchers were asked to document reports and observations about emotions within young people's sexual partnerships, the kind of words youth used to describe their emotions, what they meant when they used the ambiguous terms *kupenda* and *kutogwa*, and whether their meanings ever seemed similar to Western notions of romantic love.

Despite these efforts, we found it difficult to collect unambiguous data about young people's emotions within their relationships. Respondents had little experience describing their feelings in a narrative way, and their vocabulary, comfort, and ease in doing this was very limited. Some young men also may have downplayed their emotional attachment to a partner to appear more masculine, and either partner may have downplayed it after a breakup. Many young people's formal interview reports about their emotions were thus brief and difficult to interpret.

During participant observation, researchers were present on many occasions when young people informally discussed their sexual relationships with same-sexed peers, but these conversations usually did not address the emotions of the individuals involved. Emotions also did not lend themselves easily to observation as sexual partners had quite limited contact with one another in public, and when they did, they usually made an effort to be discreet. Even when there was evidence of emotions it was not always clear how to interpret them. For example, a range of emotions might be involved in a couple's jealous confrontation, such as hurt pride, anger over material loss, or betrayed love. The challenge of collecting and interpreting data on emotions is not unusual. As Thomas and Cole (2009, 2) noted in their book on love in

Africa, "Methodologically, how does one know if the word that informants use to signal passion or affect really maps on to the same conceptual and emotional field as 'love'?"

As noted earlier, the existence and importance of romantic love in sub-Saharan Africa has been the subject of some debate historically, and this discussion has had renewed interest in recent years. Some have suggested that romantic love—and the freely chosen, idealized form of monogamy that it suggests—are imperialist and/or Christian introductions in low income countries (Povinelli 2006; British Broadcasting Corporation 2010b; Fihlani 2010). This argument raises questions about the cultural appropriateness of HIV/AIDS interventions which promote long-term, mutual monogamy (Vaughan 2009).

In contrast, in a global review of ethnographic literature, folklore, and music from 166 societies, Jankowiak and Fischer (1992) found that 20 of 26 studied African societies had recorded evidence of romantic love, such as historical accounts depicting personal anguish and longing; love songs or folklore that highlighted the motivations behind romantic involvement; elopement due to mutual affection; native accounts affirming the existence of passionate love; or an ethnographer's documentation of romantic love. Some may question whether those criteria provide sufficient evidence of romantic love, for example, whether eloping due to mutual affection necessarily represents a passionate, idealized belief about a particular partner. Nonetheless, those authors and others have made strong arguments that romantic love may have existed in societies for which there is no prior documentation of it, although its prevalence was likely to have been variable depending on shifting factors such as kinship practices, gender ideologies, and political economies (Jankowiak and Fischer 1992; Rosenwein 2002; Smith 2009; Thomas and Cole 2009; Vaughan 2009).

In our study, triangulation of data from all sources found desire, possessiveness, and affection were not unusual in premarital relationships, but there was little evidence of romantic love. A young man might flatter and declare his passion, liking or love for a girl when first negotiating sex, and both partners usually expected the other to be monogamous, so jealousy and anger were typical if infidelity was discovered. In most villages there were also people who were so devoted to a particular lover that others believed they had been bewitched by "love medicine." Cory (1949) reported similar beliefs in his anthropological work amongst the Sukuma in the early twentieth century. Generally, however, we found that most young people's sexual relationships did not seem to involve much emotional intimacy. Varying degrees of emotional attachment were evident in some long-term premarital sexual partnerships, but there were no accounts of idealized relationships in which individuals passionately believed that their partner's character uniquely complemented their own. Similarly, in focus group discussions with young people aged 14–19 years in Malawi, Undie, and colleagues (2007) found that participants conceived of sex as natural, utilitarian, pleasurable, and passionate, but there was little evidence that they valued or experienced much emotional intimacy within their relationships.

Monogamy

Monogamy was a sexual norm or ideal behavior shared by most villagers in rural Mwanza, and many unmarried young people wanted to be in mutually monogamous relationships. Most young people were sexually active for several years before they married, but few were in exclusive, long-term (greater than one year) sexual relationships with partners who were also monogamous. This may be because, if a couple reached a stage when they sought such a relationship, they almost invariably married. Young people's decision to marry and their sexual fidelity in marriage will be discussed in chapter 9. Before deciding to marry, most young people instead had a series of monogamous relationships that lasted a few days, weeks or months, or concurrent relationships of varying length.

Fast, serial monogamy, in which a young person went from one short-term relationship to another in quick succession, was fairly common in our study population. This was particularly true for young people who had reached an age when they were sexually active on a frequent (such as weekly) basis, typically by the mid-teens for most girls and late teens for most boys. If possible, sexually active young men did not want to go long without satisfying their desire through vaginal intercourse, and young women similarly did not want to go long without the material exchange they had come to regularly rely upon for both basic needs and small luxuries.

Serial monogamy does not pose the same general sexual health risk as concurrency, as a later partner's infection cannot be passed to an earlier partner. However, it can still involve substantial risk to sexual health, particularly if someone has many short-term relationships, increasing the chance that they have contact with someone with a sexually transmitted infection. In addition, if there is only a short period of time between sequential sexual relationships, there is a greater chance of transmitting infections received from one partner on to a subsequent partner, including bacterial infections which have a limited period of infectivity, or viral infections which have an initially brief, intense period of infectivity, such as HIV (Kraut-Becher and Aral 2003; Pilcher et al. 2004; Wawer et al. 2005).

Concurrency and Sexual Mixing Patterns

Monogamy was considered to be an ideal behavior in rural Mwanza, as noted above, but in practice secretive, concurrent sexual relationships were fairly common for unmarried young people of either sex. Similarly conflicting norms and expectations related to monogamy and concurrency have been documented elsewhere in sub-Saharan Africa (Pickering et al. 1997; Meekers and Calvès 1997; Nnko et al. 2004; Carter et al. 2007; Helleringer and Kohler 2007; Izugbara and Modo 2007; Rweyemamu and Fuglesang 2008; Research to Prevention 2009; Selikow et al. 2009; Harrison and O'Sullivan 2010). In our study, a number of factors seemed to promote concurrency amongst unmarried youth, including sexual desire and relative wealth (for males), relative economic need (for females), an absent or unavailable partner, and secrecy about sexual relationships.

Importantly, some young people considered themselves to be faithful to a main partner even though they had occasional, opportunistic sexual encounters with other individuals. Other recent research in sub-Saharan Africa has also found that young people and adults sometimes interpret "faithfulness" in different ways than is typically assumed within HIV prevention interventions (Painter et al. 2007; Lillie, Pulerwitz, and Curbow 2009; Leclerc-Madlala 2009). In many other cases, however, we found that young people with concurrent sexual relationships considered themselves to be "unfaithful" but did not feel conflicted about this as long as they could keep it secret, even though they highly valued and prioritized their partners' fidelity.

The recent research focus on romantic love in sub-Saharan Africa implicitly relates to the role it may have in mutual monogamy and sexual risk reduction. In the absence of a romantic belief that two individuals are uniquely suited to one another, it may be that each partner feels less desire or obligation to practice monogamy or to stay in a relationship if problems arise. However, a study in South Africa suggests that romantic ideals taken to an extreme may also involve higher risk (Harrison et al. 2006). That study found that young women who were "hyperromantic"—that is, who strongly expressed beliefs in an intimate relationship's importance, such as "I cannot live without my partner for even one day"—reported significantly more sexual partners in the last three months than other women. The authors postulated that young women with such extreme romantic beliefs had higher numbers of partners because they were desperate to experience an emotional connection within an intimate relationship at all times.

Early research on concurrency in the sub-Saharan African HIV epidemic suggested that urban men with concurrent partners were central to the spread of HIV (Caldwell, Caldwell, and Quiggin 1989). However, there is increasing evidence that sizeable proportions of female populations may also engage in concurrent partnerships (Nnko et al. 2004; Hattori and Dodoo 2007; Tawfik and Watkins 2007; Harrison and O'Sullivan 2010). This has critical implications for sexual health at a population level, as settings in which both males and females have concurrent partnerships are those most likely to create widespread or generalized epidemics (Shelton 2007). In addition, there is increasing evidence that sexual networks in rural areas may neither be as sparse nor as low risk as previously assumed (Cowan et al. 2005; Gouws et al. 2005; Béné and Merten 2008). For example, one recent study conducted with 18–35-year-olds in rural Malawi found that more than 25 percent of sexually active respondents were linked through multiple and independent chains of sexual relations (Helleringer and Kohler 2007).

Our study was only able to draw indicative conclusions about average numbers of sexual partners and the prevalence of concurrency in rural Mwanza. However, data from many villages over three years broadly suggest that many if not most young men and women had experienced concurrent partnerships by their late teens or early twenties. Young men were more open about their concurrent relationships than young women, particularly in discussions with other boys and men. However, this did not necessarily mean young men had more such partnerships, because stigma associated with young women's concurrency may have led them to hide it more.

It does seem possible, however, that on average unmarried young men did indeed have a higher number of brief, concurrent relationships with acquaintances or strangers than was typical of unmarried young women. In contrast, when unmarried young women had concurrent partnerships they generally seemed to be longer-term than young men's. If young women had fewer but longer-term concurrent partnerships overall, they could involve equal or greater sexual health risk, particularly given the low probability of HIV transmission in one encounter and the likelihood that a longer period of relationship overlap resulted in more cumulative sexual acts which could infect partners in either direction (Halperin 2004).

Our study's findings on sexual mixing were similar to those of studies conducted elsewhere in Mwanza Region and sub-Saharan Africa. Young men tended to have sexual partners who were about the same age or younger, while young women commonly had relationships with men ranging from the same age to ten years older than themselves (Gregson et al. 2002; Buvé 2006). In addition, men who travelled regularly often had serial and overlapping sexual partnerships in both their home village and elsewhere (Lagarde et al. 2003; Nyanzi et al. 2004), and the partners they left behind in their village seemed to be more likely than other villagers to engage in concurrency (Pickering et al. 1997; Lurie et al. 2003; Nnko et al. 2004; Vissers et al. 2008; Research to Prevention 2009). In our study, it is likely that the traveling member of a couple—usually the man—engaged in sex with higher risk partners, because travel away from villages usually involved going to larger towns, fishing camps, or mines where prevalences of sexually transmitted infections were higher, particularly amongst the women who men were likely to meet in guesthouses, food stalls, and bars (Schapink et al. 2001; Desmond et al. 2005).

The Challenge of Research on Sexual Relationships

In this study we found it challenging to accurately assess many aspects of young people's sexual relationships, including lifetime numbers of partners, concurrency, and the emotional nature of partnerships. Respondents often had problems correctly recalling the exact duration and timing of sexual relationships and sometimes were biased in underestimating both the number and the overlap of their sexual partners. Self-reported sexual behavior data thus were often difficult to interpret.

For example, many young people reported very early ages at first sex, but such reports were unlikely to reflect widespread sexual abuse of prepubescent children. We found very little evidence of such abuse, as will be discussed more in the next chapter. Some reports of sex at very early ages may instead have resulted from miscalculation. Many young people could only roughly estimate their current age, as described in box 2.1, and limited recall and math skills may have made it even more difficult to accurately estimate an earlier age.

Other reports of very early ages at first vaginal intercourse clearly referred to prepubescent sexual play, as already discussed. In his early twentieth century research with the Sukuma, Tanner (1955b, 238) similarly found that, "Men in their own affairs do not distinguish between prepuberty and postpuberty sexual activity, but emphasise [sic] very clearly that the real distinction is between before and after the time of actual potency . . . where the distinction must be entirely theoretical." In our study we found that young men's reported onset of sexual activity could also be difficult to interpret as some teenagers with relatively little sexual experience considered prepubescent sexual relationships to be part of their sexual history, but then a few years later—when they had had far more sexual encounters—they no longer perceived them in that way. Such a change in perspective may be one of several reasons why adolescent sexual behavior reports can be notoriously inconsistent.

Other researchers have faced similar challenges trying to collect information on sexual relationships elsewhere in eastern and southern Africa (Mavhu et al. 2008; Beguy et al. 2009; Minnis et al. 2009; Turner et al. 2009). For example, in a different area of Mwanza Region, Nnko and colleagues (2004) found it difficult to interpret survey data which they had collected on "continuing" relationships because, regardless of timing of last intercourse, partners might base their reports subjectively on their feeling of commitment to a partner, the expectation that intercourse may occur again, or whether a key event had occurred, such as residence change.

We found that the complex nature of sexual partnerships made it difficult to collect accurate, full relationship histories even within formal and informal in-depth interviews focused on this subject. Given the brief and structured nature of survey interviews, they seem even less likely to elicit comprehensive and valid information on topics like concurrency. Nonetheless, the few studies in sub-Saharan Africa which have attempted to assess concurrency in young people's sexual relationships have mainly relied on large-scale surveys. This raises questions about the validity of associations which have been found between concurrency and HIV to date, and highlights the importance of more in-depth qualitative research on this topic (Lagarde et al. 2001; Kapiga and Lugalla 2002; Mishra and Bignami-Van Assche 2009; Lurie and Rosenthal 2010).

CONCLUSION

In this chapter we have considered macro-social patterns of relationships for unmarried young people in rural Mwanza. In the next chapter we will closely examine some of the micro-social, interpersonal aspects of relationships which were raised here, including material exchange, negotiation and coercion within sexual relationships. Later, in chapter 9, we will return to broader relationship patterns when considering how sexual partnerships change once young people marry.

Chapter Seven

Sexual Negotiation, Exchange, and Coercion[1]

In this chapter we will move beyond broad patterns in young people's sexual relationships to examine unmarried couples' personal interactions, and particularly their negotiation of sexual encounters. Such negotiation determined whether a sexual relationship started, and, if it did, how long it subsequently lasted. To understand sexual negotiation, it is important to first consider women's and men's motivations to have sex. In chapters 5 and 6 we discussed how young men's motivations were mainly pleasure and masculine esteem, while young women's were mainly material gain. Sexual negotiation and decision making thus almost always involved monetary consideration, so we will closely examine the transactional nature of sex here. In doing so, however, we do not wish to suggest that material exchange excluded other, overlapping, motives, such as physical pleasure, reproduction, self-esteem or emotional attachment.

The exchange of sex for money or gifts has been widely reported in sub-Saharan Africa. Early in the HIV epidemic an anthropological review referred to "predominantly neutral" attitudes to prostitution in sub-Saharan Africa, and "a relatively instrumental view of sex within marriage. . . . It is the filiation of children rather than payment in cash which distinguishes wives, prostitutes, and others" (Day 1988, 424). Others described sex as a service which women rendered to men in return for cash and support (Caldwell, Caldwell, and Quiggin 1989).

Transactional sex generally is interpreted as a consequence of women's poverty and economic dependence on men (Schoepf 1991; Schoepf 1992a; Seeley et al. 1994; Balmer et al. 1997; Hunter 2002; Dunkle et al. 2004). Studies have also found that impoverishment may deter women from negotiating safer sex (Baylies et al. 2000; Kaufman and Stavrou 2004; Luke 2003; Dunkle et al. 2004; Longfield et al. 2004), and make younger women vulnerable to the enticements of older men or "sugar daddies" (Haram 1995; Mensch et al. 1999; Hunter 2002; Luke 2003; Longfield et al. 2004). For example, a recent South African study of 4,800 youth aged 14–22 years found that young women who had maternal financial support for their school fees, uniforms, and other clothing were more likely to report having used a condom at last sex than other young women (Camlin and Snow 2008).

However, several studies have also suggested that transactional sex is not always engaged in due to immediate material need (e.g., Béné and Merten 2008; Hunter 2009). Many Senegalese prostitutes in the Gambia were reported to be from non-impoverished families (Pickering et al. 1992), while Tanzanian Haya women practicing prostitution were reported to be both poor and relatively well-off (Kaijage 1993). In southern Uganda, secondary school girls were reported to exchange sex for money to pay for necessities their parents could not afford, but half of them reported that, whatever their affluence, they would not have sex for free. They reported that this would be humiliating because a gift "rubs off the cheapness of being used" (Nyanzi et al. 2001, 88).

In Tanzania, girls have been found to negotiate sexual relationships to their advantage in Mwanza (Nnko and Pool 1997; Maganja et al. 2007; Wamoyi, Fenwick et al. 2010). For example, in Dar es Salaam some young women who had experienced abortions were found to be "active social agents, entrepreneurs who deliberately exploit their partner(s)" (Silberschmidt and Rasch 2001, 1822). One study in rural Malawi found that policy makers considered transactional sex to be driven by survival needs, but this differed from the views of rural women themselves, who said that they were also motivated by attractive consumer goods, passion, and revenge (Tawfik and Watkins 2007). This ethnographic research found that, "transactional sex is not only about women's poverty but also about . . . women who are not desperately poor, but who aspire to social mobility, economic independence, or simply a life enhanced by soap and lotions" (Swidler and Watkins 2007, 157). Hunter (2002) argued that transactional sex in KwaZulu-Natal, South Africa was attributable to men and women's material inequalities, a particular construction of masculinity, and "the agency of women themselves" (Hunter 2002, 101). In a study in Durban, South Africa, Leclerc-Madlala (2003) argued that women saw transactional sex as a "normal" part of sexual relationships, motivated by a desire to acquire modern commodities.

In a review of quantitative and qualitative studies of age and economic asymmetries in young women's sexual relationships in sub-Saharan Africa, Luke (2003, 67) concluded that

> girls have considerable negotiating power over certain aspects of sexual relationships with older men, including partnership formation and continuation;

however, they have little control over sexual practices within partnerships, including condom use and violence.

De Zalduondo and Bernard (1995) further argued that, to attribute transactional sex solely to economic adversity

> implies an apology for sexual-economic exchange where none is needed. . . . The inference that all instances of sexual-economic exchange are inherently demeaning (and thus probably involuntary) seems to underlie an undifferentiated treatment of the topic in the public health literature. (De Zalduondo and Bernard 1995, 158)

Early research on transactional sex in sub-Saharan Africa focused on urban areas and commercial sex work (Day 1988), and very few studies have involved participant observation (Leclerc-Madlala 2003; Swidler and Watkins 2007). However, quantitative studies of sexual behavior rarely investigate the type of gifts provided or the context of gift-giving, so there is only limited understanding of the nature of transactions and the extent to which they are specifically inducements for sexual access (Luke 2003). Furthermore, as discussed in chapter 1 much of the qualitative research of adolescents' sexual behavior in rural areas has been conducted with secondary school students, who are not typical, and/or it has relied on group discussions, which are likely to be biased towards participants' normative beliefs rather than their actual behavior.

In this chapter we will examine how macro-social factors empowered men over women in sexual negotiation, but also how, at a micro-social level, individuals' attributes and their specific circumstances could strengthen the bargaining power of either sex. While we found a degree of choice and agency for both sexes, in some cases women's ability to negotiate clearly was limited by coercion, so we will describe that in depth as well.

FINDINGS

The Central Importance of Material Exchange

In all study villages, informants of both sexes almost always said that material gain was unmarried young women's main motive to engage in sex and to stay in ongoing relationships. When other motivations specifically were investigated in group discussions, some young women reported that sexual desire could be a motive, along with peer pressure, wishing to conceive, or wanting to convince a man to marry. However, these were considered relatively minor and/or uncommon motives compared with material exchange. Findings from participant observation were similar. For example, an 18-year-old woman who had had several sexual partners "said that she enjoys having sex, but the important thing for her is being given money. She explained, 'What use is pleasure when there is no money?'" [PO-01-C-2-6f]

Results from the 1998 *MEMA kwa Vijana* assisted self-completion questionnaire survey give some indication of the prevalence of transactional sex. For males, but not females, sexual experience was associated with earning money, even after adjustment for age (Plummer, Wight et al. 2004). Of those who reported having had sex, 75 percent of females reported receiving a gift or money at first intercourse, while only 43 percent of males reported giving something. This difference probably reflected how some girls first had sex with older sexual partners who could afford gifts, while some school boys could not afford them for their first encounter. Only approximately one-quarter of both sexes reported that a girl was not obliged to have sex if she had received a gift from a boy.

Commonly reported gifts for sexual encounters were sugar cane, peanuts, soap, body lotion, underwear, and underskirts. If money was exchanged it was generally between Tshs 200 ($0.24) and Tshs 1,500 ($1.80), although occasionally the range extended from Tshs 50 ($0.06) to Tshs 5,000 ($6). The amount of money was particularly high for a girl's first sexual encounter if it was with an out-of-school youth or man. Several informants reported that the acceptable amount had recently fallen due to general economic circumstances, such as one young woman who laughingly said: "For many, now that money has become scarce, even Tshs 200 ($0.24) is enough." [PO-99-C-8-2f] The type of gift or amount of money varied from one encounter to another according to negotiation.

Girls' Motivations to Exchange Sex for Money or Gifts

Poverty

In many cases transactional sex clearly was motivated by extreme poverty, to procure essential clothing, hygiene requirements, food to stave off hunger, or school necessities. As noted in chapter 3, hunger was a common aspect of daily life in rural Mwanza, particularly during the planting season when most families did not have their first meal of the day until 3:00 p.m. or 5:00 p.m. Many adolescent girls thus used money from their sexual partners to purchase a small amount of peanuts or sugar cane at school to calm their hunger.

Parents rarely provided underwear, soap, or body lotion for their teenaged children, apart from occasionally after the harvest. A 16-year-old Year 6 girl was typical in stating: "My parents don't buy underwear and body oil for me, and I have to take care of this on my own" [PO-00-C-3-2f]. Obtaining these items was thus a common motive for sex. School girls also commonly reported that they spent money they received for sex on school requirements, such as books, pens, shoes, uniforms, and school fees. This 17-year-old girl in Year 5, who was dressed in a tattered blouse during the interview, reported:

> *R:* [My sexual partner] gives me money. I buy body lotion, exercise books, and pencils. . . . A teacher may perhaps find you without shoes, [so] you are beaten. Perhaps your [uniform's] blouse is torn, so you have put on a dress [not a uniform]: you are beaten, just like that. Perhaps you don't have exercise books: you are also beaten. Therefore I decided to do it [have sex]. [II-99-I-68-f]

Most unmarried young women either did not reveal to their parents the gifts they received for sex, or they claimed they obtained them in a different way. For example, a 23-year-old woman

> said she was recently bought a brand new manufactured dress for Christmas, but [she] was not asked where it came from by her parents, because she has a small business selling local beer. When they see her with new things . . . they assume she bought them with the profit from her beer business. [PO-99-I-1-2f]

However, as already noted, some parents tolerated their daughters' discreet relationships, and a few encouraged them if this helped support the household. One female informant reported of a peer: "Sometimes when they don't have money, her mother even allows her to bring men home to make love with them to get money for expenses" [PO-00-I-4-4f]. There were also a few reports of grandmothers directly or indirectly encouraging their granddaughters to have sex. One young man said of a young woman in his village: "If her grandmother is given a bar of soap, she allows her to go out with that man or boy" [PO-00-I-4-1m]. Similarly, two married women in their thirties described how a woman responded when the granddaughters she supported requested soap: "When will you ever grow up and start having men to give you money and soap?" [PO-99-I-1-2f].

Tamaa *(Desire) and Peer Expectations to Consume*

Although many young women had sexual relationships to meet their subsistence needs, sex was also often exchanged in order to gain beauty products or clothes which were not essential for survival. However, the distinction between essential and nonessential items based on supposed biological necessity was not clear-cut. Interpretation of this often varied at an individual level, so exchanged materials could be perceived as a continuum from subsistence needs to consumer desires, with a large area of overlap. This will be discussed more later in the chapter.

The majority of young men said that girls had sex due to *tamaa* for money. *Tamaa*, which literally means "longing," "greed," or "lust," was used in this context in two ways: female desire for nice things, and male desire or lust for sex. Young women's *tamaa* for commodities and their readiness to have sex to acquire them was influenced strongly by shared expectations amongst female peers, whether they were family, friends, or acquaintances. Some girls learned from observing their older sisters and peers that desirable things such as attractive clothes, shoes, scented body lotion, and soap could be obtained as gifts from sexual partners. Young women usually wished to dress as nicely as any others in their village, and transactional sex was one of the easiest ways to achieve this. A 19-year-old unmarried woman who ran a food kiosk observed:

> Girls entirely depend on their parents, and if a girl has *tamaa* then it becomes a problem for her, because she will desire things that her parents cannot afford, or that are not useful. . . . This will leave her with the option of looking for men, who can give her as little as Tshs 200 ($0.24) [for sex]. [PO-99-C-5-2f]

Young women's consumption was particularly focused on self-presentation. For example, one of the most popular brands of soap was strongly scented and came in several different colors, costing Tshs 200 ($0.24) per bar, which was four times the cost of the cheapest soap. Young women showed off such gifts to their friends, and particularly valued washing thoroughly and applying scented body lotion before going out in public. One 17-year-girl in Year 4 explained, "At times I am bought expensive body oil that has a nice scent, and when I apply it while going to school, most pupils comment on it and admire it" [PO-99-I-1-2f].

Some girls who had not had sex borrowed clothes and lotion from their sexually active friends, but their peers rarely were prepared to share their possessions for long if they felt a girl could obtain them herself through her own sexual activity. A 16-year-old boy in Year 7 commented that peer pressure amongst girls led girls to start exchanging sex for money or gifts:

> R: At 10 am, during break, [girls] go to buy peanuts or buns and eat. The girl [without money] will begin thinking, "How?" By then the other girls will already know how, because in the village or center they may have boyfriends, and they will tell the other girl: "How long are you going to remain like this? . . . We get money, we eat buns or peanuts, but you just sit there." And therefore they advise her how to do so too [have a sexual partner]. And definitely a boy will then approach her. [II-99-I-42-m]

Many informants noted that when a girl began having sex they became cleaner and started dressing more nicely. Many young women discussed what they received from their partners with their close female friends, and experienced considerable pressure from them to maximize the money they received from sex. Those who received little or nothing were regarded as fools for being conned, and could be disparaged. A 14-year-old girl in Year 5 described how a girl who received nothing for sex would be perceived by her peers: "They will shout at her. They will laugh at her. . . . Possibly those girls will sit in groups just gossiping about her, and she will have no comfort, she will stay lonely" [II-99-C-51-f].

Young women judged what their peers had received from sexual partners by the type of clothes they wore and, for those still in school, by their ability to afford food. A young woman who left school due to pregnancy explained: "If the girl is not given money, other girls laugh at her at school. Girls knew those who were not given money by their boyfriends, by seeing that they never had money and were unable to afford fried rice cakes and other food during break time" [PO-01-I-1-2f]. We found no evidence to suggest that ridiculing those who received very little from their sexual partners was a collective attempt to maintain a higher price for sex.

Due to *tamaa*, girls and women were said to readily agree to have sex with those perceived to have money. For example, a 23-year-old woman was heard telling another woman that, "she would rather have sex with a man who has two wives, but who could give her a piece of soap when she needs it, rather than having sex with young men who do not have wives but would give her nothing" [PO-99-C-5-2f].

It was difficult to distinguish between the motivation to seek money or gifts for subsistence rather than for nonessential consumption. Women and men rarely made this distinction themselves. Rather, women tended to present their motivation in terms of subsistence needs, while men tended to attribute women's motivation to *tamaa*, and these two perspectives seemed to reinforce their respective bargaining positions. In practice the two motivations were sometimes inseparable, since for a young woman to attract a sexual partner to meet her subsistence needs, she might need clothing and beauty products to look attractive. This was illustrated by the importance of scented soaps and lotions, which had several interrelated uses: to avoid diseases associated with poor hygiene, to clean oneself, to be presentable, to impress female peers, to remain attractive to one's sexual partner, and to attract new sexual partners. As one young woman commented: "Now a **msimbe** like me, a man cannot cheat me. Does it mean I don't wash or apply lotion? He must give me money for soap and body lotion, so that when I come from [having sex with him], I can wash" [PO-99-C-5-2f].

Capital for Small Businesses

A few enterprising young women engaged in transactional sex to accumulate capital to start a business, such as trading food products, preparing and selling snacks, or operating food kiosks, as illustrated in case study 2.1.

They considered this a better use of money received from sex than buying commodities. A 19-year-old unmarried woman described how

> when a man gave her Tshs 2,000 ($2.40), she added it to what she had got from others [sexual partners] and started her food kiosk business. She said a woman has to be clever in spending the money given to her by men. Otherwise you will always spend everything they give you and end up borrowing every day. [PO-99-C-5-2f]

However, while transactional sex sometimes enabled young women to start a business, such businesses sometimes also provided increased opportunities for transactional sex. Some young women used their small business work as an excuse to meet sexual partners and, as already noted, to explain to their parents how new clothes or money were acquired.

Farm Labor

During participant observation there were also reports of young women in mixed-sex *rika* having sex with male *rika* members in exchange for assistance completing their portions of farm work. It was not unusual for a young woman in mixed-sex *rika* to have a partner within the group who assisted her in completing her portion of the farm work. It was not always clear, however, whether such couples specifically negotiated sexual activity in exchange for farming assistance. More overt arrangements were reported in a village close to a large, company-owned cotton plantation, where young people were paid by piece work. A 19-year-old out-of-school woman explained: "Usually boys complete their portion [of the plantation work] before girls and some offer to help them. Some women agree . . . and immediately after cultivation, they enter the bushes and have sex there before going home" [PO-01-I-1-2f].

The Process of Negotiation

Explicit sexual negotiation was almost always initiated by men, although girls and women sometimes discreetly encouraged it. The statement "*Naku-penda*" was often accompanied with some reference to material exchange to persuade a girl or woman to have sex. A 16-year-old boy in Year 7 described what he said to negotiate sex: "The main words are simply . . . 'If you agree, I shall give you a certain amount of money'" [II-99-I-42-m]. According to many women, a man sometimes asked a woman to specify how much money she wanted for sex as soon as he approached her. If the man did not mention gifts in his seduction, some girls or women raised it themselves. For example, women frequently asked for a loan or for a soda, not literally meaning a soft drink (which would have cost Tshs 200 or $0.24), but indirectly asking for money without appearing to be *wahuni*. Most women said that ultimately the onus was on them to remind their sexual partners of what they wanted before they agreed to sex. For example, a 23-year-old woman said: "These men pretend that they are not aware that you bathe or apply [body lotion]: you have to tell them" [PO-99-C-5-2f]. Similarly, when a male informant visited his girlfriend one night, he explained, "Immediately after I entered she asked me, 'Where is my soda?'" [PO-01-I-1-2f]. Others did not refer to material exchange at all, but delayed agreeing to have sex until they were given, or were promised, money or gifts.

Sexual negotiation sometimes involved explicit bargaining between potential sexual partners, as related by a young man:

> When I told the girl that I wanted to have sex with her, she told me to give her Tshs 2,000 ($2.40). I told her that I did not have that amount of money and the girl said I should then give her Tshs 1,500 ($1.80). I told the girl that I did not have that amount, but I could give her Tshs 700 ($0.84). The girl said that the money was not enough, and after long negotiations we agreed that I should give her Tshs 1,000 ($1.20). [PO-01-C-2-1m]

Awareness and use of condoms in study villages was extremely low; this will be discussed in depth in chapter 10. On the rare occasion when condom use was raised during sexual negotiation, boys and men typically felt it was not good value for their money. As this 15-year-old girl in Year 4 said: "Most men who give money to their lovers don't agree to use condoms. When it happens that a woman insists on using a condom, [the men] refuse and demand to be paid back their money" [PO-00-C-3-3m].

Gifts and money were not always given before sex took place. For example, when a girl asked a male informant for Tshs 1,000 ($1.20) before they had sex, he told her, "I don't do such business, I only give money after the act [of having sex]" [PO-99-C-5-2f]. In ongoing relationships, sex was sometimes provided on credit, some young women being understanding of their partners' financial difficulties, as explained by this young man:

> If the boy doesn't have money and the girl demands it, the boy asks the girl to lend it to him, that is, he makes love with her and gives her money on another day. In fact after some days or a week, the boy pays the girl her money. [PO-00-I-4-4f]

The vast majority of young men reported that they had at some point involved intermediaries in their sexual negotiation, often when they were first becoming sexually active. Intermediaries were referred to as *posta* (literally "post office" or "mail") and were individuals close to either the man or the woman, such as close relatives, friends, or fellow *rika* members. A *posta* encouraged a girl or woman to like a particular man, and facilitated him giving her gifts. If affiliated with the boy or man the *posta* was likely to encourage the girl to agree to sex for only limited money or gifts, while if affiliated with the girl, the *posta* was likely to help her negotiate more money or gifts. Each of the female researchers was approached by *posta* many times while in study villages. For example, a young woman who spoke with a 25-year-old fieldworker: "She asked me whether I would also like to have a lover. She told me that if I took a lover, he would help me meet my daily requirements" [PO-99-C-5-2f]. On numerous occasions, young men also told the male researchers that they could arrange for them to have sex with local girls if they liked.

A *posta*'s efforts, and those of others who helped facilitate an encounter, were sometimes rewarded with small gifts, usually from the man. The fieldworkers also noted many examples of a younger sibling or relative being given a small amount of money to keep a sexual relationship secret and enable it to happen by locking or unlocking doors, or allowing a couple to have sex in a shared sleeping room. An example provided by a 17-year-old woman who had recently finished primary school:

> She said that her 35-year-old sister brings male friends into the house that they share at night. She said when her sister's boyfriend comes, she chats with him before he goes to sleep in the bedroom with her sister. She said that when she was in lower primary school she was given Tshs 200 ($0.24) as a bribe to sleep in the sitting room instead of the bedroom. Now that she sometimes sneaks out to meet a boyfriend herself, she doesn't receive any payment for this. [PO-00-C-3-2f]

Attributes, Circumstances, and Bargaining Power

The amount of money or kind of gift exchanged was shaped by the relative bargaining power of two sexual partners. Each partner's individual attributes and particular circumstances could influence this.

One commonly reported attribute that made a young woman desirable, and therefore able to demand greater compensation, was her physical attractiveness, in particular a pretty face, light skin color, and large buttocks, and her appearance in terms of clean, attractive clothing and styled hair. In addition, as discussed in chapter 5, the greater a young woman's respectability, the more desirable she was to her potential partner and the more she had to lose by agreeing to sex, which usually meant that more valuable gifts were exchanged. A young woman's bargaining skills also played a role in the amount of money or kinds of gifts she received.

The most important attribute shaping the desirability of a male partner was his perceived earning capacity, as described in chapters 5 and 6. Young women also sometimes reported liking boys and men who were polite and respectful, or who wooed them with declarations of desire or liking/love. Physical characteristics which commonly were considered to be attractive included a man being well dressed or "somewhat fat" (healthy/attractive). If a man was perceived to be attractive, a young woman might accept a more modest payment for sex, while if unattractive he was likely to be refused unless he offered a lot more. However, physical attractiveness rarely seemed to be the most important factor in determining a man's appeal for a woman. There was a common saying that "there are no ugly men, and if there are, then they are those without money."

As noted in chapter 6, newcomers to a village of both sexes were perceived as highly attractive sexual partners, because of novelty, urban style, and/or perceived affluence. Women who were known locally as **wasimbe** or *wahuni* also preferred male newcomers as partners because such men were ignorant of their sexual reputations, which could strengthen their bargaining power. Male villagers sometimes competed with each other to have sex with a female newcomer, but such a woman's sexual attractiveness and bargaining power was likely to wane as soon as she was known to have been seduced locally, particularly if she had relationships with more than one man.

Whatever their attributes, partners' current circumstances also shaped their bargaining power, in particular women's immediate material needs, men's access to ready cash, and the stage of their relationship. As a 19-year-old unmarried woman observed, to the affirmation of another:

> If a man realises that a girl has no source of income he takes advantage of her and can even have sex with her for Tshs 100 ($0.12). . . . If you just wait for men they make fun of you, like goodness knows what. They will really show you contempt. It is better that you have your own small source of income, and if a sexual partner adds to your capital, you just continue with it. [PO-99-C-5-2f]

As noted in chapter 4, farmers were at their most affluent shortly after harvest when they sold their cash crops, and their available money then dwindled until the next harvest, unless they found employment as laborers during the planting season. The frequency of sex and the payment accepted for sex thus varied seasonally. During the rainy season, sex could be negotiated for as little as Tshs 200 ($0.24), while after harvest this could increase to as much as Tshs 1,000 ($1.20). Similarly, fishermen were more likely to agree to pay large sums for sex when they had just returned from a fishing trip and had ready cash. In lakeshore villages a few young women targeted fishermen when they had just returned from a catch by strolling about on the beach in tight-fitting dresses. These women were said to "skin a goat," meaning lure the men into having sex for ample money.

As a relationship developed, bargaining power tended to increase for the man or boy. A Year 7 school girl explained:

> In the beginning of a relationship the man gives relatively more money. But as the relationship continues he reduces it, or even becomes sly so as to have sex for free. . . . [When] I met my boyfriend for the first . . . [sexual encounter] he gave me Tshs 1,500 ($1.80); this was reduced to Tshs 1,000 ($1.20) the second time. [PO-01-I-1-2f]

Finally, as already noted, sexual negotiation and activity increased and transactional sex was more explicit at special events such as weekly markets, weddings, funerals, *ngoma* competitions, and holidays, usually taking the form of "*Halleluya*" exchanges (figure 7.1). Young men tended to save up money for these occasions, and young women tried to obtain new and attractive clothing in preparation for them. For instance, as Christmas approached a 17-year-old Year 5 girl, "was thinking of asking her boyfriend to give her Tshs 1,000 ($1.20) so that she can add to what she has and go to [the district capital] to buy shoes" [PO-99-I-1-2f]. Similarly, a young woman reported, "I was given money by my partner in order to buy socks for the choir at the *Saba saba* inauguration" [PO-00-I-4-4f].

Alcohol use also increased around many special events, particularly for men in their late teens and older, and this influenced sexual negotiation in a number of ways. Young women who wanted to try alcohol usually would obtain it by agreeing to sex with a man. Intoxication was also likely to impair sexual decision-making for both young men and women, so that they were more likely to engage in sexual activity that would not have taken place otherwise, such as sex with a particular partner, sex with more than one partner, and/or sexual violence, as will be described more below.

Figure 7.2 is a simple diagram that illustrates how male and female attributes and circumstances influenced sexual negotiation.

**Figure 7.1.
People mingling at a traditional drumming-dance (*ngoma*) event.**

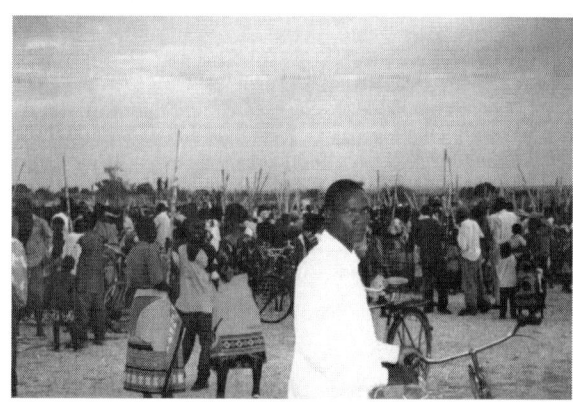

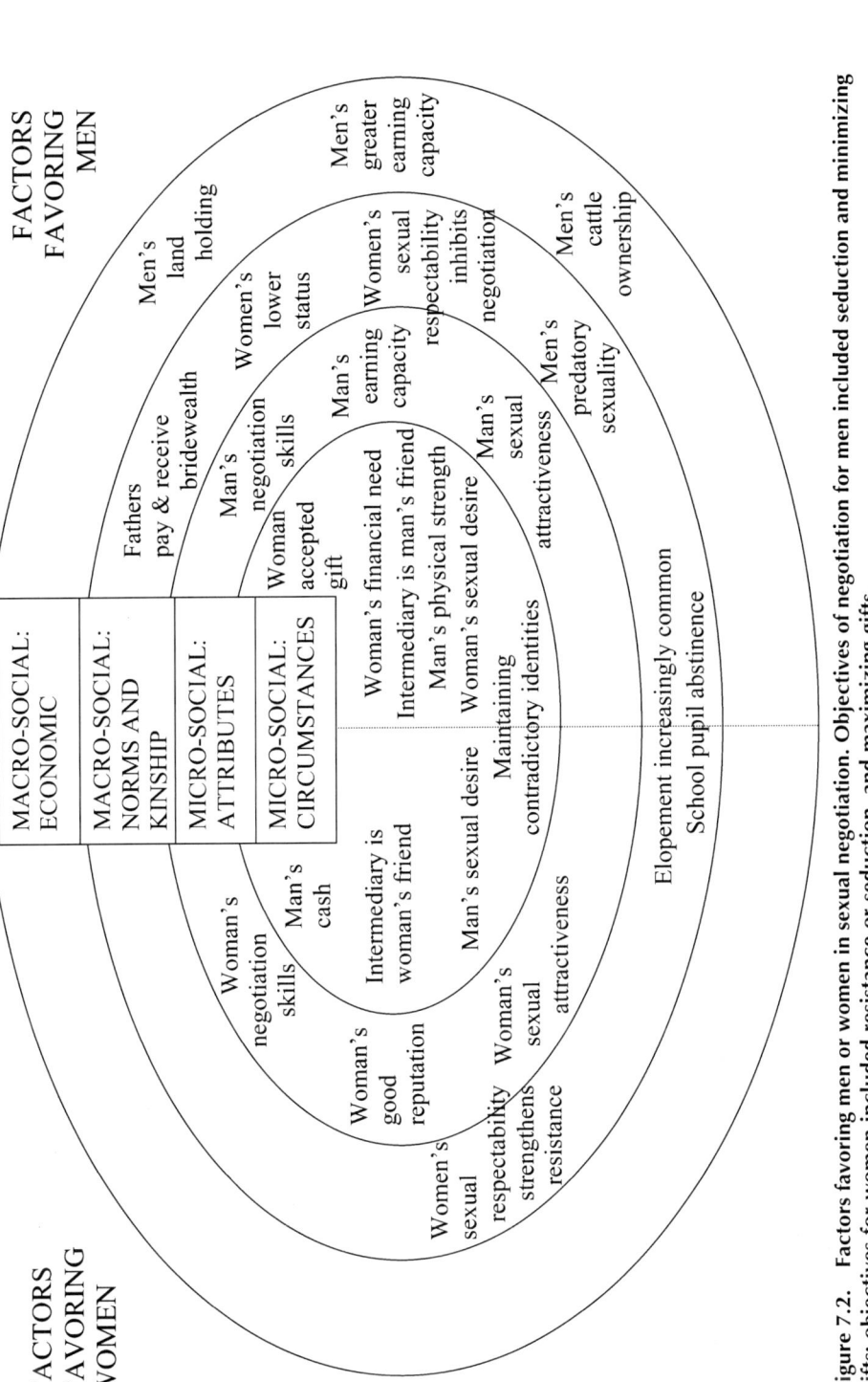

Figure 7.2. Factors favoring men or women in sexual negotiation. Objectives of negotiation for men included seduction and minimizing gifts; objectives for women included resistance or seduction, and maximizing gifts.

Different Kinds of Coercion

Young women in rural Mwanza often exercised some degree of choice and agency in negotiating whether or not to have sex and how they would be materially rewarded, even if their bargaining position was compromised by their attributes or circumstances. However, there were various ways in which men sometimes manipulated girls' or women's circumstances to strengthen their negotiating position, used threats, or, occasionally, resorted to physical coercion to have sex.

Pilot studies suggested that villagers typically only used the terms *kubaka* and **kupondya** (rape) for violent sexual assaults involving prepubescent or early adolescent girls which resulted in quasi-judicial proceedings. To better understand coercive sex more broadly, young people in surveys, group discussions, and in-depth interviews were asked about sex in which the girl or woman was forced, or it took place against her will. This seemed a clear concept for women and they readily gave examples of forced sex that they, or people they knew, had experienced.

However, men often stressed the ambiguity of this concept. They argued that it was nearly always necessary to feign a bit of force before an unmarried woman agreed to have sex, because her respectability required her to initially refuse sexual advances, even if she desired sex and planned to consent. For example, a 54-year-old man:

> He said that when he was a young man, even if a woman categorically agreed to have sex with a man, she would "refuse" until the man applied some kind of force to make her "comply." He said that in such struggles a young man would have his knees bruised as he tried to "force" the woman to have sex. [PO-00-I-4-1m]

Categorizing different forms of sexual coercion is problematic. Adopting a continuum from entirely consensual sex to violent rape, with various degrees of force or violence in between, implies that physical resistance indicates less willingness to have sex. However, an unwilling woman may not physically resist, for example, if she is frightened. Emotional trauma may also relate to other factors beyond violence, such as the woman's relationship with the perpetrator. Despite the limitations of any simple typology, we have identified six forms of coercion below which probably would have been recognized by most women in rural Mwanza, if not men. These include bullying and tricks, pressure by higher status third parties, teacher sexual abuse of pupils, coercion when drunk or drugged, forced sex other than that labeled "rape," and publicly recognized rape. Importantly, none of these categories are mutually exclusive, and in fact many incidents fell into two or more of them.

Bullying and Tricks

Most threats or force to make a young woman have sex occurred when she was thought to have reneged on an explicit or implicit agreement to have sex in return for a gift. A few sexually inexperienced girls might genuinely have not known what was expected when they received a gift from an unrelated man, but generally this was well understood. As one unmarried woman said, "A man buys you tea or soda, he gives you money, he cunningly pleases you. He can cater for your costs first before propositioning you" [PO-99-C-8-2f]. Some girls and young women instead accepted money or a gift believing that they could later avoid the sexual obligation, or repay whatever they had received, but they were not always able to do so. Having given a woman something, a man typically felt entitled to exert great pressure on her to have sex. This could include threats to inform the girl's parents that she had taken gifts, to beat her, or to snatch her *kanga* off her waist in public. Occasionally, men were also reported to bully women into agreeing to sex by fabricating stories about prior gifts. A 13-year-old girl in Year 5 reported: "He gives her, like, Tshs 20 ($0.02) for sugar cane, then he wants to beat her if she refuses [sex]. If asked by people why he wants to hit her, he says she ate [took] his money worth Tshs 2,000 ($2.40)" [PO-99-C-5-2f]. Young women sometimes agreed to sex in such cases to avoid embarrassment and protracted disputes.

Another common trick was for a man to use an intermediary to get a young woman to accept a gift indirectly. For instance, a few food kiosk owners reported that men had paid them to serve food to particular women, implying it was the kiosk owner's gift. Such women were then indebted to the men who paid for the food, and those men were in a strong position to insist on sex. Some girls and women instead described being deceived with false promises of future compensation. A young female informant bitterly described her boyfriend as "sly": "He tells you, 'Tomorrow, when tomorrow comes [I will give you money].' He says, 'Tomorrow,' like that, and you continue to have sex with him. Eventually a month is over without being paid your money" [PO-99-C-5-2f]. Failure to fulfill such promises could lead to considerable animosity, both for the woman and for her relatives if they knew about it, particularly if they benefited from the sexual exchange. Men were sometimes compelled to honor promises of payment, as explained by a 31-year-old male kiosk owner, who reported:

> When a boy agrees to give a girl money for sex, and then afterwards doesn't do so, that girl tells her grandmother. The grandmother gets very annoyed that the boy is making a fool of her grandchild . . . and looks for traditional medicines to make the boy "become a woman" [impotent], that is . . . he loses the power to have sex. . . . The young man discovers the change and goes to a

traditional healer who tells him that he is impotent because he did not give the girl her money after having sex with her. That boy goes to seek forgiveness from the girl, and gives her much more money than they had agreed previously. [PO-00-I-4-4f]

Pressure by Higher Status Third Parties

Intermediaries in sexual negotiation were sometimes someone older who had authority over the young woman, such as an elder sister, aunt, employer, or parent. In such cases the young woman might have sex out of trust or respect for the person, or a sense of obligation. An example provided by a group discussion participant:

> P: Your sister talks with a man, [and he says], "Now, if I could get your little sister, Lord! It would be fresh [good]. And you, you will drink beer, and she will drink also." And she comes to you, "My younger sister, that man has money, and I have already told you about his father and that his mother is a nurse. You agree [to have sex with him], and we will be drinking. Lord! What do you say, my younger sister? Let's go." And you will force yourself to go, following the respect you have for your sister. [GD-00-C-10-1f]

In another example, a 31-year-old mother of six reported that her first sexual experience took place when she was a school girl and an older female cousin invited two men into their shared sleeping room at night:

> She said that her cousin used to bring men home to their sleeping room. It happened one night that she told two men to come. One was her boyfriend while the other one was the boyfriend's friend. Her cousin only whispered to her about it as she was opening the door for the men, telling her that the second man would like to be her boyfriend. My informant said that it was dark and she only felt someone caressing her and then sex followed. Her cousin was busy next to her with the other man. After the intercourse the man gave her Tshs 500 ($0.60), which was a lot of money to her at the time. [PO-99-I-1-2f]

In a third example, a 21-year-old mother of two reported how, when she was 14 years old and in Year 6, her uncle directed her to become sexually involved with the man who eventually became her husband:

> [Her future husband] often tried to seduce her but she rejected him. . . . Then one night when she was asleep at her uncle's home, her uncle woke her up . . . and told her that there was a man outside waiting for her. When she went outside her uncle closed the door and told her that she should go with the man and come back the next morning. She reluctantly went to the man's home, where they had

sex. . . . She said he was older than her and she feared him. On the first day she wasn't pleased with him but after getting used to him she started enjoying sex with him and loving him . . . they continued meeting about three times per week for sex for a year before they got married. [PO-02-C-3-3m]

Three female respondents who sold drinks in fishing village bars said that their employers sometimes pressured them to have sex with a third party. The man interested in having sex might first buy the bar owner beer or give him money, and the employer would then tell the woman to leave her work to entertain the man.

As already described, in most villages there were occasional first- or third-person reports of mothers or other female guardians who actively encouraged their unmarried daughters to engage in material exchange for sex, in order to help support the household. Participant observation suggested that it was rare for fathers to overtly encourage their daughters to have premarital sex, although many if not most expected their teenage daughters to provide for many of their own material needs.

Teacher Sexual Abuse of Pupils

In the second series of in-depth interviews, one-third (22/62) of randomly selected respondents reported that at least one teacher in their school had had a sexual relationship with a female pupil in recent years. In addition, 4 of 33 randomly selected girls described being pressured sexually by a teacher themselves. There was also strong evidence of sexual relationships between male teachers and female pupils in eight of the nine participant observation villages, which were equally *MEMA kwa Vijana* control and intervention villages. These involved accounts of one or two male teachers per village who in recent years had impregnated school girls (four schools), had been caught having sex with pupils (three schools), and/or had pressured girls to have sex (three schools). Several of these accounts were known and discussed by the wider public, because teachers were dismissed, transferred, suspended, fined, left the village voluntarily, and/or married the pupil soon after she finished school.

Generally such sexual abuse began when a teacher isolated a girl in his office or home, where he had assigned the girl chores. The teacher then threatened the girl with punishment and/or offered her special privileges to pressure her for sex, as illustrated in case study 1.4. If a girl refused sex, some teachers made excuses to verbally abuse or beat her over subsequent months, interspersed with further attempts to seduce her. This is illustrated by case study 2.1 and the following example, in which a 17-year-old girl in Year 4 reported she had sex with her teacher for Tshs 1,000 ($1.20) on Christmas Eve, and then again for 500 ($0.60) Tshs on Christmas Day:

> [Earlier in the year] the teacher told her that he loved her and wanted her to be his girlfriend. She refused. She said that throughout the term the teacher caned her without reason and she thinks it was because of her refusal. . . . She said she only agreed [to have sex] twice, because he had pestered her over a long time. . . . She said it was in [her shared bedroom] . . . and she assumes, since it was dark, her 12-year-old sister did not see that it was their teacher [PO-99-I-1-2f].

Sometimes adults seemed aware of a teacher's sexual abuse of a school girl but did not act to prevent it, because they lacked evidence, they felt little recourse, or they believed it did not affect them or their family personally. For example, a 22-year-old nursery teacher

> said that [a certain] teacher openly has sex with school girls and that other teachers know about it but don't do anything. She said that she observed the teacher sending a girl to his house and then he followed. . . . She said that most teachers at the primary school are known to befriend [have sex with] school girls, including the head teacher. [PO-00-C-3-2f]

If parents had strong evidence that a teacher had a sexual relationship with a school girl, he sometimes transferred to another school on his own initiative or that of an authority. One example was told by a 25-year-old man:

> One night [a pupil] went to the teacher's house. . . . Since there were rumors that she was having an affair with the teacher, her father went straight to the teacher's home. . . . The matter was heard before local authorities the following day, and the teacher was fined Tshs 15,000 ($18). Later the teacher sought a transfer. [PO-00-I-4-1m]

During participant observation, we only learned of one teacher sexual abuse case that led to a formal prosecution. It involved a pregnant Year 5 girl and was resolved two weeks prior to a participant observation visit. A researcher later recorded:

> The girl's parents asked the head teacher if he was responsible and what he was ready to offer them. . . . He denied responsibility. The parents sold one of their cows and took the case to court in the village. The head teacher bribed the magistrate, who judged unfairly . . . The parents sold another cow to take the case to a higher court. . . . The head teacher was found guilty and moved away from the village. [PO-99-C-5-2f]

In one village, sexual abuse of girls by teachers seemed commonplace, as there were numerous, plausible first- and third-person reports that five of the six male teachers pressured different girls for sex.

Women Coerced when Drunk or Drugged

In almost every participant observation village there were reports of a local man sexually assaulting a drunken woman at some point in the past. If the woman had been drinking with the man before the assault—particularly if he had paid for her drinks—then she was considered to be at least partly responsible for any subsequent sexual encounter. In villages in each of the four study districts there were also reports of a practice called *kuliwa susa*, which referred to multiple men having intercourse with one woman during one sexual encounter. Some incidents of *kuliwa susa* were considered by villagers to be rape, but some were not. Usually descriptions of *kuliwa susa* involved men taking sexual advantage of a drunken woman, but occasionally it was also reported as a punishment for a woman's infidelity. One Village Executive Officer gave an example:

> He said *kuliwa susa* occurs when a woman is very drunk and several men remove her from the drinking place and have sex with her in turn, one after the other. . . . He said last year it happened that one woman was raped in that way and reported those men with whom she was drinking beer. They were arrested and charged in court. He said they were in a great deal of trouble, but in the end they paid a bribe and the case was closed. [PO-01-I-4-5f]

During a participant observation visit to one remote and almost entirely Sukuma village, there were widespread reports that numerous women had experienced a type of sexual assault done by men called **bagindu**. Most accounts described **bagindu** as two or more young men who entered a household at night, sprayed the inhabitants with a traditional medicine that drugged them into a trance, had sex with one or more of the women, and then stole items as trophies, such as the beads the women wore around their waists. Household members typically did not remember the experience but evidence was discovered the next day, for example, if a woman had lost her beads, or if her vagina was sore and had semen in it even though she had not had sex with her husband the previous night. All of the villagers who told researchers about **bagindu** were male, including a man in his 40s who worked for a nonprofit health organization, a 25-year-old house builder, and a 16-year-old pupil.

Authorities' responses to claims about **bagindu** varied. In one reported incident, young men were arrested by the **sungusungu**, interrogated by the Village Executive Officer, confessed by showing him a basin full of women's beads, and then revealed that they had been given the ***bagindu*** medicine by two local traditional healers. Later in the same participant observation visit village leaders held a village-wide meeting at which all adults were asked to secretly record on paper who they thought were ***bagindu***, thieves, or witches, with the assistance of literate villagers as necessary. At the end of the meeting no one was accused publicly, but the leaders said they would review the listed names later.

Other authority figures did not take reports of ***bagindu*** seriously. In one reported case secondary school girls were found undressed outside of their boarding school one morning:

> The secondary school teachers reported the incident to the District Commissioner, who denied ***bagindu*** existed. The teachers and students felt the District Commissioner was refusing to deal with that issue, so one night they caned the old women who they suspected were witches [who helped the ***bagindu***]. Later the District Commissioner scolded the teachers like they were small children. The villagers complained very much after he did that, because he appeared to be defending witchcraft. [PO-02-I-4-5f]

Forced Sex Other than that Labeled as "Rape"

During participant observation, researchers learned of numerous incidents of sexual violence which may not have been recognized as rape by the general public if they were known, even though they involved women having sex against their will, sometimes in violent circumstances. For example, one incident of *kuliwa susa* was not considered to be rape, even though a group of fishermen reportedly violently forced an unmarried young woman to have sex after learning that she had had two of them as concurrent sexual partners.

There were two important reasons why girls and women may not have disclosed sexual assaults. First, there was the concern that they might be blamed for the incident. Case study 1.4 provides one such example, in which a girl was assaulted violently while delivering food to a man's house, but she did not tell her parents because she thought they would blame her for going to his house. Another young woman reported that she did not tell her parents of an assault because she thought her father might punish both her and her mother:

> *R:* I was held down the first time I had sex. It was at the cemetery, where there is a small path going to the milling machine. . . . There were two of them, but after subduing me by force one left. . . . Afterwards I felt pain in my private parts. I went home and told my sister, "I had sex with someone . . . without wanting to." I made the decision not to tell anyone else. If my mother told my father, she could even have been beaten. Father had two wives then and had become very bad tempered at home. So mother would have been beaten. So, the two of us,

me and my sister, we just stayed like that. . . . That man was never seen in my village again. [II-02-I-290-f]

The second factor discouraging disclosure was that sometimes an authority figure, an older relative, or trusted friend had acted as the intermediary in incidents of forced sex. To report it would challenge the person's authority, and/or the victim might feel at fault for trusting the friend. One group discussion participant told how her aunt had sent her and her sisters to different men's houses on errands, having previously arranged that the men would have sex with them. When the men forced themselves on the girls, the girls tried to scream but were threatened with violence and were reduced to crying until the men finished. Another woman in a group discussion recounted how her friend had deceived her into visiting a man. When they got to the man's house her friend left to go to the toilet and the man locked the door and assaulted her. They fought and she beat on the door to escape, and the woman believed that her friend heard her but did not go for help. Eventually, the woman said, "that man forced me. He choked me until I fell down. He lifted and threw me on to the bed. . . . I mean it was a war in there. Finally, it was two hours later and my energy was spent. Then work [sex] took place." [GD-00-C-10-1f]

"Rape"

The examples above generally were not described as "rape" by study participants. An event was more likely to be perceived as rape by villagers, and thus be the focus of judicial or quasi-judicial proceedings, if the victim had no prior sexual relationship with the man, if she was prepubescent or in early adolescence, if she had not received any gift from him, if the man was a close relative, if he was believed to have raped women before, and/or if he was mentally ill, drunk, or high on illegal drugs at the time, and the woman was not. In contrast, if the man had a good reputation then people were more likely to assume the woman contributed to the incident. If she had taken money or a gift from him in advance, many would see his use of force to have sex as unfortunate but justified.

The following three incidents are examples of rape as universally defined by villagers: a 10-year-old girl was raped by a 20-year-old cousin who was caught and then fled the village; an early adolescent girl was raped when sent to a man's home on an errand, resulting in him paying a fine of cows to her parents; and a customer in a compound where alcohol was brewed and sold attempted to rape a school girl he did not know. In the last example, the girl screamed, the man ran, and the *sungusungu* arrested him the next day. After a public hearing the man escaped and the *sungusungu* caught and beat him before taking him to a distant town, where he was believed to have bribed the police to secure his release a few days later. In most villages, there were similar first- or third-person reports about drunken men who had tried to sexually assault girls or women.

In most villages there were also one or two men who were widely believed to have raped women on multiple occasions. The rapist described in case study 1.4 is one example, as many villagers discussed rumors that that man had raped multiple girls, but he was never publicly accused of it. However, the female researcher spoke with one other girl who described being raped by him in a similar way, after he isolated her at his house when she went there to purchase tomatoes from him.

Sometimes, such individuals were caught and beaten by the *sungusungu* and/or paid a fine for having raped a woman. A few of them were believed to have mental or emotional problems, such as one young man who also was caught having sex with a calf. Others were not believed to have such problems but were nonetheless considered to be potentially dangerous, so girls were warned to stay away from them, or to scream if they were ever somehow caught alone with them.

For example, in one village three researchers heard multiple independent reports about a man in his late 30s who was believed to have assaulted multiple women, including two of his adolescent daughters. That man reportedly was beaten after trying to rape one woman, but only paid a fine when he was publicly accused of raping his out-of-school 15-year-old daughter. A researcher described that reported incident of incest below:

> The man is said to have raped his daughter when his wife [the girl's mother] was attending a relative's funeral in a neighboring village. . . . He went to where his daughter was sleeping . . . and told her if she did not have sex with him, he would beat her. The daughter was frightened and agreed. The next day she reported the matter to the Village Chairman and refused to go back home. . . . The informant said that when the girl's mother returned she did not do anything about the rape. The girl then moved to live with relatives in another village. [PO-01-C-2-1m]

Many informants reported that this man either paid a bribe to the Village Chairman to drop the matter, or paid a fine of one to two cows which were slaughtered so that the meat could be distributed amongst villagers.

When an incident was likely to be perceived as rape, the man typically fled the village, either temporarily or for several years. If caught soon after an incident, a fleeing rapist usually was beaten. Ultimately village authorities and communal decision-making usually played a role in resolving such incidents, sometimes through the conciliatory process of *kusuluhisha*, in which the rapist was made to apologize formally and to pay a fine. There was only one reported case of a man going to prison after being accused of rape, and even in that incident the man was not prosecuted. Instead, after the man raped a secondary school girl, he was taken to a police station and was then imprisoned for seven months while his case was pending. In the interim the girl's family decided to withdraw their complaint, because they were concerned about their relationship with the man's family in the village, so the man was released.

Condemnation of Sexual Coercion

Use of physical force in sex generally was condemned in rural Mwanza, and violent incidents defined as rape were condemned universally. However, five factors led coercive sex to be more tolerated than this generalization suggests. First, being pressured into having sex against one's will through tricks or deference to a superior was regarded as normal by both men and women, if it did not involve violence. Second, many men interpreted a girl or woman's initial resistance as pretence only.

Third, any suggestion that a woman initially signified her consent to sex, including accepting money or a gift from a man, made it far less likely to be treated as rape. Since much of sexual negotiation was nonverbal, such as accepting gifts or accompanying a man to his house, and even consensual sex often involved a verbal pretence of refusal, men could often claim that a woman had agreed to sex. For example, in the group discussions, participants reported an incident in which a woman received several drinks from a man and then refused to have sex with him, after which he attacked her, knocking out three of her teeth. Others intervened before the man raped her, but the village authorities later dismissed the case because the woman was perceived to have conned the man.

Fourth, even when an incident was recognized as rape the rapist might experience only minor consequences, and achieving conciliation between the victim's family and the rapist generally was more important to authorities than prosecuting or imprisoning the man. Thus when an unmarried young woman was found to have been raped, payment of a fine to her parents generally was considered an adequate sanction. Often, however, authorities did not even become involved and the man experienced no consequences. In one violent incident, for example, a Year 6 pupil was raped by a truck driver who had rented a room in the same house where she and her mother lived, but no authorities were notified. The woman explained:

R: After he did it I kept quiet, but later I cried and told our neighbor. She told me, "Just keep quiet, because it is over now." . . . So I kept quiet. . . . But when my mother came home that evening I told her. She rebuked that man and he took his vehicle and left. He stayed away for several months. [GDII-00-C-10-5f]

Finally, moral condemnation of rape was tempered by an unwillingness to pursue justice after the immediate outrage had passed, except sometimes amongst the injured family. Often villagers were unwilling to discuss cases of rape openly and seemed to want to forget them. During participant observation the researchers learned of one accused rapist fleeing a village but then returning seemingly without consequence several months later. In a different incident a man was not held accountable for raping a woman because he seemed to be mentally ill during and immediately after assaulting her, even though he returned to his normal behavior soon afterwards.

Because of these different issues, coercion and specifically rape largely seemed to go unacknowledged and unpunished in rural Mwanza. However, there were also findings which suggested that, occasionally, men who were caught having consensual sex with a woman were falsely accused of rape. No young woman reported falsely accusing a man of rape, but some young men reported having been the subject of false rape accusations. In one case, a father caught his daughters reportedly having consensual sex with two men and brought rape charges against the men. The matter was only resolved after one of the men married one of his daughters. Another example involved a 15-year-old school girl who reportedly

> brought her lover to her sleeping room at night. She was then found red-handed having sex with him by her mother. The man was beaten and taken to the police with an allegation of rape, but later when told to testify about being raped, the 15-year-old girl said she liked/loved the man. The man was set free and later eloped with the girl. [PO-01-I-1-2f]

Some claims of assault by *bagindu* also began when girls or women were caught in compromising circumstances, such as the secondary school girls who were found undressed outside of their dormitories, or the wives whose waist beads were missing. It is possible some of those women consented to sex but later claimed to have been drugged and assaulted, in order to maintain their sexual respectability and to avoid punishment.

Similarly, in one village a Year 7 school girl was widely reported by her peers to have many partners, including a long-term sexual relationship with a certain married man, but when her grandmother caught her having sex with that man the girl claimed that he raped her. Some villagers believed the man had indeed raped her, whether she had an existing or prior sexual relationship with him or not, but according to the man's sister-in-law, a 34-year-old mother of six, the accusation of rape was false:

> She said that young woman had a sexual relationship with her brother-in-law for a long time. . . . [One day] the young woman was on her way to spend the

night at her grandmother's place with her younger siblings, when she met him and they decided to enter a maize field to have sex. She left her siblings by the path, and her grandmother came by . . . and asked the children where the young woman had gone. . . . Her grandmother entered the maize field to look for her and . . . the man ran away. The young woman told her grandmother that he had grabbed her and dragged her in the field. . . . The case went on for two months while the man stayed in remand [until] his wives sold their crops to pay for his release. . . . Afterwards, the young woman continued having an affair with him. [PO-02-I-1-2f]

The reports above suggest that occasionally men may have been falsely accused of rape. Importantly, however, there was far more evidence of genuine coercion which was never publicly acknowledged, and for which men were not held accountable, as will be discussed below.

Prevalence of Coercive Sex

We found it difficult to estimate how widespread coercive sex was in study villages. Survey data from the *MEMA kwa Vijana* trial suggested that one-third of sexually active school girls had experienced forced sex. For example, in the 1998 assisted self-completion questionnaire, of the 21 percent of females who reported having had sex, 34 percent reported that they had been forced to have sex at some time in the past (Plummer, Wight et al. 2004). However, it is not clear how accurate such results are given general problems with self-reported survey data validity, as described in chapters 1, 2, and 6, and possibly more specific problems if participants interpreted "forced sex" in a variety of ways.

Based on their cumulative participant observation research, female field researchers tentatively estimated that 20–30 percent of sexually active young women had received gifts and then been blackmailed or pressured into having sex, and about half had been coerced into having sex through intermediaries. Male field workers in turn estimated that about 60–70 percent of sexually active boys lied to trick a girl into having sex, for instance, saying he would marry her or give her money at a later date when he did not intend to actually do so.

School girls in rural Mwanza were vulnerable to teacher sexual abuse because of the frequent, long-term contact they had with teachers, and the persistent, diverse, and exploitative ways a determined teacher could pressure a girl to have sex. While most school girls did not experience this, there was strong evidence that a minority in almost all study schools did. With respect to overtly violent coercion, school girls were generally less vulnerable than out-of-school women, because men were afraid of school girls' parents and the possibility of quasi-judicial punishments.

The group discussions with unmarried women in their early 20s suggested that about half had experienced physical violence within a sexual relationship at some time. Both men and women in group discussions said that publicly recognized "rape" was rare in their villages, and they took time to recall the last incident. In all of the participant observation villages there were reports of publicly recognized rapes that occurred within the last two to three years, and researchers were resident in villages several times when rapes were reported to have happened. There were only a few reports of incest in the entire study area, and similarly only a few reports of sexual abuse of small, prepubescent children.

DISCUSSION

The Ubiquity of Transactional Sex

We found that young people's negotiation of sex in rural Mwanza was almost inextricably linked to the negotiation of material exchange, confirming earlier findings from group discussion research in the same area (Nnko and Pool 1997). Young women actively used their sexuality as an economic resource, and, within the constraints of macro- and micro-social factors, often willingly entered into relationships primarily for economic gain. By focusing on material transactions in this chapter we do not mean to suggest that girls and women did not have other motives for sex. Indeed, we have noted that other factors such as a man's physical attractiveness or a woman's affection for him could override material considerations, as has also been found elsewhere in Tanzania (Setel 1999b). Furthermore, the generosity and consistency of gifts sometimes symbolized a man's emotional attachment or intention to support his partner long-term. However, our data do not suggest that the material exchange was primarily symbolic, as Nyanzi and colleagues (2001) found for Ugandan secondary school pupils. In most of the premarital sexual relationships in our study, the gifts or money received for sex met young women's immediate material desires or needs. Nonetheless, to have sex and *not* to receive material compensation would have had serious symbolic implications for young women, suggesting that they did not value themselves.

The material motivations for women to have sex were diverse, ranging, for example, from staving off hunger to buying a new dress for a festival. Clearly, subsistence needs were a great concern for young women in the study area, a context in which school girls menstruated on rags and typically had only one or two well worn pairs of underwear; where they might have nothing to eat all day; where—if they did not get their own soap—they had to borrow soap from others who preferred not to share, or bathe without it; and where they easily could be beaten and thrown out of school if they did not wear shoes, or shoes to a teachers' liking.

In this context, the distinction between "legitimate financial needs" (Longfield et al. 2004, 128) and an optional "enhancement" (Swidler and Watkins 2007, 157) was very difficult to assess. Young women in this study nearly always explained material exchange in terms of their needs. Importantly, people often experience poverty subjectively as exclusion from normal social life in a particular setting (Townsend 1979). For example, if a young woman's peers have new dresses at Christmas she might experience her own lack of a new dress as poverty, but she might not have experienced it that way if no one else had new dresses. In practice, for a young woman in rural Mwanza to attract a sexual partner to meet her subsistence needs, she generally also required commodities to look attractive. We thus consider it fruitless to attempt to distinguish between "absolute poverty" and "relative poverty," particularly as it implies that transactional sex is somehow more legitimate with the former (de Zalduondo and Bernard 1995; Thomas and Cole 2009).

While premarital sexual relationships in Mwanza were often condemned by older adults, there was no evidence that the linking of sex with money or gifts was regarded as immoral in itself, as has also been found elsewhere in sub-Saharan Africa (Helle-Valle 1999). In his study within the Merina People of Madagascar, Bloch (1989) noted that the restricted use of money in Euro-American culture can make transactional sex problematic for westerners, when this is not the case in many African cultures:

> In Europe the linking of monetary exchange and sexual or familial exchange is seen as typically immoral or as a source of humour or dissonance. By contrast, in Madagascar the need to keep the two areas separate is not present. The right thing for a man to do is to give his lover a present of money or goods after sexual intercourse. . . . It is thus clear that if the Merina attitude to money strikes us . . . as needing elucidation it is because the symbolism of money is powerful, not in Merina culture, but in European culture. (Bloch 1989, 166–67)

In rural Mwanza, the different factors shaping sexual partners' relative bargaining power sometimes led to apparent contradictions in the amount exchanged for sex. For instance, sex with school girls was either relatively cheap, because they welcomed even very small gifts, or relatively expensive, because they were perceived to be virtuous and unattainable to adult men. Similarly, greater material need might lead a girl or woman to have sex for a relatively small amount, but some girls negotiated relatively large amounts from their partners specifically because they did not have financial support from their parents.

Villagers' views about transactional sex illustrated the contradictory norms around young people's sexual behavior described in chapter 5. Some parents exercised discretion and kept different social realms separate, condemning premarital sexual relationships but also telling their daughters to support themselves, knowing how this was done in practice, or they readily shared the gifts provided by daughters, as has been found in some other African studies (Nyanzi, Pool and Kinsman 2001; Boileau et al. 2008). Conversely, women's negotiations were severely constrained by the need to maintain their reputations, even though transactional sex was almost ubiquitous. To ask for payment explicitly was disreputable, but so too was receiving nothing for sex, which was considered demeaning. As a result, most women protected their reputation by not asking for gifts or money directly, but delayed agreement to have sex until they were given or promised something.

Underlying Factors in Transactional Sex

A fundamental principle behind material exchange for sex was the norm of reciprocity, that is, that a gift is never free but involves an obligation to provide something in return (Setel 1999b; Mauss 2002). Villagers often referred to this explicitly, and it was reflected in young women's indignation when a gift was not given for sex, or young men's indignation when a gift was not returned in sexual favors. Although the principle does not necessarily require immediate reciprocity, in many young people's sexual negotiations little delay was tolerated.

This obligation of reciprocity may have indirectly related to bridewealth, which still determined the nature of marriage in rural Mwanza during our study. Traditionally amongst the Sukuma, bridewealth was exchanged for important rights, which included rights to a woman's domestic and farming labor, to her reproductive capacity, and to sexual access to her (Cory 1953; Varkevisser 1973). The illegitimacy of sex before marriage related in part to relatively little or no payment being made to the woman's family for access to sex and, in some cases, reproductive ability. Material exchange for premarital sex could thus be seen as a modification of conventional norms: the contentious issue was not the material exchange, but that the woman's family did not benefit, or may have lost potential income if she was considered less marriageable because she was known to have had premarital sex.

Elsewhere in northern Tanzania, unmarried women's strategic calculations to maximize their long-term economic interests led some to intentionally seek serial partners rather than to marry (Haram 2004). In our study, we also found many young women changed premarital sexual partners if gifts and money received from one partner reduced over time. However, we did not find evidence that such partner change was an intentional, long-term choice as an alternative to marriage.

Several reasons combined may explain why less was exchanged for sex after first sex within a relationship. The young woman might have become less desirable to her partner, the prestige of seduction having been achieved and fantasies of sexual contact realized. Meanwhile, the woman's respectability had been undermined by her succumbing to the man's pressure to have sex. Furthermore, most men were unable to maintain the gifts offered for first sex.

On the basis of ethnographic data from Malawi, Swidler, and Watkins (2007) have argued that transactional sex and concurrent relationships should be seen as one form of broader patron-client relationships that are pervasive throughout sub-Saharan Africa. In this entrenched system of "unequal interdependence" (Swidler and Watkins 2007, 157), the authors suggested that affluent men were expected to share their wealth with poorer women, thus becoming patrons (sexual partners) of multiple women out of a "moral obligation to support the needy" (Swidler and Watkins 2007, 147). Women, in turn, were expected to reciprocate with sexual favors, and saw economic and social advantages in having more than one male patron. Our study found that young women in rural Mwanza experienced similar motivations and practices. In contrast, however, we found that affluent men with multiple unmarried partners were overwhelmingly motivated by sexual desire and opportunity. In our study there was little evidence to suggest they were also motivated by an underlying sense of moral obligation to share their wealth.

HIV Risk and Transactional Sex

Our findings suggest that material exchange for sex may have increased the risk of transmission of HIV and other sexually transmitted infections in five ways. Most obviously, material need or desire were young women's main motivations to have transactional sex, and this encouraged sexual activity that might not have occurred if young women had had more lucrative sources of income or goods. Second, material exchange for sex provided a dynamic for partner change, as new partners tended to give more valuable gifts. Third, the transactional nature of sex meant that men's desirability as sexual partners was closely related to their perceived affluence. The most affluent and desirable men were more likely to be HIV-infected, either because they came from more urban areas, or because they were villagers who could afford to maintain more than one partner and to change them frequently.

A fourth link between transactional sex and HIV was that it could create a barrier to condom use, as men generally had very negative attitudes towards condoms and refused to give much or any money in exchange for intercourse with a condom. The fifth connection between transactional sex and HIV infection relates to vaginal lubrication. If there is little lubrication during intercourse, there is a greater likelihood of abrasions and therefore infection. The group discussions revealed a general preference for lubricated vaginal intercourse, and sexual foreplay was often intended not only to please the woman but to arouse her enough that she would be naturally lubricated, as will be discussed in the next chapter. When girls or women had sex purely for material gain, however, and had little attraction for a particular partner, limited physical desire may have resulted in limited vaginal lubrication.

Unequal Power in Sexual Negotiation and Coercion

Men and women in our study often entered into sexual negotiation with different objectives. For men these included seduction and minimizing gifts, while for women they included resistance, seduction, and maximizing gifts. We found that the relative power women and men had in negotiating sexual encounters were shaped by factors at both the macro- and micro-level. Figure 7.2 illustrates how macro-level economic, kinship, and normative factors created the material and ideological conditions that encouraged transactional sex and overwhelmingly benefited men in sexual negotiation. Young men had more, and greater, economic opportunities than young women. They were more likely to have their own agricultural plots, more likely to own livestock, and there were more occupations open to them. Furthermore, they had far fewer domestic duties to compete with paid work. The most relevant social norms related to women's inferior status and to sexual culture as described in chapter 5. While young women regarded their sexuality as an asset to be exploited, they were nonetheless greatly concerned to maintain their sexual respectability. This was particularly important in the negotiation of transactional sex.

While these factors structured the broader context for sexual encounters, they also operated at a micro-social level, shaping people's motivations to engage in sexual relationships and the negotiation that occurred within them. Potential sexual partners' negotiating power for specific encounters largely was shaped by their individual attributes and their immediate circumstances, both of which could persist over time. At this level the different dimensions of power sometimes benefited women, as illustrated in figure 7.2. For example, a woman's physical attractiveness or her prestige as a sexual partner might improve her bargaining power, as has also been found elsewhere (Vanwesenbeeck et al. 1999; Tschann et al. 2002; Luke 2003). Both parties could also be disempowered by their need to present themselves differently in different social realms, as discussed in chapter 1. For instance, unmarried young women might wish to present themselves as sexually available to seducers but they also needed to ensure that they concealed sexual experience from their parents.

Immediate, circumstantial factors were also important: material need, the threat of physical force, or strong affection reduced a woman's bargaining power, while strong affection or intense sexual desire reduced a man's. In some circumstances, women or girls' scope to negotiate was severely constrained by men or boys' coercion, both nonviolent and, less commonly, violent. It is very difficult to collect representative and valid data on sexual coercion, primarily because of problems in clarifying local understandings of coercion and in overcoming inhibitions to disclose such experiences. Our findings broadly suggest, however, that sexual encounters in which a young woman did not want to have sex but was coerced were fairly common, especially when she previously had accepted a gift from the boy or man, or when an intermediary was involved in the coercion, particularly an authority figure.

In our study there was considerable evidence that the use of physical force in sexual encounters happened at least occasionally, but assaults that came to be dealt with in a quasi-judicial way as "rape" were rare. We also collected strong evidence that a minority of school girls experienced teacher sexual abuse in most schools; some of the implications of this widespread practice within the school system were discussed in chapter 4. In contrast, reports of incest and/or sexual abuse of small, prepubescent girls or boys were very rare in our study. In her anthropological work in rural Mwanza in the late 1960s, Varkevisser (1973) similarly recorded only one case of attempted rape of child under 10 years of age, noting that villagers perceived the perpetrator as foolish rather than evil. While our findings suggest that such practices almost never took place in the study area at the beginning of the twenty-first century, we cannot draw definitive conclusions about this. Sexual abuse of small children would have been considered so unacceptable locally that, if it occurred, it probably would have been extremely well hidden from researchers and villagers alike.

CONCLUSION

In this book, we have moved from examination of broad social norms shaping sexual culture (chapter 5), to consider patterns of relationships for unmarried young people (chapter 6), to then concentrate on the interpersonal level of sexual negotiation and coercion in this chapter. In the next chapter we will focus on the specific sexual activities which were common within young people's sexual relationships in rural Mwanza, and the implications which they have for HIV risk.

NOTE

1. Some material in this chapter was adapted from Wamoyi, Joyce M., Danny Wight, Mary Plummer, Gerry Hillary Mshana, and David Ross. 2010. Transactional sex amongst young people in rural northern Tanzania: An ethnography of young women's motivations and negotiation. *Reproductive Health* 7:2.

Chapter Eight

Sexual Practices

A large body of research on sexual behavior in sub-Saharan Africa has been assembled over the last three decades, largely prompted by the HIV epidemic. Numerous studies have examined the specific sexual practices of highly vulnerable groups, such as commercial sex workers or migrant laborers. In contrast, as discussed in chapter 6, research with the general population usually has focused on self-reported survey variables such as age at first sex, or number of sexual partners in the last year. With the exception of condom use—or lack thereof—little is known about what people in the general population actually do during sexual encounters. This is probably due to several interrelated factors, including: the widespread norm that it is improper to talk about sex explicitly; researchers' reluctance to investigate beyond the standard measures of sexual behavior for fear of being seen as intrusive or prurient; and concern that research findings would be perceived as offensive. It is striking, for instance, that studies focused on young men's abstinence rarely investigate masturbation, that is, the manual stimulation of one's own genitals, although this may be a main way of managing sexual desire without sexual intercourse (e.g., Izugbara 2007).

Detailed knowledge of sexual practices is important for several reasons. First, it is critical to understanding people's exposure to sexually transmitted infections and also to interpreting why the HIV epidemic is so virulent in sub-Saharan Africa. For example, a few researchers have postulated that widespread but unacknowledged anal intercourse has contributed to the intensity of the African epidemic (Brody and Potterat 2003). However, few studies have examined this practice in the general population, so it is difficult to draw firm conclusions about it. Second, detailed information about sexual practices helps us understand how the power imbalance between the genders works itself out in sexual encounters (e.g., Tamale 2006), and why some people might be motivated to change their sexual partners. Third, such knowledge is important in assessing what kind of biomedical or behavior change interventions might be realistic and effective. For example, to what extent could unprotected vaginal intercourse be substituted by other, lower risk sexual activities? And are there any practices intended to enhance vaginal intercourse which may positively or negatively influence disease transmission, such as shaving pubic hair, or avoiding intercourse during menstruation? And how might men's and women's preferences for vaginal lubrication affect their use of a microbicide gel to prevent HIV transmission during intercourse?

Prior to the recent spate of sexual research in sub-Saharan Africa, anthropological studies suggested that sexuality was almost exclusively linked to vaginal intercourse and the possibility of reproduction (Caldwell, Caldwell, and Quiggin 1989; Setel 1999b; Maticka-Tyndale, Tiemoko, and Makinwa-Adebusoye 2007). The most legitimate sexual relationships were those in which a couple intended to reproduce. While many ethnic groups considered pleasure to be acceptable or desirable within such relationships, non-procreative sexual activities generally were considered improper. In a review of literature on sexual behavior in sub-Saharan Africa, Caldwell and colleagues (1989) summarized: "[Sex] does not imply elaborate sexual activities . . . Reports are consistent . . . that most sexual relations are confined to the sexual act, with little foreplay or titillation." (Caldwell, Caldwell, and Quiggin 1989, 196)

HISTORICAL LITERATURE ON SUKUMA SEXUALITY

Some African societies have or once had initiation ceremonies, that is, ritualized events which marked formal admission to adulthood; these sometimes included instruction on sexual matters. Particular African initiation ceremonies have been described as educational, empowering, or important to the social cohesion and moral code of communities (Kenyatta 1938; Caldwell, Caldwell, and Quiggin 1989; Rwebangira and Liljestrom 1998; Hudson 1999). However, such ceremonies have rarely been a part of Sukuma culture, with the main exception being particular spirit societies (Stroeken 2006). Most anthropologists have attributed this to the relatively recent origin of this ethnic group. However, researchers have also noted that, historically, older girls and boys informally learned about sexual matters in their same-sex dormitories, and Sukuma mothers sometimes instructed their daughters in how to satisfy their husbands before they married (Cory 1953; Abrahams 1967; Varkevisser 1967; Allen 2000).

In the mid-twentieth century Tanner (1955b) conducted a study of sexual mores amongst married Sukumas. He described Sukuma sexuality as both "a matter of appetite" and "a means of ensuring their own survival through the continuation of the lineage in their legitimate children" (Tanner 1955b, 238). In comparison with some other African ethnic groups, sexual prohibitions and prescriptions were not very formalized, and there was no clear initiation into sexual life or marked end to it. However, after menopause women's sexual activity was believed to decline rapidly. Postmenopausal wives usually moved to share their sleeping quarters with their children, rather than their husbands, clearly illustrating the reproductive rationale for sex.

In his study Tanner (1955b) noted that a woman's personal hygiene was considered important to her sexual attractiveness, and to maintain this Sukuma women bathed regularly, plucked out armpit hairs to reduce odor, and plucked out pubic hairs because these were believed to cut men during sex. In Tanner's research, there was no taboo against sex during menstruation but it was restricted on the grounds of cleanliness. Tanner (1955b) also noted that sexually active girls or women wore strings of colored beads around their thighs, and these could serve multiple purposes, including sexually attracting men and holding traditional medicines intended to prevent conception or promote fertility.

This early ethnographic research described Sukuma sexual activity as largely restricted to vaginal intercourse, which reportedly was practiced with the man on top of the woman, lying side by side, or standing up "for surreptitious occasions" (Tanner 1955b, 240). For the man to enter the woman's vagina from behind was seen as insulting to the woman. Fondling was only practiced as a preliminary to penetration, usually taking the form of touching the breasts and stomach, but not the genitals, and the lips were not used for kissing on the mouth or any other body part.

Tanner (1955b) noted that Sukuma women were expected to be passive in sexual encounters to avoid association with prostitutes. However, he also reported that Sukuma men sought to excite and satisfy their partners during sex, specifically delaying their orgasm until their partner also climaxed, in order to increase their own desire and to prevent the woman seeking satisfaction elsewhere. Not waiting for the woman's orgasm was said to lead women to gossip about a man as "making love like a chicken" (Tanner 1955b, 239–40). Shortly after marriage it was considered unremarkable for a couple to have intercourse four or five times during one night, but this frequency was believed to decline as marriage went on. Later it was considered rare for a married couple to have intercourse every day, and if they did this might be seen as indulgent and detrimental to health.

RECENT RESEARCH ON SEXUAL PRACTICES
IN SUB-SAHARAN AFRICA

Very little research in sub-Saharan Africa has examined the range of sexual activities engaged in by prepubescent or adolescent youth. In high income countries, masturbation is generally boys' first sexual activity and young couples typically engage in what are regarded as progressively more intimate sexual activities over a series of encounters before they engage in vaginal intercourse (Gagnon and Simon 1974; Laumann et al. 1994; Wight and Henderson 2004). The extent to which this also takes place in sub-Saharan Africa is unclear.

In the case of masturbation, research findings are highly variable. For example, Kazaura and Masatu (2009) found that none of a sample of 2,749 unmarried 10–19-year-old Tanzanians reported masturbation unless they had also experienced vaginal intercourse; specifically, of those reporting vaginal intercourse, 36 percent of males and 17 percent of females reported masturbation. In a self-completion questionnaire survey of 12–24-year-old primary and secondary school students in Mwanza Region, Matasha and colleagues (1998) found participants had very little knowledge and few positive feelings about masturbation. In Zambia, secondary school pupils were found to have widespread misconceptions about the dangers of masturbation (Warenius et al. 2007), and in Zimbabwe a diverse sample of women and men reported little knowledge or practice of masturbation (Vos 1994). However, in contrast to these findings Setel (1999b) reports that masturbation was common and considered unproblematic amongst pubescent boys in Kilimanjaro, Tanzania. In Kenya, adolescents in an in-depth qualitative study reported experience of masturbation, and some of the older youth claimed to be "experts" in it, but they associated masturbation with embarrassment and shame (Balmer et al. 1997).

Studies in sub-Saharan Africa in the last two decades have largely confirmed that vaginal intercourse is the predominant sexual activity between couples, and sexuality is intrinsically linked to the possibility of procreation (Maticka-Tyndale, Tiemoko, and Makinwa-Adebusoye 2007; Bagnol and Mariano 2008). A preference for "dry" vaginal intercourse has been documented in some parts of Africa, for instance Malawi (Woodsong and Alleman 2008; Bisika 2009), Mozambique (Bagnol and Mariano 2008), Zimbabwe (Woodsong and Alleman 2008) and South Africa (Scorgie et al. 2009). Research on this topic suggests that the term "dry" (a translation from local languages) is not always meant literally, and instead may refer to a preferred state of a vagina as tight, warm, and/or not excessively moist during intercourse (Hilber et al. 2010). However, in some contexts women actively seek to reduce vaginal lubrication using herbs, powders, commercial products, or other substances. People who engage in such practices have reported that they increase men's pleasure as well as enhance women's sense of agency and identity, the sexual well-being of both sexes, and men's fidelity (Bagnol and Mariano 2008; Scorgie et al. 2009; Hilber et al. 2010). Nonetheless, some researchers have raised the concern that actively drying vaginas in such ways may increase the possibility of disease transmission through increased friction and abrasion (Brown and Brown 2000; Myer et al. 2005).

There is little evidence of the use of substances for "dry" sex in northern Tanzania. A multi-method study of intra-vaginal practices amongst women at high risk of HIV infection in Mwanza City found that women and their partners preferred a tight vagina, which was associated with virginity and fidelity (Montgomery et al. 2008). When water and privacy allowed, women cleaned their vaginas with fingers, soap, and water before and after intercourse, and/or wiped them dry with a cloth (Allen et al. 2010). However, only 5 percent of participants reported otherwise attempting to "dry" their vaginas, usually through the use of lemon juice, which has been associated with cervical abrasion and cell damage that may increase the risk of HIV transmission (Allen et al. 2010). In several research sites, including Mwanza, the lubrication provided by a vaginal microbicide gel was widely liked, particularly by women, many of whom say it improved their sexual pleasure (Woodsong and Alleman 2008; Montgomery et al. 2010).

The limited research on oral sex amongst young people in sub-Saharan Africa has rarely clarified whether it is assessing fellatio (the licking or sucking of a penis) or cunnilingus (the licking or sucking of a woman's genitals) (e.g., Bond and Dover 1997; Kazaura and Masatu 2009). This research suggests that oral sex is not common, and when it is practiced it is mainly as a supplement to vaginal intercourse rather than as an alternative. In Kazaura and Masatu's Tanzanian sample, 9 percent of males and 6 percent of females who reported vaginal intercourse also reported experience of oral sex, but none reported oral sex and not vaginal intercourse. In Zambia both masturbation and oral sex were perceived as perverse wastes of semen, in the understanding that ejaculation should only be for reproduction (Bond and Dover 1997). In marked contrast, in the self-administered questionnaire study by Matasha and colleagues (1998) 40 percent of sexually active primary school pupils reported that their first sexual act was oral sex. However, the authors noted that some primary school participants probably misunderstood the term and overreported oral sex, especially as only 4 percent of sexually active secondary school students in the same study reported it as their first sexual act.

Research on anal intercourse amongst general populations in sub-Saharan Africa has found it to be rare and widely condemned (Vos 1994; Bond and Dover 1997; Setel 1999b; Allen 2007; Mavhu et al. 2008; Ndinda et al. 2008). However, there is increasing evidence that heterosexual and homosexual anal intercourse are practiced to a limited extent. For instance, in Kazaura and Masatu's (2009) study of 10–19-year-old Tanzanians, 9 percent of males and 5 percent of females who had experienced vaginal intercourse also reported experience of anal intercourse, although it is unclear whether this was heterosexual or homosexual. Matasha and colleague's (1998) study found relatively high reports of anal sex amongst sexually active primary school pupils (9 percent) but not amongst sexually active secondary school students (0.4 percent), again suggesting those findings were biased by primary school pupils' misunderstanding and overreporting. Generally reports of anal intercourse have been highest amongst specific populations such as sex workers and their clients. For example, 41 percent of female sex workers in a Kenyan study reported having had anal intercourse (Schwandt et al. 2006), while 42 percent of truck drivers visiting sex workers in South Africa reported having experienced it (Ramjee and Gouws 2002).

In our study we found it challenging to collect detailed information on sexual practices during in-depth interviews with pupils and participant observation, so six group discussions and twelve follow-up in-depth interviews were conducted specifically on this topic within the broader series with young adults described in chapter 2. The next section will summarize our findings on the nature and prevalence of vaginal intercourse, foreplay, vaginal lubrication and drying practices, genital hygiene, other practices intended to enhance vaginal intercourse, heterosexual oral and anal sex, and male and female homosexual activity.

FINDINGS

Learning about Sexual Practices

In earlier chapters we mentioned several of the common ways that young people in rural Mwanza learned about sexual activities. Direct observation was one of the most important of these. Given the limited nature of housing, many small children shared rooms with their parents, and many older children and adolescents shared rooms with their older siblings and cousins. In almost every village multiple informants of both sexes mentioned having witnessed sexual intercourse in such a setting, sometimes on many occasions, and this made children sexually aware at very young ages.

For example, a Year 7 pupil explained why he started to bring girls to his room for sex at night: "He said that his elder brother's habit of bringing a girl to the house for sex was really causing him a lot of trouble, particularly when he heard them having sex and his body became excited and his penis became erect" [PO-00-C-3-3m]. Similarly, the 16-year-old daughter of a Village Chairman described how she frequently had sex in the presence of a younger sibling: "She said that she has sex with her boyfriend three times per week at home in the kitchen, where she sleeps with her 6-year-old sister. She said that her boyfriend comes at 10:00 p.m. and stays until about 5:00 a.m., but she thinks her little sister just sleeps through it" [PO-00-C-3-2f].

Beyond such experiences young people primarily learned about sexual activities from their friends, peers, and siblings. As described in chapter 6, prepubescent children often learned about sex while playing games in which they pretended to be adults and attempted to engage in intercourse. Once children reached their teens, peers often acted as role models to those who were reputedly less sexually experienced, by sharing, discussing and demonstrating their knowledge of sexual acts.

In addition, in all-male settings men sometimes talked informally about sex in front of boys, as a male researcher observed in the blacksmith's workshop in one village: "I heard how the blacksmiths spoke about sexual acts freely, regardless of their age. This made me think that the young boys who were present learn about sexual acts by overhearing what their elders say" [PO-01-I-1-3m]. As discussed in chapters 4 and 5, parents generally did not discuss sexual issues with their children. However, there were rare exceptions, such as when fathers discussed sexual matters in front of their sons around a *kikome* fire, or older women within a household advised adolescent girls and unmarried women on contraception.

In our study, very few adolescents in *MEMA kwa Vijana* trial control communities reported ever having learned about sex in a school program or other formal settings. Tanzania established guidelines for implementing HIV/AIDS and life skills education in schools in the mid-1990s (United Republic of Tanzania 2002). During the trial, however, process evaluation surveys found that such education only consisted of brief and superficial sessions in a minority of rural Mwanza primary schools.

Vaginal Intercourse

The data from all research methods suggested that, for most young people, first sexual encounters involved vaginal intercourse, or at least an attempt at it. Most girls and young women reported experiencing pain during their first experience of vaginal intercourse, clarifying that the pain went away within a day or two. However, a couple of young women said that their first experience was so painful that it led them to abstain from sex for several years afterwards.

In participant observation and in-depth interviews, boys who reported vaginal intercourse before adolescence said they felt pleasure even though they did not ejaculate. Numerous young men said that during their first vaginal intercourse they also experienced **kuchunyukila**, a painful tearing of the foreskin. Youths who experienced this typically were uncircumcised and/ or fairly young (prepubescent or early adolescent) at first intercourse. All of these informants reported this happened only once and that their foreskin healed soon afterwards.

Both young men and women considered vaginal intercourse to be the only normal form of sex. Some said it was beneficial for the health of men and women. For example, female respondents in different villages reported that male blood or semen from intercourse caused a woman to gain weight, to become more attractive, and/or to "sparkle" [PO-01-I-7-5f].

It was unusual for a couple to have a sexual encounter that did not involve vaginal intercourse. As one male group discussion participant explained:

P: I have only heard about one couple who just held each other, just touching each other, and then he left her. Afterwards he told me, "I went to my *geto* with that woman and I just held her and she touched me a little bit, ah, then we just left." I didn't understand why they left each other like that. [GD-00-C-12-3m]

Group discussion participants mentioned different positions that might be used for vaginal intercourse. Most thought that the woman lying on her back with the man on top was the most common position. In male group discussions this was said to be the position women enjoyed most, although some referred to it as "cockroach's death," because cockroaches turn on their backs when they die. Other positions mentioned were couples lying on their sides, or a woman bending while a man entered her from behind, which was referred to as "plucking vegetables" or "bending over" sex. Women in their 20s in one of the group discussions said that a man used this position if he did not like the woman. However, in participant observation a couple of male and female informants mentioned this position as a practical option when having sex outdoors, for example, when unable to lie down because the ground was wet after rain. In group discussions, female participants referred to a wider range of positions than men, including the woman being on top of the man. Women described this as "dipping oneself" or "measuring oneself." They explained it was done with a man with an exceptionally large penis, so that the woman could control the extent to which his penis entered her vagina and avoid discomfort or pain.

Although a woman's feigned resistance or passivity could be considered desirable during sexual negotiation, most young men praised women who were active during vaginal intercourse, for example, who caressed the man's body, said his name aloud, or moved their waists and hips. Unmarried young men ideally liked to have multiple orgasms during one sexual encounter, for example, to have vaginal intercourse and ejaculate two to four times in the course of several hours spent with a partner at night. Many young men reported experience of this, particularly when they were with a new partner. For example, a 19-year-old in Year 6 "said that every time he experiences his first orgasm during an encounter, which he said usually happens fast, he just continues until he has a second orgasm, and that is when he withdraws and they relax" [PO-01-C-3-3m].

Only rarely did young men report being impotent during a sexual encounter, and this was considered to be a very disturbing experience. For example, a different 19-year-old in Year 6:

> He told me about a day which he perceived as very bad, one which he will never forget. He said on that day he failed to have intercourse with his new lover after suddenly becoming impotent. He said they went to have sex after school but his penis did not become erect even when he caressed his lover. He said later he managed to have intercourse with her on "LY" Day. [PO-00-C-3-3m]

The use of condoms to prevent pregnancy or disease transmission during intercourse was rare in rural Mwanza at the time of the study. Findings related to condom use will be presented in chapter 10.

Foreplay

As already noted, it was unusual for young people to engage in sexual activity without having vaginal intercourse, and many encounters seemed to involve vaginal intercourse only, with very little other contact between the partners. However, young people sometimes also engaged in non-penetrative sexual activity as foreplay before intercourse. This was most typical of older youth and young adults who were more sexually experienced than early to mid-adolescents, and who also typically had more time and more conducive settings for a sexual encounter, for example, a partner's home at night rather than a field during a school break. Some people in relatively long-term relationships said that with more time they had learned more about their partners' desires and engaged in more foreplay, enhancing their mutual pleasure (*raha*).

Foreplay typically was reported to include caressing of breasts, waist (particularly where a woman might wear a string of beads), thighs, buttocks, vagina and/or penis. Both men and women usually reported liking such foreplay, and generally considered a sexual partner who engaged in it to be more experienced and enjoyable. For example, a Year 7 pupil described one of his most memorable sexual experiences:

> He was very happy on that day . . . because the girl was not shy, so they engaged in foreplay before they began intercourse. The girl touched his penis and other parts of his body, which made him feel much happier than he had

felt with his former lovers. He said they were so absorbed that they even forget
about the time, and his mother nearly discovered that he had a girl in his *maji*.
[PO-00-C-3-3m]

Similarly, women praised men who engaged in foreplay. For example, a
25-year-old woman who had a reputation as a *daladala*:

> She said sex with men from town is different from sex with those from the vil-
> lage, for in town a man entices you while men here just pound away and don't
> know how to caress or seduce. She said when a village man gets a woman, he
> pulls her and forcibly undresses her, sometimes even tearing her underwear in
> his hurry to have sex. [PO-00-I-4-4f]

Kissing on the mouth or sucking body parts, such as a woman's ears or
breasts, was unusual. As a 30-year-old single mother of two children explained:

> She said that Sukuma men in the village mainly touch breasts before or dur-
> ing sexual intercourse. She said a few who have travelled to towns know other
> sexual techniques like sucking the breasts, kissing the ears, or fondling other
> parts of the body. She said she thinks she would not enjoy sex with a man who
> kissed her on the mouth, and if she started a sexual relationship with one who
> did, she would end it. [PO-00-C-3-2f]

In the group discussions most young men also said that kissing was not
common in their village and it would appear very strange to kiss a village
girl in public or private. One man explained: "If you kiss a village girl, truly
she will be startled. She could run away" [GD-00-C-10-3m]. However, in one
village a few young men argued that it had become more acceptable to kiss
a girl in recent years, saying, for example, that a boy could kiss a girl's hand
during sexual negotiation.

Increasing Lubrication

Findings from all research methods suggested that villagers typically preferred the vagina to be moderately lubricated during intercourse. Many specifically said that the foreplay was to arouse and naturally lubricate a woman
in this way. As one young woman described: "He plays with her. Then if she
gets aroused, she gets a bit wet" [GD-00-C-12-f]. Similarly, a male group
discussion participant explained: "When you bring her inside your room,
first you have to start caressing her . . . on every part of her body so that she
becomes aroused. Yes, then you do it [have intercourse]" [GD-00-C-10-m].

In one female and two male group discussions, participants mentioned a
practice called *katelelo*, which they described as a way to arouse a woman
prior to intercourse that was practiced by members of the Haya, Zinza and

Longo ethnic groups. In *katelelo* a man was said to rub his penis against a woman's clitoris, stimulating the production of vaginal fluid until he was close to ejaculation himself, when they would have intercourse. Male participants specified that *katelelo* is done with the woman sitting on the man's thighs while they face each other. Male participants said that Haya, Zinza or Longo men or women sometimes taught *katelelo* to sexual partners from other ethnic groups, but this did not seem to be common.

Only a few villagers reported having experienced problems with excessively dry vaginal intercourse. They reportedly disliked this experience because it reduced sexual pleasure for both partners and possibly caused the girl or woman pain. For example, a young man in Year 7: "He told the other youth that he dropped his girlfriend [a 15-year-old Year 6 pupil] because she is dry as a log of wood during sex, so there is no sweetness/pleasure in the experience" [PO-99-I-1-2f].

Some young men and women said that if a woman's natural lubrication was insufficient then partners could use artificial lubrication instead. In all three villages group discussion participants said that the leaves of a certain plant were sometimes used to produce a slippery fluid that would lubricate a cow's vagina when it is unable to give birth, or a woman's vagina when it was too dry for intercourse. Use of such lubricants was reportedly uncommon and mainly done to reduce the possibility of painful intercourse if a girl was a virgin, her vagina was particularly small, or the boy or man's penis was particularly large. Participants reported that men who had sex with young adolescent girls might use this, and female participants gave an example of a teacher who was said to have applied such plant fluids to the vagina of a Year 1 pupil prior to intercourse.

Decreasing Lubrication

In both group discussions and participant observation, young men were much more likely to report problems with too much vaginal lubrication during intercourse rather than too little. Young women discussed their own lubrication preferences primarily in terms of men's tastes, as if their partner's pleasure or dissatisfaction determined their own. Young men made jokes and complained about intercourse with a woman who had a lot of vaginal fluid, saying it could be noisy, messy, and smelly, the penis might accidentally slip out of the vagina, and afterwards they disliked the need to wash themselves. For example, a 27-year-old milling machine operator:

> He said he did not care that [his girlfriend] has a new partner in the village because he had had sex with her many times before she moved away, and even again recently when she came back for the Christmas holidays. He said he noticed then that her vagina had become very large and too wet. He said that she

has lost her sexual attractiveness for him, and that when having sex with her the last time he had to think of his other girlfriend to be aroused enough to finish. [PO-99-C-2-1m]

Many group discussion participants commented that over-lubrication was disliked during vaginal intercourse, but the process of intentionally and thoroughly drying the genital area for "dry sex" rarely seemed to be practiced in rural Mwanza. Female participants said they did not believe there was any treatment for excessive lubrication, except to interrupt intercourse to wipe away fluid from the couple's genitals. Some male participants said that women could reduce vaginal fluid by putting lemon juice inside their vaginas, and two female participants mentioned this was a way to stop menstrual blood flow prior to intercourse, one of whom reported having done it herself.

Genital Hygiene Practices

Young people generally liked to bathe at home once per day using soap and water that had been carried to the household from a local water source. Some instead washed themselves at the water source itself, such as Lake Victoria or a hand-dug pond. Young people typically tried to clean their genitals more often if they were menstruating (for women) or sexually active (before and/ or after intercourse). However, the extent to which they were able to do this varied greatly depending on privacy and access to water. Limited access to water also influenced the extent to which villagers could clean themselves after urinating or defecating. Most people did not use anything to clean themselves after urinating or defecating, or they used a leaf taken from a nearby bush. Occasionally people instead used water, or paper torn from an exercise book. Old newspapers and manufactured toilet paper were very rarely available or used for this purpose.

Several common genital hygiene practices were intended specifically to make vaginal intercourse more enjoyable, including washing the genitals shortly before sex, pubic hair shaving or cutting, and avoidance of intercourse during menstruation. Less commonly, a minority of young men chose to be circumcised for this reason.

Most women and some men reported that they liked to wash in advance of an anticipated sexual encounter, although this often was not possible given many encounters were spontaneous, and access to water and soap was limited, as noted above. Occasionally, villagers reported that they had had vaginal intercourse while the woman was menstruating, as in the example above when a woman used lemon juice to reduce her menstrual flow. However, most young people said they did not have sex when a woman was menstruating because it was considered unclean and unpleasant. Occasionally, men also reported that this practice was dangerous because it could expose a man to disease. Instead, most couples said they did not have sex and simply slept together when a woman was menstruating, or occasionally had sex using non-penetrative methods (e.g., rubbing or fellatio) to relieve a man's sexual desire, as will be discussed in the next section. Some young men also reported seeking out a different sexual partner when their first-choice partner was menstruating.

Partway through the second series of in-depth interviews, spontaneous comments by respondents revealed that some youth shaved their pubic hair with a razor blade or cut it with scissors. To better understand these practices respondents were asked about them in the remaining ten male and sixteen female interviews (average age 19 and 18, respectively), in which seven males and four females reported shaving their pubic hair, and another two males and five females reported cutting it. Respondents who reported these practices were all Christian or had no reported religion. Some also said that their sexual partners cut or shaved their pubic hair. These respondents had all been randomly selected for in-depth interviews, with the exception of two HIV-positive women and one HIV-positive man.

When respondents were asked why they cut or shaved their pubic hair, most had difficulty explaining it, although they generally implied it was an issue of genital hygiene and/or sexual attractiveness. When asked what would happened if he stopped, for example, one young man laughed and said, "Hah—it would be dangerous! Yes, my hair would grow too much" [II-02-C-276-m]. Another reported that shaving pubic hair prevented scabies, an infection caused by a contagious parasitic mite:

R: You find that if he uses a—what—a razor blade, it helps to prevent scabies. Now if he uses a razor blade, a razor blade shaves it all off, it finishes everything. When hair start to grow again they cause scabies, and some people do not want to have scabies because it bothers them." [II-02-I-280-m]

Most of the respondents who said they did not cut or shave their pubic hair said they eventually would but had not yet done so because they were too young. The following excerpts from a 22-year-old man and then an 18-year-old woman illustrate how these practices were taken for granted:

I: Have you ever used a razor blade for any purpose?

R: Of course, I have used a razor blade to shave my pubic hair.

I: And do other people do so also?

R: Other people? Of course they do.

I: Even the children?

R: No . . . only older people are allowed to do so. [II-02-I-297-m]

R: I have used a razor blade to shave hair . . . on my private parts.

I: Do you know whether many people shave their pubic hair?

R: Yes.

I: Why do they do it?

R: I don't know.

I: Mm, and why do you do it?

R: Aah, I just shave myself. . . .

I: How old are the people who shave?

R: Maybe they begin when they reach 12 years of age, or later. [II-02-C-271-f]

The reported frequency of cutting or shaving pubic hair varied widely, from once per week to once every several months for both methods. Half of those who shaved or cut their pubic hair reported at least once accidentally cutting pubic skin while doing this, and bleeding a little as a result. For example, one young woman said, "I cut myself once and bled a little. It was not a wound, it was just a small cut. It healed by itself" [II-02-C-269-f]. Similarly, the HIV-positive woman described later in the book in case study 3.2 reported that she once cut herself with a razor blade while shaving her pubic hair, and afterwards she developed a genital rash around that area.

Razor blades were purchased for Tshs 20 ($0.02) each, were not shared, and were disposed of in a latrine after several uses. Scissors usually were a household pair that was shared by different family members.

Finally, in in-depth interviews and participant observation a small minority of male youths reported that they chose to be circumcised, or planned to be, because they believed this was more sexually attractive and hygienic, and/or it would reduce the possibility that they might become infected with a sexually transmitted disease. For example, a 21-year-old young man:

> He said that he has decided to be circumcised in order to avoid the shame that he feels when he is having sex with his partners. He said that if a partner discovers you are not circumcised, she refuses to hold the penis and insert it in her vagina, a situation which forces him to insert it himself. [PO-01-C-3-3m]

Similarly, during participant observation a few young women reported that they preferred to have sex with circumcised rather than uncircumcised men, but none reported the opposite. Young people's attitudes and practices related to circumcision will be discussed more in chapter 11.

Other Practices to Enhance Vaginal Intercourse

As in the early twentieth century, young Sukuma women in our study commonly wore a string of beads to attract men sexually and sometimes to prevent conception or increase fertility. These strings were almost always worn around the waist, not the thighs. Young women's waist beads were said to be a source of pride for them, and men were reported to be strongly attracted to women wearing beads and to become highly aroused when touching the beads during sex. For example, a 25-year-old unmarried man "said that because his lover is sexually experienced and wears beads, during their last sexual encounter he ejaculated four times" [PO-01-C-3-3m]. Similarly, a health educator in his 40s "said that the majority of women in the village wear beads in order to make their men feel good when they have sex. He said that if a woman is wearing beads then a man would caress them while having sex, and this would stimulate him to want more sex" [PO-02-I-4-1m].

A few young male respondents reported taking pills to enhance their experience of vaginal intercourse. These pills were said to be marketed to treat stomach ailments but had a side effect of long-lasting erections. They were purchased for Tshs 50 ($0.06) per pill in pharmacies in a district capital. A 22-year-old bicycle taxi driver explained how he used the pills in order to have sex with two girls one Christmas Day:

> He said he met one girl at the village center around 4 pm and convinced her to go with him to his home, where they had sex until around 5 pm. . . . Then at night he had sex with the daughter of the deputy head teacher. . . . He took her to his house where they had sex from around 9 pm to 2 am. . . . He told me that he ejaculated once with the first girl and three times with the second girl. I asked him if he felt very tired afterwards, and he said he did not because he has great stamina and he used a pill known as "Zentos" to enhance his sexual performance and power. [PO-99-C-2-1m]

Other Heterosexual Activity

In the group discussions, participants described occasional circumstances when a man and woman might engage in sexual activities without also engaging in vaginal intercourse. One woman said that when she menstruated her partner chose to do other activities, such as rubbing his penis between her breasts, in her armpit or against her navel. Other participants in that group said this was something that would only happen between emotionally intimate or committed

partners. In another group discussion there were third-person reports of a boy
or man rubbing his penis between a girl's thighs without penetrating her, particularly a man who was reported to do this to a child when his wife was away.

Female group discussion participants also described how on rare occasions a man might use his fingers, or an object like a bottle, to penetrate his
partner's vagina. One participant said she had a friend whose partner used his
fingers in this way because he was impotent. Generally, however, the women
believed that if a man used his fingers or an object rather than his penis he
had disdain for a woman, and he must believe her vagina to be dirty. Some
women reported that men sometimes smelled their fingers after touching
vaginal fluids, which made the girl or woman feel degraded.

Oral Sex

Oral sex was mentioned by male and female participants in all discussion
groups, usually referred to as sucking or licking of the genitals. Generally
participants were referring to fellatio, which everyone agreed was unusual.
They said it might only take place if a woman is menstruating or the man
specifically asks for it. Female participants generally agreed that women did
not enjoy performing oral sex on a man. However, women evaluated it in
contrasting ways, either as an expression of great intimacy or as a somewhat
degrading act. Some said it was only practiced by people who loved each
other very much, and one said it was used to arouse a man prior to vaginal
intercourse. One single woman said she had a married sexual partner who
gave her money to perform oral sex on him. Several other participants distanced themselves from the practice, saying it is something that town girls or
white people did, and that African men only had learned about it from white
people's videos. The most explicit condemnation of oral sex came from the
discussion group with younger female participants. One said people who
practiced oral sex were immoral. She gave an example of a girl who used to
go to discos who men in the village were said to fear because she liked sucking a penis during sex.

Most male group discussion participants also attributed fellatio to imitation
of pornographic movies or magazines. One young man said:

> *P:* I think it is just an issue of imitation. When we watch those X-rated movies,
> a young man decides to do what? To imitate. That is why these days young
> men tell you, "For me, if a woman does not massage my penis and put it in her
> mouth, truly I won't feel good." [GD-00-C-10-m]

Oral sex performed by a man on a woman was mentioned only briefly in
group discussions, and was reported to be extremely rare. A few female participants said that women enjoyed it, while most male participants thought it

would be unhygienic, particularly since vaginas are near the anus. They said they would not perform oral sex on a woman themselves.

Anal Intercourse

Heterosexual anal intercourse was mentioned in group discussions with both sexes in all three villages. A variety of expressions were used to describe it, such as "putting it in the back/rear" and "doing it in the anus." All the data sources suggested that anal intercourse was rare in remote Sukuma villages and was practiced only by a very small minority in larger, multiethnic villages, particularly fishing villages. A number of factors may have contributed to the relatively high prevalence of heterosexual anal intercourse in fishing villages, including the influence of sexual practices in nearby fishing camps, which will be discussed later in this chapter.

Female participants said that men sometimes wanted anal intercourse because they became dissatisfied with vaginal intercourse or wanted to try a new experience, for example, saying: "I'm used to here in the front, but let me now try it there in the back" [GD-00-C-11-f]. Some younger women said that anal intercourse could happen when a girl was tired of vaginal intercourse but the man wanted to have more sex, and another woman gave an example of a friend having anal intercourse because her partner wanted sex when she was menstruating.

Participants also said that men learned about anal intercourse by watching the pornographic movies occasionally brought to villages, and they were interested in trying it themselves afterwards. One participant gave an example of a drunkard who tried to have anal intercourse with his wife after watching a film, which became the subject of much village gossip. In addition, some female participants in the fishing village said that men sometimes used anal intercourse to punish or humiliate a woman:

> *P:* There are some men who see it in the video and think, "Today I'm going to try this with my woman." There is another one who does this to you with the purpose of shaming you, thinking, "Today I will teach her a lesson that she completely learns." [GD-00-C-10-f]

A couple of female participants reported that a woman might want to have anal intercourse because, if male blood or semen entered a woman through her anus, it was rumored that she might develop larger, more attractive buttocks. However, all female group discussion participants were personally negative about anal intercourse, typically saying that it was painful for a woman and that the purpose of the anus was for defecation, not sex. Some male participants also said this. Women often stated that if a man wanted to have anal intercourse with a girl or woman he must have contempt for her.

Generally male and female group discussion participants reported that the few women who engaged in anal intercourse were **wasimbe**, *wahuni* or *malaya* who did it for a lot of money or because they liked sex in general. One young man said, "It is mainly women who stay in towns who do things like that. Very few people from the villages could do things like that" [GD-00-C-10-m]. However, the few women who reported experience of anal intercourse described their partner either coercing or forcing them, in some instances when they were still in school, and universally reported the experience was painful. One female group discussion participant from a remote village reported that a sexual partner once asked her to have anal intercourse, but she refused. Three from the fishing village discussion said that they had engaged in it after insistence by a partner. One said that her partner told her it was not possible to transmit an infection via the anus, so unprotected anal intercourse was safe, unlike unprotected vaginal intercourse. However, she felt pain during the experience and this led her to end the relationship:

> *P:* He told me, "Listen, you know, Lord, we do it quickly there in front, but there at the back it is not even easy to get diseases. It's better to try. . . . Yes, now it is necessary to do it a different way." We had understood and respected each other for a long time, so I listened to him, but truly it really hurt me. Truly I was not satisfied with him. It forced us to completely give up on each other. [GD-00-C-10-f]

Two women from the same village said that they were forced to have anal intercourse by previous partners who were of Arab origin. One of the women was in Year 6 at the time and said that her anus was torn and painful for days afterwards, making it difficult for her to control her bowel movements. Some women from this village mentioned that a few men paid women a lot of money for anal intercourse. They said that such women had to bear the pain of the experience, because if they refused the men would demand their money back. One explained:

> *P:* There are even some men who can give you a lot of money to have sex there in the back. If you tell him, "Don't do it to me there," he tells you, "Am I your spare part? I gave you my money, and I'm not asking for it back. I just want it there [in the anus], at least a little bit." [GD-00-C-10-f]

In this quote, "spare part" refers to something kept as a back-up, suggesting the woman does not adequately value the man or his money.

Women's Sexual Pleasure and Masturbation

In the group discussions there were both implicit and explicit references to women's sexual comfort and pleasure by both men and women, for instance, when talking about women's preferred sexual activities and positions. In everyday social interactions during participant observation research, young women were much less likely than young men to discuss sex explicitly. However, in female company young women occasionally joked and talked frankly about sexual acts and their own satisfaction. Although women's potential for sexual desire and pleasure was recognized by both sexes, only a small minority believed that women primarily "make love to quench their lust" [PO-01-I-4-5f] rather than for material gain.

In each of the research methods, young men and women occasionally referred directly to the clitoris and its importance in women's sexual pleasure, as shown, for example, in the comments of the young man in case study 1.1. In the female group discussions some women described the intense pleasure felt when "finishing" having sex, which was a term commonly used to refer to orgasm for both men and women. Experience of orgasm seemed to be highly variable between women and for individual women at different times or with different partners. For example:

I: When you are with your boyfriends, do you have intercourse until you finish [have an orgasm]?

R: Mm, only once in a while.

I: Often you don't finish?

R: Mm . . . very rarely. I find that such a thing only happens with the boyfriend that I like/love a lot. [GDII-00-C-10-5f]

Female group discussion participants agreed that women were more likely to experience pleasure when more sexually experienced and when in long term relationships. Adolescent girls were considered the least likely to experience pleasure due to their physical immaturity, sexual inexperience, and the hurried nature of many of their sexual encounters.

Female participants in all of the group discussions mentioned various techniques that some women used to reduce or satisfy their sexual desires on their own. These included engaging in strenuous manual work, washing their genitals with cold water, or, the most widely mentioned option, splashing warm water on their genitals or wiping/rubbing them with a warm, moist cloth. When describing this last activity they used an expression that was otherwise used for wiping oneself after using a toilet. In the fishing village women said that some girls stood in the lake with their legs apart when they felt sexual desire, so that the waves touched their genitals. One reported that she had heard another girl saying: "When it itches me, I go to the lake to be beaten by a wave, pwa! pwa!" [GD-00-C-10-f]. In two villages it was reported that some women apply snuff or powdered tobacco to their vaginas to reduce their sexual desire. However, in both groups there was an argument as to whether this was actually a treatment for intestinal worms.

In two villages male and female group discussion participants reported that some women used their hands or an object to masturbate. One male participant explained, "Women penetrate themselves with their fingers, and move them in and out a bit like a penis" [GD-00-C-11-m]. Women also said that some use green bananas to penetrate themselves while masturbating, although this was uncommon and was attributed to particular *wasimbe*. In the fishing village, male and female participants also mentioned women using a shaped piece of wood to masturbate.

Male Masturbation

Taken together, the different data sources suggest that male masturbation was not uncommon in rural Mwanza, especially amongst adolescent boys, but unlike other common sexual practices it rarely was discussed amongst boys and young men, and when it was it was generally disparaged. Male group discussion participants varied greatly in their opinion about the degrees to which male masturbation was common or acceptable. For example, these issues were debated at length in the discussion in the most remote, inland village. The following excerpt highlights eight comments from that discussion, but some individuals may have commented more than once:

P1: Now I think that every man did it [masturbated] when he was still a boy. You can't say, "We just hear about people doing it elsewhere," because every boy does it. . . .

P2: I agree with him. Many boys do it before they begin sleeping with girls. . . .

P3: In this area, many boys masturbate, but in towns not many do it because it is easy to find a girl there. . . .

P4: For many people to know that there is such a thing, it has to be taking place everywhere. . . . Because how does one know about it if he hasn't done it himself? . . .

P5: It's very common. . . . And it's good because it doesn't affect someone's health, or anyone else's. . . .

P6: Actually, it can be a very bad thing. If it is truly done by almost all of the population, then that nation will be degraded. It should not be allowed . . . and if such a person is discovered, legal actions should be taken against him. . . . Because there is a man and a woman, and people should do it like that, in pairs. . . .

P7: I agree [that it is bad], because . . . if you masturbate, you will definitely find that you make yourself weak. . . . Your penis will become erect, but you won't be able to get a child.

P8: The people who do such a thing are very few, and they should know that it is a sin. . . . And in most cases girls will look down upon them. They will say, "Ah, if you go with this man, you will just sleep [without having sex]." He can't even do anything. [GD-00-C-11-3m]

Most young men considered masturbation to be primarily a response to failing to seduce a girl or woman. Some said it was done by boys who were too shy to seduce a girl or woman, and others said it might be practiced by any boy or man who had not had vaginal intercourse for a long period of time. One male participant said: "I myself may look for a girl and fail to get one. When it becomes evening, yes, then I have to do it that way. After I ejaculate, I don't have a desire for a woman any more" [GD-00-C-10-3m].

Few young men specifically said masturbation was sinful, but many perceived it very negatively, asking, for example, "Why do that? Why not look for a woman instead, even an *msimbe*?" [GDII-00-C-12-7m] As illustrated in the excerpt above, some youths believed male masturbation might sap a man's virility. One young man likened it to having sex with a goat:

R: I cannot do it. I might dream of having sex with a woman and startle myself awake only to find I have already ejaculated . . . you cannot blame yourself for that. But to touch there and do that thing on purpose, aah . . . you cannot do it until you ejaculate. In my opinion, it is a very bad thing. [Others do it] perhaps because they miss a lover and fail to tolerate it, like when someone rapes a goat. [GDII-00-C-10-6m]

Young women hardly mentioned male masturbation, beyond one group discussion participant saying that she had heard that men use soap for masturbation.

Sex between Males

Some male and female villagers said that they had never heard of the possibility of men having sex with men. It rarely came up in general conversation, although in several villages participant observation researchers were present when anal intercourse between males was mentioned during angry arguments. Each time, a man or a woman told another man that he should be sodomized, not meaning this as a threat but rather as a great insult.

In most villages the practice of intercourse between males seemed very rare. Almost all accounts about it involved one of three contexts: fishing camps, prisons, or unusual circumstances in people's homes. These accounts usually described situations in which the active partner was unable to have vaginal intercourse, which was his first choice for sexual satisfaction. As one participant explained: "Even when things are bad for a lion, it will eat grass" [GD-00-C-10-3m]. In such accounts, the receptive partner typically was described as being coerced or forced, and was believed to be weakened and to lose sexual prowess in the course of the act.

During both participant observation and group discussions, researchers heard rumors about men having anal intercourse in fishing villages and camps. For example, during an exchange between a Village Executive Officer, a teacher, and a photographer at a fishing village bar:

> One of them said that it is common for men to have anal intercourse at fishermen's camps. He said, "If you want to see the incredible things that fishermen do, you just go to the fishing camps on the islands." He said that here in this village there are also a few men who engage in anal intercourse, but few compared to the big fishermen's camps. [PO-01-I-7-5f]

On another occasion in the same village, the same female researcher was present when the subject of fishermen men having anal intercourse came up again. At that time, a Sub-Village Chairman was talking with a man whose wife had refused to have sex with him:

> They said that if your wife refuses to have sex with you, you might as well go to live at the fishermen's camps where the men have anal intercourse. When I asked if this was true, they said, "Even here in the village, people have anal intercourse. Don't you walk about at night?" They laughed very much then and said, "If you are willing to wear a pair of trousers [to appear like a man], we will take you to watch one night, if you are bold enough." I declined to do so. [PO-01-I-7-5f]

In the male group discussion in a fishing village, participants also reported that men and boys had anal intercourse in the nearest fishing camp. They said that boys went to fishing camps looking for employment, such as hauling nets or preparing food, and were either paid small amounts of money or were just given food and a place to sleep at night. It was said that fishermen who had stayed in the camps for long periods without having sex with women developed a great sexual desire and might have sex with these boys, sometimes raping them.

Men in this group discussion recounted several stories related to this. For example: "Among the fishermen you find that there are adult men and then there are boys. Now those boys are the ones who it is done to. It happens. My father was a fisherman and he told me about another fisherman who dared to do such a thing to a boy" [GD-00-C-10-m]. It was reported that men might threaten to expel a boy from the camps or to deny him food if he refused to have sex with them. One participant described this: "He tells him, 'Today if you don't want [sex], I will throw you out and you will fail to get a place to sleep'" [GD-00-C-10-m]. Some participants also mentioned the use of alcohol in such encounters, with fishermen buying boys *gongo* or other strong drinks and then raping them once they became drunk. One explained:

P: You find it is just a boy, one who is maybe 11 years old or older. You find he is already a drunkard, and the man makes him take *gongo* with one thing in mind: 'Wait until he gets drunk.' When they leave the *gongo* place, he drags him, and when they reach the bushes he finishes his problem. [GD-00-C-10-m]

In each of the male group discussions, participants also reported that anal intercourse was common in prisons based on what they had heard from others, some of whom had been incarcerated. In prison some men were reported to "turn other men into women" forcing them to have anal intercourse because they did not have access to women. For example:

P: There is one person who came from the prison who said he faced a very sad event there. When he first arrived he was given soft porridge and he ate it. Afterwards a man came and told him, "You have eaten another man's porridge so that man is going to sodomize you tonight." He was indeed placed together with that man and really that man used all his strength, yes, and his fellow prisoners assisted him in holding [the new prisoner] down while he was [sodomized]. [GD-00-C-12-3m]

Finally, two male group discussion participants from different villages mentioned a third setting in which sex between males might take place, not necessarily involving penetration. This was in homes in which a man or older boy attempted to have sex with a younger boy. One participant reported that his 10-year-old brother had told him his 14-year-old brother had attempted to have anal intercourse with him one night when the participant was away fishing on the lake. The younger brother woke up and reportedly avoided it. A similar account was given in another group discussion:

P: My brother told me that once when he was staying at my uncle's house in another village a neighbor came and slept in the same room, because he did not have a house on his land. . . . My brother woke up during the night, and . . . he saw that man going outside to the toilet. He looked on his thighs and found that he was totally wet, that is to say, he had the semen of another man on his behind and his thighs. [GD-00-C-12-3m]

In the female group discussions, participants also reported that male-to-male anal intercourse was not common in their villages, but they had heard that it happened in prisons. Some women in the fishing village said a few local men were believed to exclusively have sex with boys and men, and paid other men or boys to engage in it.

Sex between Females

The participants in the three female group discussions said that they had never heard of girls or women having sex together in their villages. However, participants in each of the three male group discussions described incidents in which girls or women were believed to have engaged in sexual "play" together, although they disputed whether this activity was simply practice for sex with men or sexually satisfying in itself.

One male participant said that his sister-in-law had told him how she used to have sex with a female friend:

> *P:* Let us not think that [same-sex sexual activities] are for men only, for women also do them. Because my sister-in-law once told me, "In the past, when we were children, I had sex with another girl." Then I asked her, "How could you have sex with a girl?" She said, "In fact one lies on her back and the other one goes on top. . . . We were teaching each other. One tells the other, 'Do this, do that,' you see. But one day mother found us, and we ran." [GD-00-C-10-m]

Similarly, another male participant described how he once found some girls having sex with each other outside. He said:

> *P:* We were coming from the farm around 4 pm. . . . We walked in the grass and we found some girls sitting there. They were naked, they had spread their legs like this. Now we said, "Let's wait and see clearly what they are doing." We found that indeed they were coming near each other in order to have sex. . . . So we said to them, "And what are you doing there?" Well, they had to run away. [GD-00-C-10-m]

DISCUSSION

Our findings on young people's sexual practices in rural Mwanza confirm several features of sexual behavior previously documented across sub-Saharan Africa. These include that vaginal intercourse was the most common and acceptable sexual act, that sex was almost always linked to the potential for reproduction, that the male sex drive was perceived as an essential biological urge, and that "deviant" sexual activities such as anal or oral sex were associated with external influences. The study also highlighted practices which are relevant to sexual health research and intervention work but which have received little or no prior attention. These include activities which may increase risk, such as the relatively high prevalence of unprotected anal intercourse in fishing camps and villages, or the common practice of shaving or cutting pubic hair in all types of villages. They also include low risk activities which may be widely practiced despite negative attitudes and misconceptions about them, most notably male masturbation. We will discuss each of these issues below.

Vaginal Intercourse

In our study it was reported that sexual activities such as stroking and caressing almost invariably led to vaginal intercourse in the same encounter, while oral sex and other non-procreative activities were unusual and generally viewed negatively, as has been found elsewhere in sub-Saharan Africa (Maticka-Tyndale, Tiemoko, and Makinwa-Adebusoye 2007). Even those prepubescent children who played at having sex attempted to have vaginal intercourse, perhaps influenced by having observed it in shared sleeping rooms. The finding that young people generally preferred moderately lubricated vaginal intercourse was in keeping with much of the research elsewhere in sub-Saharan Africa. No young people in our study expressed a preference for very dry vaginal intercourse, which has been reported to be desirable amongst several ethnic groups in southern African countries, and there were few reports of substances being inserted specifically to dry the vagina prior to intercourse.

We found that male sexuality was understood by both sexes to be driven by a fundamental biological urge: young men were believed to need intercourse on a fairly frequent basis, and when in exceptional circumstances women were not available for extended periods of time, men might resort to anal intercourse with other men. The belief that sexual desire is central to men's essence has been found across sub-Saharan Africa, including Sudan (Allen 2007), Zambia (Bond and Dover 1997), Zimbabwe (Vos 1994) and South Africa (Scorgie et al. 2009). However, we have seen little prior research that documents men's sense of virility and pleasure relating to how many times they have intercourse and ejaculate within one sexual encounter, beyond a couple of incidental mentions in broader accounts (Schapink et al. 2001; Steinberg 2009). Our finding that young men preferred to have intercourse multiple times within one encounter suggests there may be a greater exchange of fluids than typically assumed in survey questions about the frequency of encounters. It also has implications for condom use, if, for example, a young man needs to use three condoms to prevent disease transmission during one encounter. These findings highlight the need for more exact data about sexual practices when assessing risk behaviors.

In their review of research on sexual behavior in sub-Saharan Africa, Caldwell and colleagues (1989, 198) commented on the role of women's pleasure:

> A contrast may exist between the cultural regions in the extent to which women enjoy sex, especially within marriage, but the evidence is so scattered that any

certainty is impossible. The point is important because it may bear some connection to the frequency of relations in sexual networks and to the speed of
transmission of sexually transmitted diseases. For East Africa there are a number of descriptions of female enjoyment of sex within marriage and the assumption of their husbands that this must be so and that even traditional husbands
must ensure this.

In our study, when young people were asked about pleasure during sexual
encounters, it was not unusual for both men and women to report experience
of it, particularly women in their twenties, who typically had more sexual
experience and freedom than teenage girls. When questioned, young villagers often described foreplay as specifically intended to arouse the woman
and increase vaginal lubrication to make intercourse more comfortable and
enjoyable for both sexes. In group discussions some men expressed their concern to avoid pain for women and sometimes also voiced an expectation that
both partners would experience orgasm during an encounter. In the women's
group discussions, some participants talked about their own sexual pleasure
and described sexual encounters in which they took the initiative in deciding
on the activity or position. These findings that young rural women sometimes
successfully communicated and asserted themselves in having their desires
met during sexual encounters are promising, suggesting a potential to reori-
ent such communication and negotiation skills within intervention programs
towards safer sexual practices.

However, these observations are qualified by findings that many women
perceived their partners' pleasure as more important than their own. For
example, women's accounts of engaging in sexual activities other than
vaginal intercourse to satisfy their partners when they were menstruating
suggested they were having sex due to men's desire, not their own. These
findings are similar to those elsewhere in sub-Saharan Africa, in which
women reported that their first concern was to please their partner sexually
in order to encourage his fidelity and related economic and health benefits
(Woodsong and Alleman 2008; Mlangwa 2009; Montgomery et al. 2010;
Hilber et al. 2010). Furthermore, men and women's discussion of the use
of lubricants for men's sex with young females suggests a lack of mutual
arousal and, possibly, consent.

Anal Intercourse

Our study's findings on anal intercourse were limited, as most reports were
third-hand and there were only a few first-person reports by women who
had experienced it, and none by men who sought or practiced it with either
women or men. Nonetheless, given the sparse research on this practice to

date, our findings offer some new insights on it within general African populations. Young men and women reported that heterosexual anal intercourse was rare but could occur for different reasons, such as a man's dissatisfaction with vaginal intercourse, his wish to punish or abuse a woman, or his desire to experiment after seeing a pornographic video. Notably, one woman in the group discussions was persuaded to try anal intercourse by a man who claimed it did not transmit infections like vaginal intercourse. All the women who reported experience of anal intercourse said they felt substantial pain or discomfort during and afterwards, and more generally women said that a man who wants to engage in anal sex has contempt for the woman. This is in line with previous research with Kenyan sex workers that found women did not initiate anal intercourse and associated it with coercion (Schwandt et al. 2006).

The tendency in rural Mwanza to associate "deviant" sexual activities, such as anal or oral sex, with urban life, prostitutes, and/or Western pornographic videos is in line with South African research showing that knowledge about anal intercourse is increasing due to the influence of television programs (Ndinda et al. 2008). In our study anal intercourse between men was also believed to be fairly common in all-male settings such as prisons and fishing camps, where the receptive partner typically was coerced or forced. In our study villages, most accounts of heterosexual and homosexual anal intercourse came from large, multiethnic fishing villages where immigration, emigration, wealth, video show frequency, and fishing camp experience were higher than in more remote and conventional villages. As discussed in chapter 6, fishing villages also seemed to have a higher prevalence of other sexual risk practices, such as multiple and/or concurrent partnerships for both men and women. Our findings thus support a recent review that has identified fishing communities as particularly high risk rural settings in sub-Saharan Africa (Béné and Merten 2008).

Low-Risk Sexual Activities

Study of sexual practices should not only highlight areas of potential risk but also whether low risk activities may be common or acceptable, as this can be important in the development of culturally appropriate sexual health interventions. Our finding that some young couples occasionally engaged in non-penetrative sex, such as rubbing a penis against a woman's body when she was menstruating, suggests that there is potential to promote such activities as low-risk alternatives to unprotected vaginal intercourse.

We were unable to determine the prevalence of male masturbation in our study population, but overall our findings suggest this was a fairly common but very private practice for adolescent males. Although it was probably practiced by many boys and young men, negative attitudes and misunderstandings about it were widespread, such as the belief that it reduced a man's virility and potential to reproduce. Few young people seemed to perceive masturbation positively as a safe and potentially satisfying alternative to unprotected vaginal intercourse, and some instead perceived it as more harmful. These findings emphasize the need for sexual health interventions to directly address both high and low risk sexual practices, to ensure that participants have an accurate understanding of their relative risk.

Genital Hygiene Practices

Until the recent research on the feasibility and acceptability of vaginal microbicides, few studies examined genital hygiene practices in sub-Saharan Africa. At the beginning of the twenty-first century, we found that very limited access to water, soap and paper in most rural settings made maintenance of genital hygiene and cleanliness difficult. Some existing genital hygiene practices may have reduced sexual health risk (e.g., avoidance of intercourse during menstruation) while some may have increased it (e.g., regular use of razors to shave pubic hair). Notably, the practice of reducing pubic hair to enhance sexual encounters seems to have been common amongst the Sukuma at least since the mid-twentieth century (Tanner 1955b). However, the technique has changed from plucking hair to cutting or shaving it. The practice of entirely removing public hair may increase the risk of disease transmission during intercourse through increased roughness and abrasion, e.g., from contact with stubble, or through cuts introduced by razors. As such, it warrants further study.

CONCLUSION

In the preceding chapters our examination of the sexual behavior of unmarried youth in rural Mwanza moved from the macro-social to the micro-social level, first addressing norms and then relationships before considering negotiation and specific activities. We will now turn to married young people's sexual relationships, beginning with four case studies which describe typical young people's experiences of marriage and/or divorce. In the final chapters of the book we will then examine broader beliefs and practices related to reproduction and sexually transmitted infection.

Case Study Series 2

"He Told Me, 'Just Come and Live at My House'"

Typical Young People's Experience of Marriage and Divorce

This case study series focuses on the lives of four young people who married and/or divorced during the course of our study. It describes their family and school backgrounds, socioeconomic activities, and sexual relationship histories in detail, as well as their experiences of married life. Bahati's case study (2.1) describes a poor young woman who engaged in premarital sex primarily to meet her subsistence needs. She later met a man and within a month formally became engaged and married him in the hopes of creating a more financially secure future. Joseph's case study (2.2) details the elopement of a 25-year-old man and a 16-year-old girl, particularly the preparation that took place within the groom's parents' household before the elopement. Zawadi's case study (2.3) describes how a single young woman became pregnant and then married simply by moving in with her most recent sexual partner. Her experiences also illustrate other important themes, such as the poor diagnosis, treatment, and prevention of sexually transmitted infections, and how a young woman's concurrent sexual relationships could bridge different populations of men. Finally, Tereza's case study (2.4) provides an example of the greater sexual freedom and social stigma that young, childless women often experienced after divorce.

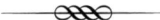

2.1. BAHATI: A YOUNG WOMAN'S TRANSITION FROM SCHOOL TO MARRIAGE

The first time Bahati was interviewed she was 15 years old and in Year 5 of a *MEMA kwa Vijana* control community primary school. She participated in a paired interview with her friend, Asha, a 14-year-old who was also in Year 5. The same interviewer then interviewed Bahati again alone two and one half years later, when Bahati was out of school and married.

259

Bahati was her mother's first child and her only child with Bahati's father, who Bahati had never known. Bahati's mother was a Zinza farmer and beer brewer. She had remarried and had five other children, and was expecting a seventh child at the time of the interview. Bahati's stepfather was a drunkard who beat both Bahati and her mother. As Bahati described: "When he comes back home from a beer shop, he starts beating me without good reason. . . . He beats my mother even if she is pregnant, he has no mercy, he just beats her" [II-99-C-51-f]. Such extreme domestic violence was unusual in rural areas.

Because of problems with her stepfather, at the time of the first interview Bahati was living in a maternal aunt's household. Bahati's polygynous uncle was the head of that household of eleven people, which included another co-wife. Within her uncle's household Bahati carried out the domestic and farming responsibilities typically expected of adolescent girls. She also cultivated and sold cotton on her own, from which she had earned Tshs 780 ($0.94) in the most recent season, which she used to buy two blouses and a skirt. During her first interview Bahati said that she liked school very much and that she hoped to go to secondary school. One day she said she also hoped to marry "a religious man who does not drink liquor or cause chaos or constantly abuse and beat his wife or children" [II-99-C-51-f].

During that interview Bahati said that she had a boyfriend who recently began attending her Seventh Day Adventist church. The boy wrote her letters stating that he liked/loved her and hoped to marry her. Bahati said that they had not had sex, and she intended to remain abstinent until she married, because this was what was dictated by her faith. She and Asha, who was also a Seventh Day Adventist, discussed this during the interview:

B: The bible does not allow adultery.

A: The bible does not allow it, but we just do it.

B: You shouldn't commit adultery.

I: You just do it?

A: Yes.

I: Bahati . . . did you ever have the desire to do it, but the bible did not allow it?

B: Yes. . . .

I: Whenever you strongly feel like doing it, what do you normally do? . . .

B: I just live with it. [II-99-C-51-f]

During her second interview Bahati said that she and the boy she had liked during the first interview had begun to have sex when she was 16 years old and in Year 6. That sexual relationship continued for over a year. The first time they had sex under a tree near her house in the evening and he gave her Tshs 2,500 ($3) which he had earned from fishing. After years of refusing his and others' sexual requests, she explained why she finally consented:

B: During that period at school we were always being asked about uniforms and shoes, and, moreover, I was a prefect [so expectations of her were high]. . . . The teacher wouldn't like to see a uniform with a hole. If he discovered that it was torn he would tell you to go to buy a new uniform. If he saw our shoes were tattered . . . we were beaten and sent back home. I just had to have sex to get that money, so that I could buy shoes. [II-02-C-251-f]

Bahati said that the second time she had sex with that boy he gave her Tshs 1,500 ($1.80), which she used as capital to start a fish frying business. Her business became profitable and she used what she earned from it for required school supplies and to build a stall in the village center, where she sold peanuts, *mandazi* and *uji* that she and her aunt prepared at home. The third time that they had sex the boy did not give her money but gave her a pair of *kanga* instead. They continued to meet for sex about once per week over the next 1–2 years, often meeting in his room during the night. Bahati said that she feared getting pregnant during that time but she never attempted to prevent pregnancy as she did not know any birth control methods. She said that after they became sexually involved this young man no longer spoke of marrying her. He also increasingly travelled as a fisherman so he was away from the village a lot. When she learned one day that he had another sexual partner, she ended the relationship.

During her second interview Bahati reported that the boy described above was her only sexual partner before she got married at the end of Year 7. However, her sexual knowledge increased in other ways during her final year of school. For example, when she was going on an errand to a larger village she was asked by a friend of her brother's to purchase a pack of 12 condoms for him, for a price of Tshs 500 ($0.60):

B: At that time I didn't know that it was condoms, he just told me to go to buy him *Salama* [the condom brand name]. . . . At the shop I saw the word "*Salama*" and "condom" on the cover. I thought, "Mm! Ooh! So condoms are like this." I didn't open them. . . . The shopkeeper asked me, "Do you use condoms?" Mm, I asked him, "What are they used for?" He said, "You buy them without knowing their use?" I told him, "But I . . . I have only been sent, I didn't know what they were." Ee, he gave them to me and I took them to my brother's friend. [II-02-C-251-f]

Bahati reported that she was approached by a number of boys and men who sought to seduce her during her final year of school but that she refused them all. This included one teacher who verbally abused her in class after she rejected him:

B: He tried to seduce me, but I refused, so he uttered some filthy words about me in class. And then when he heard that I had become engaged he continued behaving insultingly.

I: What did he say to insult you?

B: Just a lot. . . . Sometimes you are told that you are prostitutes. . . . He just insults you. But I knew that I was not the one who did something wrong. . . . He had told me that I should have sex with him, and I just refused. [II-02-C-251-f]

Five months before her second interview, Bahati had met her future husband, a fisherman and a Seventh Day Adventist from a neighboring village. They became engaged almost immediately. She explained:

> *B:* We just met . . . he was visiting a relative in my village. . . . And I was on a bicycle coming from the well. Yes, he stopped me. . . . He said he wanted to become engaged to me. Mm, I told him, you just come to my uncle's house to propose marriage. Then he named the day he would come, and I went to inform the people at my home.
>
> *I:* What did your uncle say?
>
> *B:* He said, "Let him come." [II-02-C-251-f]

Bahati's uncle and her future husband met and agreed on the marriage and the terms of bridewealth. The next day Bahati's future husband gave her uncle and mother Tshs 100,000 ($120), two cows, three goats, and one pair of *vitenge* (high quality, colored, patterned cotton cloth). Three days later, they were married at a ceremony in a Seventh Day Adventist Church.

When asked why she decided to marry when she did, Bahati said that she would have preferred to continue in school but she had not passed her Primary School Leaving Examination. She had wanted to repeat Year 7 and the examination using a false name, but her mother said she could not afford it. Moreover Bahati did not have a home where she was welcome to live long-term, because her stepfather was abusive, her uncle resented supporting her within his household, and her mother was dependent on one or the other:

> *B:* My mother was being mistreated by her husband. . . . Sometimes she was chased away, and when she was chased away, I was too. . . .
>
> *I:* So you decided to just get married?
>
> *B:* Yes. . . . My mother is poor. . . . We were living desperately there at my uncle's place. . . . When I was schooling my uncle wouldn't even give me money to buy exercise books. He said, "Your mother is the one who gave birth to you. I didn't beget you." [II-02-C-251-f]

Bahati said that she did not have sex with her husband before they married. However, she believed her husband knew she had had a prior sexual relationship and that he did not perceive it as a problem:

> *B:* Some youths were talking about me after hearing that he was going to marry me. . . . They would say, "Ee, your fiancée is already engaged [has a different sexual partner]," and he would say, "Even if a girl has already been engaged, is she finished? So what if she was engaged, because I hadn't proposed to her at that time. . . . Does it mean that if you go [have sex] with a person she becomes your wife?" Mm, he said, "An unmarried girl doesn't belong to you alone, she belongs to everybody." . . .
>
> *I:* So your husband asked you about it?
>
> *B:* No, he didn't ask me. We just remained quiet about it up until now. [II-02-C-251-f]

At the time of the second interview Bahati was living in her mother-in-law's household. Her husband was gone for extended periods fishing on Lake Victoria and nearby islands. When he was away she shared their one-room house with her sisters-in-law. During the rainy season she earned money by growing peanuts, cassava, and sweet potatoes and selling them at the market. When her husband was home he sometimes helped her cultivate their plot. She also participated in an all-female *rika* of married and unmarried women that cultivated other people's farms for a fee. During the dry season Bahati instead earned money by preparing and selling fried fish, cassava, tea, *uji*, and *mandazi* in the village center. Like many young married women in our study she referred to herself as a "newcomer" in her husband's village, and said that she had not yet made any friends, but she nonetheless seemed to be comfortable and contented with her new family and home.

Bahati had not considered contraceptive use after marrying, and she laughed when asked whether she might ever use a method to prevent sexually transmitted infections. She was uncertain about the general purpose, safety, and use of condoms, let alone the possibility of negotiating their use with her husband:

I: Will there ever be a day when you might agree to use condoms?

B: No. . . .

I: Why not?

B: [Laughter] . . . I don't know why not . . . or what they prevent. I don't know. . . . I just can't.

I: Do you think it is safe for a person to use condoms?

B: I just don't know. [II-02-C-251-f]

Despite these comments, Bahati was aware that she might be at risk of HIV/AIDS:

I: Have you ever been taught about AIDS?

B: Not yet. . . .

I: Do you think you could get AIDS?

B: Yes, perhaps I could get it.

I: Why do you think you could get it?

B: The man perhaps. . . . If my husband makes love with other women outside of marriage, and if those women perhaps have AIDS viruses. [II-02-C-251-f]

Bahati's comment that her husband might have extramarital relationships which put her at risk was astute, given that—like her first sexual partner—her husband was a fisherman, and fishermen typically engaged in more risk practices than other villagers, as described in chapters 6 and 8. In fact, when Bahati participated in the *MEMA kwa Vijana* 2001–2002 survey three months after marrying and two months before her second in-depth interview, she tested positive for Trichomonas, a sexually transmitted infection that was found in 27 percent of the young women who participated in that survey (Ross et al. 2007).

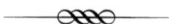

2.2. JOSEPH: A YOUNG MAN'S ELOPEMENT WITH A TEENAGE GIRL

During a participant observation visit to a *MEMA kwa Vijana* control village, a 25-year-old son (Joseph) within a Catholic Sukuma host family eloped with a 16-year-old girl (Leticia). Neither individual was a trial member because Joseph left school before the trial began, and Leticia completed Year 7 in a non-trial primary school during the trial's second year. One of the female researchers witnessed Joseph and his family prepare for the elopement for one week before it happened, and also was present when the new daughter-in-law was welcomed into the household the day afterwards. Approximately one year later, that researcher and a new female researcher returned to the household and heard details of what happened during and after the elopement from various household members, including the bride and groom.

Joseph supported himself by owning and staffing a kiosk in the district capital. He said he moved there because kiosk business in rural areas was slow and his relatives there expected to receive items from him for free. He had a child from a prior sexual relationship and he had tried to elope with a different girl at an earlier date, but she rejected him at the last minute. It is unclear how long Joseph and Leticia knew one another before their elopement. Prior to it, the only person in Joseph's family to have met Leticia was an aunt, who reportedly helped Joseph select Leticia to marry. Joseph returned to the village from the district capital one week before the elopement, in order to obtain his parents' permission and make necessary preparations.

To prepare for the elopement, Joseph sought out people who owed him money for repayment, while his younger brothers also collected money and clothing for him, and his mother planned a special meal for her new daughter-in-law's arrival. The researcher noted:

> Joseph will bring the girl on Tuesday. He went today to discuss it with her, using a plan developed by one of his aunts. Tomorrow one of his younger brothers will go to the district capital to fetch some clothes, and he has already secured a bicycle. His sister said, "Tonight my mother will not sleep at all. I think she is very happy to get a daughter-in-law." [PO-01-C-2-5f]

Throughout that week, everyone in the household talked about the planned elopement openly and often discussed the value of elopement relative to formal engagement and a wedding. Elopement was perceived as a good thing for a groom. Joseph's mother suggested that a man who eloped took more initiative and felt more attachment to his bride than a man who married formally:

Over a meal they talked about a man who had thrown out his wife. Someone asked if the man had been forced to marry that woman, but they said he had not been forced by anyone. Joseph's mother added, "If he had had a formal engagement with her, perhaps you could say that he was forced, but he liked/loved her so much that he eloped with her." Joseph laughed and said, "If you elope with a woman, does it mean that you like/love her that much?" His mother said that if you elope with a woman, it means you like/love her so much that you don't need advice from other people about whether to marry her or not. [PO-01-C-2-5f]

The likelihood that Joseph would save himself and his family a substantial amount of money by eloping rather than marrying formally may have contributed to the happy mood within the household, but this rarely was mentioned. In other discussions elopement was described in terms implicitly insulting to a bride. For example Joseph's 16-year-old sister, Pendo, described the recent elopement of an acquaintance as "a wedding escorted by dogs." [PO-01-C-2-5f] Joseph's mother made similarly disparaging comments about the likelihood that that Pendo, her daughter, would elope, claiming that no man would value her enough to ask her parents for her hand in marriage. For example:

One of Joseph's younger brothers said that he wants his own wedding to be very big, and he wondered where his parents will get the cattle for it. His mother said that when Pendo elopes they will only receive chickens. He replied, "Why should she elope and not have a formal wedding?" His mother said, "Who would become engaged to such a black [dark-skinned] girl?" . . . Several days later, Joseph's mother told me that she was sending Pendo to fetch water for one of the last times, because Pendo will leave the household as soon as she has finished school. I asked her where Pendo will be going, and she said, "She will just elope. Where else could she go?" [PO-01-C-2-5f]

The researchers learned the details of Joseph and Leticia's elopement a year later, when Leticia chatted about it with a researcher and another young woman:

Leticia said that the day she eloped she had taken a pail out in the evening, as if she were going to the drying area to collect *udaga* [pealed fermented cassava roots, used to make flour]. Her sister accompanied her. On the way, Leticia put the pail down and told her sister that she was going to the village center, and that when she came back they would then go to fetch the *udaga*. Joseph was waiting for her at the center and carried her away on a bicycle. Leticia said that they reached his village at 10 pm and all of the people in the household had already gone to bed. Her friend asked why they decided to leave so late in the evening, and Leticia replied, "Have you ever heard of anyone eloping in daylight?" [PO-02-C-2-6f]

On the day after the elopement, Joseph's younger brother and sister stayed home from school, because they wanted to meet their brother's bride, and

Joseph's mother prepared a special meal. The couple stayed there for several days before returning to Joseph's home in the district capital together. One informant said that Leticia's parents sought her out there to try to convince her to return home, but she refused. Leticia later told a researcher that her father had not spoken to her at all the first time that she visited her parents' household after the elopement.

Despite Leticia's parents' initial displeasure, an elopement fine eventually was negotiated between the two families. Joseph contributed part of the money from his own earnings. His father sold two of the household's four cows to raise the rest. Some other youths in the household resented this, because the loss of household assets meant less possible future bridewealth for them. However, they did not say this in their father's presence. Despite these efforts to pay the agreed elopement fine quickly, by the time the researchers returned to the village one year later Leticia's parents had not received most of the collected amount. In the interim, one of Joseph's brothers had died suddenly and Joseph's father reportedly used some of the money on alcohol and womanizing while he was mourning.

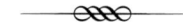

2.3. ZAWADI: A YOUNG WOMAN'S TRANSITION FROM SCHOOL, THROUGH UNMARRIED YOUNG ADULTHOOD, TO MARRIAGE

Zawadi was 16 years old and in Year 6 of a *MEMA kwa Vijana* control community school when she participated in an in-depth interview. The same researcher then interviewed her again two and one half years later, when she was living in a rented room with her husband and two-month old baby near Mwanza City.

During the first interview Zawadi reported that she had been living with a widowed maternal aunt for the previous six years. They had lived in a village center in a house made of bricks and iron sheeting, for which her aunt paid Tshs 2,000 ($2.40) per month in rent. Zawadi participated in all domestic and farming chores within her household, and her aunt paid for some of her clothing and school fees. Zawadi's father and mother had separated when she was very small and they lived in other villages. Her mother had remarried as the second wife of a polygynous traditional healer who eventually had four wives. Zawadi and her family were Catholics of Kerewe ethnicity.

The year before the first interview Zawadi had earned Tshs 19,000 ($22.80) cultivating her own cotton crop, which she used to buy a school uniform, other clothes, and a bed sheet. Zawadi enjoyed school, although she disliked sometimes being beaten by teachers, as happened once when she missed school for three days to visit a relative.

During her first interview Zawadi reported that she first had sex in an empty building near her village center when she was 14 years old and in Year 4 of primary school. Her partner was in Year 5 and their relationship continued for five months. She said that, after each sexual encounter, he would give her exercise books, pens, and/or Tshs 500 ($0.60) to Tshs 1,000 ($1.20). She broke up with him because she believed he had many sexual partners.

When Zawadi was in Year 5 she said she began a sexual relationship with an out-of-school villager that lasted over one year, until the time of the first interview. He had once told her that he also had another, out-of-school sexual partner, but she decided that was acceptable. Four months after she began her relationship with him she also began to have sex with a third man, an unemployed Mwanza City resident who sometimes visited his relatives in her village. At the time of the first interview Zawadi considered that ten-month relationship to also be ongoing, although she had not seen the man for 3–4 months. Finally, two months before the first interview Zawadi had moved to her grandmother's village, where she was receiving treatment from a traditional healer for a painful genital condition. While living there she had begun a sexual relationship with a fourth man, who ran a local kiosk. After their sexual encounters he gave her body oil, soap, laundry detergent, kerosene, and/or Tshs 1,000 ($1.20) to Tshs 2,500 ($3), which she used to purchase underwear and food. Zawadi said that none of her three current partners knew about each other.

Zawadi reported that it would be very difficult for her to ever abstain from sex, because she relied on her partners to obtain necessities and she sometimes experienced pleasure with them too. She said that she had never used contraception and at the time of the first interview she was worried that she was pregnant, because she had not menstruated for two months and some villagers had told her they thought she was pregnant. She said if she was pregnant, she wanted to abort it: "I have thought about having an abortion, but I don't know the medicine for it. . . . I would like to abort it so that I can finish school first. . . . But my traditional healer says that she cannot do it" [II-99-C-55-f].

Zawadi had never visited a health facility. Before she went to live with the traditional healer, her grandmother had sought and received permission from her head teacher to take her out of school for traditional treatment of her genital condition. Zawadi explained that her genitals were sometimes swollen, painful, and itched severely, and that she had growths (**masinza**) around her vaginal opening. She said that the growths began as small pimples that discharged a clear fluid, but then became big, and could not be burst. She believed that, if left untreated, the growths would become as long as a finger, although she had not seen them become that big herself. For Tshs 1,000 ($1.20) the traditional healer had treated Zawadi's growths by cutting them off with a razor blade. Zawadi said that during this procedure she lost a lot of blood, which the healer staunched by applying a herbal medicine. Zawadi said that the procedure was so painful that she had difficulty walking for some time afterwards. She believed, however, that the treatment had been partially effective, and she hoped to have the traditional healer repeat the procedure soon:

I: When is she going to cut you again?

Z: When I get money again. . . .

I: Where do you look for money?

Z: From my new boyfriend. . . .

I: He has said he will give it you?

Z: Yes.

I: You told him that you are suffering from this?

Z: Yes. [II-99-C-55-f]

Zawadi may have been open in discussing her condition with her new sexual partner and other villagers because she did not perceive it to be sexually transmitted. She instead believed that she had contracted it while walking on a pathway:

I: And who do you think infected you with that illness?

Z: That illness?

I: Yes.

Z: Nobody infected me.

I: Did your traditional healer tell you how you got the illness?

Z: She said that I stepped on it. . . . When someone's ***masinza*** are cut off a person goes to throw them on a path, so that if you step on them you also get the same illness. . . .

I: Is there any other girl here who is suffering from an illness like yours?

Z: Yes, just many . . . even the big [older] ones. . . .

I: Who told you that they suffer?

Z: They say so themselves. [II-99-C-55-f]

Zawadi's illness causation beliefs and treatment practices were typical of many villagers. Her description of her symptoms suggests that she might have had genital warts and/or herpes. Neither of those infections were tested during the 1998 *MEMA kwa Vijana* survey that Zawadi had participated in several months before her first in-depth interview. However, she was tested for herpes in the 2001–2002 survey conducted three months before her second in-depth interview. Like 21 percent of the young women who participated in that survey, she tested positive for it (Ross et al. 2007).

During her second in-depth interview, Zawadi told the researcher she had not in fact been pregnant as she had feared during the first interview. She did not return to school after completing the traditional treatment for her genital condition, but instead went to live with her sister in the district capital. Soon afterwards one of her former teachers recruited her to work for one of his or her relatives in Mwanza City. Zawadi then worked in domestic service for one year in Mwanza City. However, her ***masinza*** returned, so she decided to leave her job and seek treatment from the same rural traditional healer who had treated her earlier. This time the healer only provided her with a topical herbal medicine and did not cut off any growths. Zawadi complained: "She didn't even treat me. She just gave me some medicine to apply there myself, and I did not heal at all" [II-00-C-255-f]. Zawadi reported that she paid that traditional healer a total of 17,000 Tsh ($20.40) over the years, but she had come to believe that that particular healer was not competent, because her genital condition was not cured.

During her second in-depth interview Zawadi reported that she had had a lifetime total of seven sexual partners. New partners since the first interview were a pupil, a teacher trainee with whom she had an ongoing relationship during her year in Mwanza City, and her husband, who was a *dagaa* fisherman. Zawadi met and began her sexual relationship with her husband within one month of returning from Mwanza City, while she was still seeking traditional treatment for her genital condition. Every 1–2 weeks her new partner picked her up outside of her grandmother's home at night and brought her to his brother's house for sex. Soon afterwards Zawadi realized that she was pregnant. Initially she considered using traditional medicine to suspend fetal development for months or years until a more opportune time when she would take traditional medicine to resume fetal growth. She explained:

> Z: They make some medicine for it, those who know medicines, like traditional healers. The pregnancy moves here [gesturing] to the back. . . . Later on, when you want to give birth, he/she then makes the pregnancy ready for you again.
>
> I: Have you ever used that method?
>
> Z: No. They told me to do that, but I refused. . . .
>
> I: Who told you to do that?
>
> Z: Just this woman in my grandmother's village. But another one said that if you keep a pregnancy in your back for a long time it doesn't come out later. When you try to return it to the front it appears to be a real pregnancy, but then it disappears. And you can never get pregnant again . . . for the rest of your life. [II-00-C-255-f]

The belief that a pregnancy could be suspended in this way was reported in several villages and will be discussed more in chapter 10. Zawadi told her new partner that he had made her pregnant, and he suggested that they get married, which they did ten months before the second interview:

> Z: I did not even plan to get married. Then I got pregnant. He told me, "Just come and live at my house." I thought I should go and live there because I had a burden [pregnancy]. Where could I have gone? . . . Up until now, I am still with him. . . . He has a good character. For instance, he is not the type to like/love many women. If he likes/loves you then you are his one and only. . . . He is not a liar, and doesn't go around badmouthing people or giving away people's secrets. . . . And he is not harsh. [II-00-C-255-f]

Zawadi and her husband had moved between several of his relatives' households in different villages and towns. At the time of the second interview they were living with their two-month old daughter in a large lakeshore village near Mwanza City.

During her pregnancy a female acquaintance told Zawadi that she would deliver her baby through her mouth. Zawadi believed that the woman had bewitched her and that she would die if she tried to deliver her baby without receiving traditional care, so she and her husband paid Tshs 20,000 ($24) for her to receive treatment from a new traditional healer for two weeks:

> Z: The traditional healer told me, "You won't be able to give birth until I treat you. Moreover the baby is positioned badly." That is when I went to drink some medicine there. He/she treated the yellow skin that woman had put into me. I healed. And my swollen legs also healed. He/she told me, "The baby is positioned badly. You will not give birth until you are operated upon." [II-00-C-255-f]

Zawadi said that she also received prenatal care at a local health facility, but she did not seek a higher level of medical care until the traditional healer told her to do so. She first went to the nearest hospital, but they referred her to the regional hospital for her delivery. She felt she received good medical care there.

At the time of the second interview, Zawadi continued to have unpleasant genital symptoms, including many growths, severe itchiness, and a foul-smelling, white discharge. She still believed that the only way to reduce the growths was to have them cut off by a traditional healer. During her pregnancy, she had asked her new traditional healer to cut them off, but the healer had said that she needed to wait until after her delivery. Zawadi said that she still had those symptoms when she delivered her baby at the regional hospital, but the medical staff did not seem to notice them, and she did not tell them. Zawadi said that her genital condition made it difficult for her to have sex with her husband. She said they had thus abstained from sex since about one month after they met, when Zawadi first knew she was pregnant and they married.

During the second interview Zawadi said that her genital condition might be caused by witchcraft, and she reiterated her belief that it was not infectious:

> I: Do men also become ill with **masinza**?
>
> Z: No, they don't.
>
> I: Could a girl infect another person with **masinza**?
>
> Z: No.
>
> I: And what causes **masinza**?
>
> Z: It is just being trapped by bad medicine.
>
> I: Who trapped you?
>
> Z: Maybe a witch. They bewitch you on a path. You need to jump over the trap, or you become ill. [II-00-C-255-f]

Later, the interviewer specifically asked Zawadi about sexually transmitted infections. Although both Zawadi and her husband seemed to understand what sexually transmitted infections were, and that they could be treated medically, they did not associate them with Zawadi's condition:

I: What does "sexually transmitted infections" mean?

Z: If you are ill, something like a dirty discharge comes out of your genitals. . . . People infect each other with it if they have sex.

I: Have you ever had any symptoms of sexually transmitted infections? Like the dirty discharge from the genitals which you were referring to?

Z: No. . . . Never. . . .

I: And here in this village, if one gets these sexually transmitted infections, where does one go for treatment?

Z: There is a hospital in a nearby village. . . . My sister-in-law went there and was treated. . . . She had a dirty discharge coming out of her. She used to walk with her legs wide open. They used to say that she had a sexually transmitted infection.

I: Was she then treated?

Z: Yes. . . .

I: Did your husband know?

Z: Yes. [II-00-C-255-f]

Zawadi had never participated in an AIDS education program, but she understood that AIDS was sexually transmitted. She laughingly said that she might be exposed to it if her husband ever had sex with a woman who had AIDS. Zawadi knew condoms were used to prevent sexually transmitted infections and could be purchased from shops. However, she believed condom use indicated distrust or lack of fidelity, so she could not imagine using them with her husband:

I: Do you think you would ever use condoms?

Z: [Laughter] I don't think so. . . .

I: Why do you think you would never use them?

Z: Because I don't know them. . . .

I: If your husband brought a condom, would you be happy if he used it, or would you refuse?

Z: [Laughter] . . . I would refuse. . . .

I: Why would you refuse?

Z: Now why would he not have used a condom previously? Why would he suddenly want to start using it?

I: How about if someone who is just a lover asks you to use it?

Z: I would not refuse. [II-00-C-255-f]

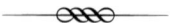

2.4. TEREZA: A YOUNG WOMAN'S EXPERIENCE OF MARRIAGE AND DIVORCE

When a female researcher met Tereza during a participant observation visit in a *MEMA kwa Vijana* control community, Tereza was 22 years old and living in her paternal aunt's household, which was also the researcher's host household. Tereza's mother tongue was Zinza, and her command of Swahili was limited. She reported that she had had difficulty understanding the subjects taught in primary school so she had dropped out some years earlier, when she was in Year 6. She thus was not a trial member. At the time of the participant observation visit she helped in her aunt's farm, bar, and food kiosk. However, she did not earn cash through that work. Instead she said she obtained her soap and body oil from her sexual partners.

During her teen years Tereza said that she had had three overlapping sexual relationships with young men in her village. She married her first husband when she was 20 years old. They had a child who died at the age of 6 months. After that her husband left for fishing work and did not return or send money back to support her. One year before the participant observation visit Tereza had moved into her aunt's household and her first marriage was considered to have ended.

Tereza's second marriage began and ended the following year. She married by moving in with a polygynous man who already had two wives. She explained why their marriage ended after six months:

> Tereza said that she separated from that man because he could not provide for her financial needs. The man was very strict and did not want her to have a boyfriend who could buy soap and body oil for her. Tereza also said she left him because he liked his first wife more than her. . . . But Tereza said that the man still seems to think they are married. . . . Tereza said she is planning to ask her aunt to talk to the man because she wants to be free to look for other men, or to respond to requests from other men. [PO-99-C-5-2f]

Most villagers perceived Tereza as a divorced single woman and thus as an **msimbe.** The disrespect accorded such a status was illustrated by an argument the researcher witnessed between Tereza and a single male cousin in his 30s:

> The man abused her, saying she was ugly. He said, "Even a tractor would pass you by. You have rusted like iron in water, so who would look at you?" Tereza replied that she was better than him because some of the most handsome men used to try to seduce her, and she named the names of the men who used to do so. She said that he instead is such a mess that he seduces old women. Tereza said he was old and unmarried and that most of his girlfriends were ugly. The man responded that she is, in fact, an **msimbe.** . . . On realizing that the chat was heading in a wrong direction, Tereza's aunt advised them to talk of something else. [PO-99-C-5-2f]

Tereza was an adult but she was a dependent in her aunt's household, so her aunt sometimes restricted her activity. Nonetheless, being unmarried and childless, Tereza had more freedom of movement than many girls who recently had left school and many women who were responsible for children and a household. Tereza sometimes left her household for hours at a time without telling anyone where she was going or where she had been, and her aunt complained about this. Tereza was markedly happy on days when her aunt travelled as she could do fewer chores and have greater independence.

Tereza enjoyed singing, dancing, and joking with both men and women, and she liked to attend video shows. The researcher accompanied her to a video show which was attended by four other women and more than thirty men. After the show Tereza flirted and bantered with different men before returning home:

> Tereza laughed as a certain man pressed her breasts. He said, "They are no longer tasty. . . . Those who came before me finished all of their sweetness." Tereza teased another man. . . . She said he gave a girl Tshs 200 ($0.24) and went to pick her up at night [to have sex] and lied that he would add to her money later. Tereza said that she would never take Tshs 200 ($0.24) from a man for sex. The man said that sometime Tereza may have sexual desire, and since she is not married he could assist her by having sex with her without giving a gift. Tereza touched her breasts and said, "These are still firm and thus you cannot have sex for free, nor for just Tshs 200 ($0.24)." [PO-99-C-5-2f]

Early in the participant observation visit Tereza told the researcher that she was no longer in a sexual relationship because she was concerned about sexually transmitted infections. However, she soon admitted that she was sexually active, as this was obvious when Tereza met different men in the company of the researcher. The researcher recorded one example that took place in Tereza's home during the day:

> The man asked Tereza whether she was going to turn in alone that night, or if he should come spend the night with her at her home. Tereza talked in low tones and told him she is sleeping in the same room as me and there is no way she was going to invite him [to have sex] in my presence. The man said, "You are a grown up. Why do you let it bother us?" . . . When Tereza's aunt appeared, the man pretended to be talking about general issues. . . . He talked loudly about the market place. Her aunt greeted him and passed by to the toilet. [PO-99-C-5-2f]

Tereza explained to the researcher that young women who shared a room together did not reveal it when one of them snuck out to meet a sexual partner at night. The researcher was present one night when a man arrived for such a liaison:

> We heard a knock at our window after we had turned off the lamp and were sleeping. . . . A voice said, "Open up." Tereza did not question who it was but opened the window and started laughing. . . . The man requested to spend the night in our

house, but Tereza told him it was impossible because they had me, a visitor, sleeping there. . . . After he left Tereza said that if he does not give her money she will not have sex with him, because most men cheat their sex partners and do not give them anything after sex. . . . She said no one buys body oil or soap for her, so she has to use her brain to get them [through sexual negotiation]. She also complained that if you are sick and do not have a boyfriend nobody bothers to take you to hospital, but if you have one he will take you. She added, "People should enjoy life before they die, right?" [PO-99-C-5-2f]

Tereza did not consider contraceptive use because she believed she was unable to become pregnant without the assistance of traditional medicine, which she had used prior to her first pregnancy. When asked if she had any plans for the future, she said she was taking a break from sexual relationships and did not plan to marry soon. Despite this statement, two weeks later Tereza's aunt discovered that Tereza and a boyfriend planned to run away together to another town. Tereza had asked a male cousin to transport her secretly to the town where she would meet her boyfriend, but the cousin told her aunt first. Her aunt in turn hid Tereza's clothes so that she could not leave, and Tereza did not run away.

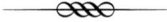

CONCLUSION

This series of case studies described young people whose experiences of marriage in rural Mwanza were fairly typical, albeit diverse. These experiences included marriage by formal proposal, elopement, or simply moving in together after conceiving a pregnancy; marriages which were monogamous or polygynous; and marriages which quickly ended in divorce. In the next chapter we will examine some of the issues raised in these case studies in more depth, including the decision to marry, different ways young people married, marital relationships, extramarital relationships, polygyny, and divorce. Later chapters will address other topics raised here, including contraception and abortion (chapter 10) and illness causation and treatment-seeking (chapter 11).

Chapter Nine

Married Young People's Sexual Relationships

Marital traditions in sub-Saharan Africa are diverse, but some broad patterns are common to many ethnic groups. Historically across sub-Saharan Africa, for example, it has been common for girls to first marry in their teen years, while men have often waited until their twenties (Caldwell, Caldwell, and Quiggin 1989; Caldwell et al. 1998; Żaba et al. 2009). Young women's age at first marriage has increased since the introduction of formal schooling, in many cases shifting from marriage at puberty to marriage several years later, but age differences of 5–10 years between husband and wife are still not unusual. For example, the 2004–2005 Tanzanian Demographic and Health Survey found that 28 percent of 15–19-year-old women and 1 percent of 15–19-year-old men were married, compared to 76 percent and 35 percent of 20–24-year-old women and men, respectively (National Bureau of Statistics and ORC Macro 2005).

As discussed in chapter 3, traditional marriage amongst the Sukuma was based on family alliances and economic considerations, such as a potential spouse's productivity or bridewealth (Cory 1953; Tanner 1955a; Varkevisser 1973; Abrahams 1981). Like most African ethnic groups, the Sukuma had a patrilocal tradition, meaning that a woman typically moved from her parents' household to her husband's upon marrying (Caldwell, Caldwell, and Quiggin 1989). Husbands and wives usually have had separate activities within their household, and largely socialized and worked with others of the same sex throughout the day. According to Sukuma custom husbands had the legally and socially acknowledged right to have extramarital sexual relationships (Cory 1953). Thus while a husband could divorce a wife on the grounds of her infidelity, a wife could not do the same if her husband took mistresses or other wives (Cory 1953).

In chapter 6 we addressed the role of love, and specifically romantic love, in unmarried youths' sexual relationships. Romantic love has often been identified as a precursor to companionate marriage, in which emotional intimacy is considered to be both the ideal foundation and the goal of marriage. Historically, anthropologists have found companionate marriage has not been common in sub-Saharan Africa, arguing that married individuals typically felt stronger bonds for their biological families than their spouses, although some have further stipulated that this is changing with modernization (Caldwell, Caldwell, and Quiggin 1989; Caldwell et al. 1998). Recently, however, some researchers have argued that emotional attachment in African marriages has been underestimated historically, noting, for example, that bridewealth itself can reflect strong sentiment (Hirsch et al. 2009; Smith 2009; Thomas and Cole 2009). As Thomas and Cole (2009, 22) argued:

> Despite . . . anthropological emphasis on rights and responsibilities, our evidence suggests that bridewealth has also included affective dimensions. For instance, one elderly Malagasy woman proudly told . . . how her former husband had "even paid a bull for her"—evidence in her mind not only of her productive and reproductive value, but also of how much that man had loved her.

Since the advent of the HIV epidemic, social scientists and epidemiologists have brought new scrutiny to marriage in sub-Saharan Africa, often through surveys of self-reported sexual behavior and health (e.g., Boerma et al. 2002; Mitsunaga et al. 2005; Hattori and Dodoo 2007; Benefo 2008; Anglewicz et al. 2010). Marriage frequently has been assumed to be protective for young adults, on the assumption that faithful married partners will not introduce new infections into a marriage, or transmit existing infections to others. Qualitative studies in some African settings have found some people strategically sought to reduce risk through marriage, including intentional selection of a low-risk spouse; communication to persuade a spouse to reform or to better understand personal risk; and divorcing a spouse who was likely to bring HIV into marriage (Reniers 2008). However, marriage may nonetheless involve relatively high risk for some individuals, particularly for women, because older, higher risk men often marry younger, lower risk women, and because extramarital sexual relationships may be common for men (Caldwell, Caldwell, and Quiggin 1989; Omorodion 1993; Ferguson et al. 2004; Helle-Valle 2004; Kimuna and Djamba 2005; Clark, Bruce, and Dude 2006; Parikh 2007; Jana, Nkambule, and Tumbo 2008; Smith 2009; Hirsch et al. 2009; Hageman et al. 2010).

While extramarital partnerships have been fairly well documented for men in sub-Saharan Africa, they have rarely been documented for women, particularly in rural areas. It is unclear whether African women indeed have less extramarital sexual activity than men or are simply more intent on hiding it because of potential stigma and punishment (Gersovitz et al. 1998; Nnko et al. 2004). There is increasing evidence that at least a small proportion of married women engage in extramarital sexual relationships. For example, in the 2004–2005 Tanzanian Demographic and Health Survey, 22 percent of men and 9 percent of women who currently were married or cohabiting with a partner reported having had sex with a nonmarital, noncohabiting partner in the past twelve months (National Bureau of Statistics and ORC Macro 2005).

Polygyny, or the practice of a husband having more than one wife at one time, is more widespread in sub-Saharan Africa than almost anywhere else globally (Caldwell, Caldwell and Quiggin 1989). This is possibly maintained by substantial age gaps between spouses, limited emphasis on a strong conjugal bond, and a great pressure on widowed and divorced women to remarry quickly (Caldwell, Caldwell and Quiggin 1989). In recent surveys in Tanzania, for example, 11–12 percent of married men and 23–24 percent of married women reported that they were in a polygynous marriage (National Bureau of Statistics and ORC Macro 2005; TACAIDS et al. 2008). The vast majority of these marriages involved two wives only. Rural and/or less educated men and women were more likely to be in polygynous unions than others, as were relatively poor women (National Bureau of Statistics and ORC Macro 2005).

By definition, polygynous marriages consist of concurrent sexual relationships, but they may be lower risk for the individuals involved than other forms of concurrency, if no spouses have sexually transmitted infections and their sexual network is closed, that is, none of them have extramarital relationships (Research to Prevention 2009). However, one study found that polygyny involved a higher risk of HIV infection, both because polygynous men had more extramarital sexual activity than monogamously married men, and because polygynous households absorbed a disproportionate number of HIV-positive women as junior wives, for example, after widowhood (Reniers and Tfaily 2008). A review of polygyny in sub-Saharan Africa also found it was associated with accelerated transmission of sexually transmitted infections, when compared to monogamous marriages, because it involved concurrent sexual partners and it correlated with low rates of condom use, poor communication between spouses, and age and power imbalances (Bove and Valeggia 2009). That review also suggested that women in polygynous marriages experienced disproportionately high levels of anxiety and depression, particularly around stressful life events.

In contrast to these individual-level findings, at a population level HIV prevalence has been found to be lower in countries where the practice of polygyny is common, and within countries, lower in areas with higher levels of polygyny (Reniers and Watkins 2010). The authors of that study suggested

that, because HIV-positive women disproportionately join polygynous marriages, they are less likely to transmit HIV outside of their small, married
sexual network and within the general population than if they remained
unmarried. They also suggested that, even within marriage, polygynous HIV-
positive women may be less likely to transmit HIV to their husbands than
monogamously married HIV-positive women, because polygnous husbands
divide their time between two or more wives and each wife is likely to have
intercourse less frequently than monogamously married women.

Our study primarily focused on young people's unmarried sexual relationships, but those relationships often led to marriage at a young age. In the
1998 *MEMA kwa Vijana* survey, for example, none of the primary school
study population was married, but at the follow-up survey approximately
three years later 3 percent of males and 29 percent of females had already
married (Lutz 2005). Young women who had married were twice as likely
to have HIV, herpes, and syphilis as young women who had never married
(Lutz 2005). When the study population was surveyed again approximately
six years later, 33 percent of males and 56 percent of females were currently
married, and an additional 3 percent and 10 percent respectively were divorced (Doyle et al. 2010).

The next section will describe our qualitative findings on the process of
marrying, relationships between husbands and wives, extramarital sexual
relationships, polygyny, and separation or divorce for young people in rural
Mwanza. Later in the chapter, we will discuss these findings in terms of
sexual health risk, both within and outside of young people's marriages.

FINDINGS

Of 63 Year 5–7 pupils who were randomly selected to participate in in-depth
interviews at the beginning of our study, 2 of 29 men and 17 of 33 women
were married when reinterviewed two to three years later. At that time one
of the men and five of the women already had one child, and some other
women were pregnant. In addition, all three of the women who were selected
for interviews because they had been pregnant in 1998 were married and had
two children in 2002.

For recent school leavers, the most common forms of marriage were either
(a) formal engagement, when a man proposed to a woman's parents and negotiated bridewealth (*mahari* or **bukwi**) in advance, or (b) elopement, when
a couple ran away together and a lesser elopement fine (**ngwekwe**) was paid
by the husband to the woman's family after the fact. Formal Christian, Muslim, or Sukuma **bukwilima** weddings only happened in a small minority of

the marriages involving engagement. Occasionally, a young woman who recently had left school became married simply by moving in with a man after it became known that he had made her pregnant. In such cases the man either did not compensate her parents or paid them a traditional fine (***nsango***) for having caused a pregnancy out-of-wedlock. Once young women had been out of school for several years or longer, almost all marriages happened either by elopement or simply moving in together, as seen in case studies 2.3 and 2.4.

The Decision to Marry

Marrying and having children soon afterwards were almost universal life goals in rural Mwanza. Girls generally were expected to marry within two years of completing school. If they did not do so their reputations usually suffered and their families were likely to receive less bridewealth if they did eventually marry. Many girls may have liked the opportunity to continue in school and some experienced family pressure to marry soon after finishing, but most genuinely desired to marry soon after completing school. Young men instead generally wanted to become more economically independent before marrying, and their parents wanted this also. Notably, by the second series of in-depth interviews, the only male respondent to have married by choice soon after leaving school, rather than in reaction to a pregnancy, was more financially secure and prepared to support a wife than most recent school leavers, as he already had a productive cotton farm and a small bicycle parts business.

For both young men and women, marriage represented an important transition to adulthood and its anticipated independence, security, status and comfort. Sex also played an important part in the decision to marry, as a way to have unlimited and exclusive sexual access to a desired partner (particularly for men) and as a way to legitimately have children (particularly for women). Many young people married after having had varied and complicated premarital sexual relationships. Some reported looking forward to having one reliable, committed partner when they married, and a few expressed hope that mutual marital fidelity would reduce their sexual health risk.

Before marriage, when young men described a desirable sexual partner they often listed physical characteristics, such as a woman who was light-skinned or "somewhat fat." When describing desirable qualities in a wife, however, most young men also mentioned a hard-working nature, politeness, and good behavior, such as sexual fidelity. One man explained, "With a girl of a certain type, you can only have a sexual relationship, you cannot marry her. To marry her is . . . not easy. It is neither good nor easy" [II-99-I-9-m].

Like men, young women often said that in addition to attractiveness a desirable husband was faithful and worked hard. Many young women also valued a man with personal wealth, achievement, and status, such as owning a kiosk or being a community leader. The more gifts or money men provided in premarital sexual relationships the more desirable they usually were considered to be as potential husbands. The size and frequency of gifts was seen to reflect a man's long-term ability to support a woman, and it was not unusual for a woman to marry a man primarily on this basis.

Although young men and women typically held such ideals about a future wife or husband, many couples married quickly and informally, before they knew one another well. Most married in-depth interview respondents reported that they had met their spouse for the first time about one month before marrying, regardless of whether they married by engagement, elopement, or simply moving in together. Case studies 2.1 and 2.3 provide examples of this. Often it did not seem necessary to know a partner well before marrying, but what was critical was for both individuals to be at a point in their lives when they wanted to marry. Compatibility of personalities was thought valuable but not essential, as the woman usually was expected to adapt herself to her husband's personality.

Some young women were believed to have difficulty attracting a husband, either because they had bad behavior or because they were believed to have the condition known as *damu nzito* that was mentioned in chapter 6. *Damu nzito* reportedly was inherited from parents or inflicted by witchcraft; in either case, it was not believed to be caused by the woman in question and traditional medicine was considered the only way to treat it. For example, a researcher recorded that a 27-year-old married man "told me that the daughter of the African Inland Church pastor has good behavior and finished primary school [one year earlier] but no one has shown interest in marrying her. He said this is her bad luck, because she has *damu nzito*" [PO-99-C-2-1m]. Occasionally, men were also reported to have *damu nzito*, so that even if they married the couple separated soon afterwards.

We found almost no evidence of people who intentionally chose never to marry, with the exception of priests and nuns, and even some priests were known to maintain informal wives and children. A small number of individuals went through adulthood without ever marrying, but this was considered unfortunate by them and other villagers. The vast majority of young people who divorced also hoped to remarry and frequently did so within a few months.

Marriage by Engagement

In the second series of in-depth interviews with randomly selected respondents, half of the married women said that they became formally engaged to a man before marrying him. Typically, the man met the woman's father or another male guardian to propose marriage and negotiate bridewealth in advance, as described in case study 2.1. It was not unusual for a man to propose marriage in this way based on the recommendations of his friends and family, having had little or no prior contact with the young woman. A 17-year-old female Year 7 pupil provided the following explanation:

> She said if an [unfamiliar] man comes to see his relative or friend in the village he will ask several people who is a suitable girl to marry. The man will then be told about a certain girl who people perceive to be good. He then goes to her home to talk to her parents. If they agree, then they proceed with other steps toward marriage. [PO-00-C-3-2f]

Young women typically had a say in accepting or rejecting marriage proposals, and it was not unusual for a woman to reject a suitor because she did not like him enough or she did not yet want to marry due to schooling, as shown in case study 1.4. However, if a young woman's father or guardian approved of a suitor and wanted her to marry him then usually she would agree to it also. For example, a 16-year-old girl in Year 7 told a researcher "she will have no control over her marriage, and if a suitor comes to propose marriage and her father decides she should marry him, then she will" [PO-00-C-3-2f].

It was rare for a young woman's father to try to force her to marry. In one example, a mother of two in her twenties strongly resisted her father's insistence that she marry a wealthy, older, married man with whom she had had several sexual encounters. It was not clear whether the man had already paid her father bridewealth:

> *R:* My father said, "Now you are going to get married even if it is by force, because I'm your parent." . . . After three days some village elders called me. They told me to marry that old man or else I should return his money back to him. . . . Mm, I said, "Now how am I to return back the money? Did I force him to marry me? I don't want him to marry me." . . . Then they called me there to my aunt's place where my father said, "If you don't want that old man to marry you, say it here before this gathering. And if you refuse to accept him, you should know that from today onwards I'm no longer your father." [GDII-00-C-10-5f]

Ultimately this young woman conceded and allowed the man who wanted to marry her to stay with her while he was visiting her village. He had moved in with her two weeks prior to the interview.

Most of the in-depth interview respondents who reported having been engaged before marriage said that they had little or no wedding celebration. However, two women from different districts had a formal Protestant (African Inland Church) ceremony. In both cases the church required the couples to be screened for infectious illnesses first. One of these women described how she came to marry her husband one month after meeting him:

> R: When he saw me [the first time], he told me he wanted to marry me. I told him to come to my house and negotiate with my parents. And he did. They told him, "Go and prepare yourself and bring the bridewealth, so that you can have the wedding." And he prepared himself. . . . [In addition to the church wedding] there were just many things, like there was a disco at home where people danced. [II-02-I-288-f]

The negotiation and payment of bridewealth or an elopement fine were critical steps in the marriage process. After such payment a husband was entitled to have sex with his wife, to make her pregnant (even if she wanted to use contraception), and to keep older children after divorce. In our study, the families of female in-depth interview respondents who married through engagement received Tshs 150,000 ($180) on average, but it usually came in the form of four to eight cows worth Tshs 20,000 ($24) each, plus additional cash. Some men were unable to pay most of the bridewealth immediately. In two of those cases the woman's parents forbade her to move to the man's household, although the couple was allowed to consummate the marriage and sleep together within her parents' household while waiting for the outstanding payment.

Both participant observation and in-depth interviews suggested that formal traditional weddings had become uncommon in rural Mwanza. Only one of the 21 married female respondents—one of those selected for an interview because she had been pregnant in 1998—reported that she had had a **bukwilima** wedding. She was a single mother when she met her husband and they married one month later. She described the festivities: "My husband called three of his friends to come, and they invited others to my home. They came, and we slaughtered goats for them. They stayed for three days" [II-02-C-301-f].

Another rare example of a traditional wedding was provided by a Jita woman in her late teens who was married to a young fisherman. Before she met her future husband, his aunt had selected her as an appropriate wife for him. The couple then met and began a discreet sexual relationship, which continued for three months before they married. She explained the wedding process:

> She said that after a [Jita] girl becomes engaged, and bridewealth of one bucket and a sheep is paid, the girl is kept indoors where she is trained by her aunt in married life and how to look after her husband, children, and guests at home. She is supposed to eat very little food during that time, so she would not need to go outside to use the latrine. She said that she herself felt so hungry after two weeks that she was dizzy when she was taken to the home of her

parents-in-law. . . . On that day there was a big celebration. . . . At night her husband collected her and took her to another house where they had sex. . . . She said, nowadays the question of [proof of] virginity no longer exists. She said in the past a white bed sheet was spread on the bed on the wedding day, and if the girl was a virgin, blood would remain on that sheet . . . but that was not done for her. [PO-01-I-7-5f]

Many rural young women reported wishing for a traditional wedding and envying the few who had one. However, few young women expected to marry in that way. For example, a 30-year-old single mother of two

> talked about a certain family she termed lucky as all girls in the family received marriage proposals and were formally married. She said that the girls got the proposals even before they completed primary school, and the suitors waited for them to complete. She added that the parents of these girls are said to be using traditional medicine to attract suitors to their daughters. [PO-00-C-3-2f]

Rural young men, in contrast, usually expressed relief that there was little pressure on them to have a formal traditional wedding because of the cost and complication involved.

Marriage by Elopement

Half of the married male and female randomly selected in-depth interview respondents reported that they had eloped (*kutorosha* or **kulehya**). When a couple eloped the girl or woman ran away from her parents' household with her partner, sometimes hiding at one of his relative's homes away from the village for days or weeks and then returning to his household to live, as shown in case study 2.2. One young woman's elopement was typical. She finished Year 7 when she was 16 years old and met her husband for the first time the same month, when he was visiting relatives in her village. She explained that they eloped two months later:

> R: We just agreed, just the two of us. I didn't inform the people in my home. I left at night. . . . Mm, I just left, just me. I didn't tell anyone. . . . [My husband] himself later brought the news to my family. . . . Then my family went to his home. They didn't say a word [to me], they just came to an understanding with my husband's family. Then his family had to pay. [II-02-C-271-f]

Eloping was less costly and time-consuming than a formal wedding, and it did not require the active involvement and approval of both sets of parents, which was important for couples who feared parental opposition. A young woman's father never knew of her plans to elope, but occasionally a young woman's mother did, particularly if the mother had already been aware of her daughter's premarital sexual relationships and knowingly had benefited from the material exchange involved. Sometimes the man's family helped him plan an elopement, and support from the man's parents could be important if he still lived in their household. Nonetheless, during participant observation there were several examples of young men bringing wives into their parents' household without forewarning.

Often elopement happened fairly spontaneously based on a couple's appeal for one another and general desire to marry. Sometimes it was the direct result of a pregnancy or a different kind of scandal. For example, a 27-year-old man (Juma) who worked at a village milling machine told a researcher how a casual sexual encounter with a teenage girl (Nyanjige) led to serious charges which in turn led them to elope. Juma explained that he and a married friend had met Nyanjige and her sister at the milling machine and the girls had agreed to meet the men for sex the next day at an isolated spot out-of-doors. The next day the girls' father discovered them in the act and the men ran away. The father beat the girls and immediately began legal proceedings against the men, accusing them of rape. The researcher recorded the outcome in his field notes:

> Juma decided to convince Nyanjige to run away. . . . She agreed and he took her to a relative's home in the district capital. [After three months], he came back to the village and . . . told the father that he had Nyanjige and intended to marry her. . . . The legal case against Juma had lost steam because the first witness [Nyanjige] was not present. The father accepted Juma's proposal and they agreed on a date when he should come back to learn the [amount of elopement fine]. Juma arranged for Nyanjige to come back to the home of a friend, where they lived as husband and wife. [PO-99-C-2-1m]

The day after an elopement, a young woman might openly be welcomed and provided with a special meal by her husband's family, or she might remain sequestered in his room for several more days before venturing out to be introduced formally to her husband's parents. By the time a young woman's parents learned of her absence and where she had gone, people widely assumed that she had consummated the relationship sexually and she was thus considered married. During one participant observation visit, for example, a 20-year-old woman eloped with a man in his early twenties. The next day the young woman's mother and sisters found her and appealed to her to return home, but she refused by saying that she had become an adult when she eloped, implying that there was no going back to unmarried girlhood.

In some cases a girl's parents reacted angrily to elopement, particularly if she was young, if the parents had expected to receive ample bridewealth, and/ or if they disapproved of her partner. However, the act of eloping effectively forced their hand. Usually, the negotiated elopement fine was lower than what would have been expected in bridewealth. For example, the average *ngwekwe* fine reported by in-depth interview respondents was Tshs 80,000 ($96), about half of the average bridewealth. *Ngwekwe* fines also usually came in the form of cows and cash, such as three cows and Tshs 20,000 ($24). Like bridewealth, these payments sometimes were not completed until years after the marriage. For example, an African Inland Church pastor in his 60s reported that he was still waiting for payment of the elopement fine that had been agreed after his 20-year-old daughter married a man in his twenties 1–2 years earlier. He told a researcher:

> After a long discussion they came to a compromise about the elopement fine but until now it had not been paid. Today he summoned his son-in-law to ask him whether he loves his daughter, and to tell him that if he does not, then he should bring her back to her parents' home. His son-in-law said that he does love her and he plans to convince his father to bring the agreed amount next month. [PO-02-C-2-5f]

Marriage after Conceiving a Pregnancy

Some couples married after the young woman became pregnant, eloping without her parents' permission as described above. Often, however, after the initial shock and upset related to an out-of-wedlock pregnancy, it sufficed for the man to take public responsibility for the pregnancy and to have the woman simply move in with him. Sometimes this involved payment of an *nsango*, especially if the young woman was in school or had recently left it when she became pregnant. Frequently, however, no payment was made.

Of the randomly selected in-depth interview respondents, the two wives and the one husband who reported neither engagement nor elopement said that they married specifically because they were expecting a child. In one example, when a young woman was asked how she came to marry, she replied:

> *R:* Me? I just got married. . . . He made me pregnant, then he married me. . . . He told me, "Since I have made you pregnant, it is better that I just take you home." And I agreed. . . . He told my parents, but they already knew. They had to agree [without compensation], since I was already pregnant. [II-02-I-257-f]

Case study 2.3 also provides an example of a young woman who married in this way, although she had been out of school and living independently of her family for a couple of years at that time. The other randomly selected respondent who married due to pregnancy reported that her family received Tshs 100,000 ($120) and a cow as the *nsango*.

Of the three schoolgirls who initially were selected for interviews because they were pregnant in 1998, only one married the man who she believed made her pregnant. The other two had their first babies and then married and had a baby with other men, one by simply moving in with him, and the other, as already mentioned, in a ***bukwilima*** wedding.

One of the two married male respondents reported that he had married because his sexual partner became pregnant. His partner secretly told him when she was three months pregnant and he then avoided her until she was six months pregnant, when her family came to notify him and his family formally. He explained why he initially avoided her, and how his own family reacted:

> *R:* I thought her family would abuse me, because . . . it was not right [to have premarital sex], it is just like stealing. . . . So they do not permit us to do so. That is why I was so afraid when she said she was pregnant. But I was lucky when they came to tell my family about the pregnancy because I was not home. . . . When I returned I ate dinner with my family and afterwards my father said, "[Some visitors] say you have made a girl pregnant." I said, "Where do they live?" He said, "I don't know where they live—you are the one who used to go there." Then my father said to my brother, "He is refusing to say where he went. Where did he used to go?" And my brother told them. They said, "Why are you denying it, when you know?" I kept quiet, not saying anything. [II-02-C-266-m]

Later, when this young man's partner was eight months pregnant, he brought her supplies and stayed in her parents' household for two weeks, sleeping with her in her room at night. At the time of the interview he had visited his wife only one other time, after her delivery some months earlier. Nonetheless he considered himself to be married to her. He explained:

> *R:* [At her home] I sleep with her in the same house.
>
> *I:* So they know that she is your wife?
>
> *R:* Yes.
>
> *I:* When did you officially get married, or when did people know that you were married?
>
> *R:* Let me say it was when I went there [when she was 8 months pregnant]. . . .
>
> *I:* Did you offer bridewealth?
>
> *R:* No. . . . I just went there to take care of the pregnancy. . . . I would say becoming engaged and offering bridewealth is not done much anymore. . . . Maybe you live with your father, and you do not have any possessions at home. You could just stay like that waiting for your parents to tell you to become engaged to someone, but they will never tell you to do so. That is why people like me use a short cut, although I did not do so willingly. [II-02-C-266-m]

Sometimes young men considered it desirable to make an unmarried, out-of-school woman pregnant, not only as a demonstration of their virility but also, as the young man above noted, as a way to marry her without paying much compensation. For example, a 21-year-old man said that he would not mind making a girl pregnant, because "many boys become very happy when they do, because it becomes easy to marry the girl without paying a large amount of bridewealth" [PO-00-C-3-3m].

Once young women had been out of school and unmarried for one or more years, it was more common for them to become pregnant and then marry a man by moving in with him. Like the young men described above, some young unmarried women specifically sought to become pregnant in the hope that it would lead to marriage.

In all of the research methods there were also plausible accounts of women who publicly attributed a pregnancy to the sexual partner who they most wanted to marry, even though a different partner may have been equally or more likely to be the biological father. This practice was common enough for a woman or man involved in such an experience to report it in almost every participant observation village. Two examples:

> *R:* When I realized I was pregnant I didn't know who made me pregnant, because I used to go with many boyfriends. . . . I claimed that the baby belonged to a certain boy. That boy took me to live in his home, but I didn't know that he was counting the number of months. Now after I gave birth he told me, "This can not be my baby, take it to its father." I moved back home. [GDII-00-C-10-5f]

> A visiting neighbor told [a 23-year-old single mother of two] that a certain man is claiming to be the father of her youngest child. The woman responded that she does not care, because several men have claimed this and she is the only one who knows who is the father of her child. She said that just because she had sex with them does not mean they made her pregnant. The two women commented that a woman can have sex with more than three boyfriends in one week, so if she becomes pregnant she assumes the one who provides her with the most money, soap and body oil is the father. [PO-99-C-5-2f]

Transition to Married Life

Young couples gained status and certain privileges and responsibilities when they married, for example, often moving from shared same-sex housing into a house of their own. The transition to married life involved the greatest change for young wives, as it often meant living in a new home with a largely unfamiliar husband and sometimes his entirely unfamiliar family and village. Young wives were expected to obey their husbands and their husbands' parents, and often they had less freedom of movement than they had had when they were unmarried. An 18-year-old woman explained:

> *R:* You see, when you are a girl you go to the market for a walk . . . The level of fun is high [Laughter]. But now that I am married, I need to ask permission. When you are refused, you can't go. Would you force your way? [Laughter]. . . .
>
> *I:* If you decide to go to the market without asking for permission first, what would happen?
>
> *R:* E-he! If he meets you when you have already gone to the market? It won't be good. It is okay if you have a husband who is not strict. He will just tell you, "You were wrong to do this and that." But that is not typical. [II-02-C-329-f]

In another example, a 20-year-old woman explained why she did not attend *ngoma* events or discos:

> *R:* My co-wife and I never go to them. We don't go to them at all.
>
> *I:* Why don't you go?
>
> *R:* Mm, we just don't go. . . . We have been forbidden.
>
> *I:* Who has forbidden you?
>
> *R:* Our husband.
>
> *I:* Does he tell you why he has forbidden you?
>
> *R:* He just wants us to stay home. [II-02-I-258-f]

For many young women, marrying meant not only building a new relationship with a husband but also with his parents and other family members when she began to live in their homestead. A young daughter-in-law typically held many domestic and farming responsibilities and had a subservient role amongst adults within a household. Many young wives seemed comfortable and satisfied with this role within their husband's parents' household, as seemed to be the case for the young woman described in case study 2.1, but some were not. A young wife complained about this during one participant observation visit:

> She said that amongst Sukumas a married woman is expected to work very hard planting acres of food to feed her in-laws if necessary. She said that husbands can relax because they are sure their wives will feed them. In her case she has planted three acres of sweet potatoes and cassava, which she goes to the farm two times a day during the rainy season with her youngest child on her back. I had also observed her farming with her three-month-old child on her back. [PO-99-C-5-2f]

In another example, a 21-year-old mother of two reported that, after living with her husband's parents for three years, she was happy when she moved to live with her husband in town:

> She said that life with her husband is good nowadays, and she feels free and much happier after leaving the home of her parents-in-law and living in her own home with her husband. She said that it is difficult to live at the home of your parents-in-law and it needs a high degree of tolerance. She said she just thanks God for leaving without quarrelling with them, and that is why she feels happy when she comes to see them now. [PO-02-C-3-3m]

Some young married couples stayed with the husband's parental home long-term, while others like the one mentioned above moved away, either within the village or to a more distant village or town to pursue a new livelihood. The status of those who stayed within a homestead typically grew over time as they cultivated their own agricultural plots in addition to the family's, built small businesses, and increasingly contributed to the economic welfare of the homestead and family.

Relationships between Young Husbands and Wives

Above we described how many young married couples only knew each other for a month before marrying. However, even those who knew each other for longer usually only had had limited opportunities to spend time together before marriage, as described in chapter 6. Once married, couples also usually spent little time together in the course of their daily lives, for both economic and social reasons. Case study 2.1 provides one example of this. Men sometimes earned money away from home in fishing, mining, trade or other activities. Many wives did not have regular paid work but had primary responsibility for farming the family plot, as described above.

Participant observation researchers occasionally observed married couples laughing together as they worked, but joint work was the exception rather than the rule and it usually was restricted to the most intensive periods of the agricultural cycle. Men also rarely assisted in domestic tasks at home, although they might help with certain chores, such as husking maize or shelling peanuts. As noted in chapter 3, men and women typically ate separate meals within a household. In public places, married couples rarely walked around together or chatted to each other. The notion of a married couple sharing leisure interests was culturally alien. Women rarely had leisure time, and when they did, the gendered segregation of activities made it unlikely that they would share it with their husbands. Having few household responsibilities, husbands usually chose to spend their free time socializing with other men. It was thus not unusual for married young men to hang out with unmarried young men in the village center in the evenings, and to attend discos or video shows there.

Young married couples that seemed most content within their marriages typically described their spouses as well behaved, faithful, hard-working and reliable. However, the few husbands who sought out and enjoyed the company of their wives during the day were sometimes disparaged as having lost control and been subjugated by their wives, and the wives were sometimes suspected of using traditional medicine to bewitch their husbands. A 25-year-old married man provided one example:

> He told me about a man who discovered that his wife had given him traditional medicine to make him obey her and just stay home. He said she got the medicines from a traditional healer and put them in his food and under his bed. The man said he discovered this after a traditional healer told him. . . . When the husband went home he found the medicine which his wife said was for her stomach problem. The couple then had a bitter quarrel and the husband decided to divorce her. [PO-02-I-4-1m]

At night, wives were expected to be sexually available to their husbands except in certain circumstances, such as when they were menstruating or they had recently delivered a child. After marriage a man usually did not provide money or gifts to his wife in exchange for a specific sexual encounter, but material support was still a very important part of marital relationships. In fact the most common reason why women were reported to have extramarital relationships, or to end a marriage, was inadequate financial support from a husband. Husbands typically provided the most for their wives early in a marriage. Long-term, wives often had to pay for many expenses and buy their own clothes, shoes, and body lotion.

Most young women were expected to conceive a child within a year of marriage so it was very rare for a couple to consider contraception before their first baby. After having one or more children some women did wish to practice contraception, particularly to space out their subsequent pregnancies. However, men typically did not wish to prevent conception within marriage, and women were expected to follow their decisions. Some wives claimed to follow their husband's wishes while discreetly using female-controlled contraceptive methods, including traditional methods, Depo provera, or oral contraceptives. Our study found almost no reports of condom use within marriage, again because husbands did not wish to prevent conception but also because condoms were disliked in general. Condom use and other contraception use will be discussed in the next chapter.

If a wife refused to have sex with her husband or was discovered to use contraception against his wishes, this could lead to public conflict and divorce. In one fishing village, for example, a young woman refused to have sex with her husband, a bar owner, after learning that he had been unfaithful. Her husband then beat her and she ran away to her parents' home. A female researcher was present when the man went to the woman's parents' home to demand her return:

> He told his mother-in-law, "My mother, you know the reason why I married my wife [for sex]. Now if she refuses when I am her husband, what do you think I should do?" . . . His wife complained very much that he had beaten her severely, but she promised to return to their home in the evening. . . . [Later] I asked him why he hit his wife, and he said, "She refused to give me sex, although she knows that I married her mainly for that. When I wanted to punish her, she ran away." . . . He said that it is a wife's duty to have sex with her husband. [PO-01-I-7-5f]

Physical abuse such as that described above seemed to be uncommon within marriage. When it did occur, it usually was not socially condoned and it could be considered adequate justification for a woman to leave her husband. However, there were occasional instances when a husband was considered justified in hitting his wife, such as when he had evidence that she was unfaithful.

Extramarital Relationships

In most participant observation villages there were first-person and third-person reports of many young husbands and a few young wives having secretive extramarital sexual relationships. Our data suggest that most men experienced at least one—and sometimes many—such relationships by the time they had been married for several years. Many of the sexual concurrency and mixing patterns described for young people's premarital relationships in chapter 6 also applied to young people's extramarital sexual relationships. For example, husbands reported being unfaithful primarily due to sexual desire and wives primarily due to economic concerns.

Secrecy was equally or more important in extramarital relationships than in premarital ones, especially for women. A 20-year-old single man explained how he expected to continue having multiple partners after marrying, but he clarified that he would be more careful to hide them:

> *R:* [My sexual activity] will change a little after marriage, but not much. I will be with her at home and also with one from outside. Yes, but sex with those from outside will have to be done very, very carefully. . . . Mmm, I will only go after them occasionally, and not in haste . . . because I will not care much about them, but I will care about the one I have at home. [II-02-C-261-m]

Fidelity seemed to be most common during the first months and years of a marriage, when husbands enjoyed novel, nightly sexual access to their wives, and wives often had their material needs met and were monitored closely within their husband's household. Men sometimes began extramarital sexual relationships when they travelled, when their wives were in late pregnancy or were recovering from delivery, or simply when they desired a different sexual partner than their wife. As with the premarital relationships, a man's extramarital affairs could take a number of different forms, including: one-off, spontaneous sexual encounters (for example, around a celebrative event); repeated clandestine, opportunistic encounters with a particular person; and semi-open, long-term relationships that might result in offspring and formal marriage eventually.

Many wives seemed to be aware of their husbands' infidelity and this often led to conflict within the marriage, but if the couple did not separate then wives typically resigned themselves to it. One young mother of two described her ambivalent feelings:

> She said she just wants to finish harvesting her peanut crop and then she will return to her parents' home to clear her mind. She said her husband is becoming a nuisance and she wants to teach him that she gets very annoyed when he goes to sleep with other women. She said men are not reliable and when her husband started seducing her he was a nice person, so she had no desire for other boys. . . . She said nowadays he doesn't care much for her, because she has become thin and her buttocks no longer shake when she walks. [PO-01-C-2-5f]

Women's extramarital sexual relationships mainly seemed to consist of secretive, open-ended and sometimes long-term involvement with one or two familiar men, rather than one-off encounters with strangers. Such relationships could involve extended periods of no extramarital sexual activity, followed by an increase when a husband travelled and/or did not provide sufficient household support. Married women most often reported taking lovers to support themselves or their families, particularly if their husbands were drunkards, had travelled for extended periods, divided limited income between different households (as in polygynous marriages), or did not contribute sufficiently to a household for some other reason. These extramarital partners provided the woman with cash or needed goods, such as fish or other food to feed the woman and her family. If an extramarital partner gave a woman a gift that would make her husband suspicious, she might give it to a girlfriend to hide for her, and several women reported keeping such items for their girlfriends. There were also occasional reports of women who had extramarital relationships due to sexual desire. Again, this was disproportionately—but not exclusively—reported by women whose husbands were sometimes absent from their household due to travel or another reason. In most villages, there were also rumors about women who took extramarital partners because they believed their husbands to be sterile and they wanted to have a child. Some men who believed their wives were infertile also did this but were relatively open about it, formally divorcing their wife, openly taking a junior wife, or having a semi-public relationship with a mistress.

While men sometimes were fairly open about their extramarital affairs, women were rarely so. If a woman was caught having an extramarital sexual relationship, her husband might beat her or divorce her, and if there was sufficient proof then her lover might also be fined. For example:

> While at the **kikome** my informants talked about a certain man who has two wives but who still likes to have sex with other women. Last year he was caught in the neighboring village having sex with someone else's wife. . . . The woman's husband had said that he would be traveling away from the village for the night . . . but he came back early and caught them. The husband took the man's clothes and shouted to call other people. The man was apprehended and the case was heard the following day. He was fined 4 cows, Tshs 30,000 ($36), and a bicycle. [PO-01-C-2-1m]

Despite possibly severe consequences, researchers occasionally observed married women who were somewhat open about having extramarital partners. One example was a woman in her early 30s (Tabia) who told a researcher of extramarital relationships she had had while married to her polygynous husband (Masele), a 59-year-old boat captain. The woman said that her husband knew about and tolerated her extramarital relationships, because she was relatively young and "still had warm blood." She nonetheless tried to be somewhat discreet and actively hid evidence of her relationships from her husband, so as not to offend or upset him unnecessarily. This woman had been sexually involved with one of her extramarital partners, Christopher, for ten years. On multiple occasions, the researcher observed Christopher giving Tabia gifts or money, and heard them make arrangements to meet for sex later. Tabia gave several reasons why she chose Christopher as a sexual partner, including that he earned good money as a fisherman, he gave her many gifts, he attracted her physically and emotionally, and his wife and children lived in a distant village. The researcher recorded:

> When Masele went on a trip recently Tabia got the opportunity to go to sleep at Christopher's place. She said that Christopher had written her letters that made her body tingle with passion when she read them, compelling her to seek him out. She said, "There are letters, if you read them, your body loses strength." . . . Tabia told me her lovers give her gifts, large fish, *dagaa*, and body oil or

lotion. Only very rarely do they buy her clothes or dresses, because she fears that Masele will ask her how she bought them. [PO-01-I-7-5f]

Tabia showed the researcher herbal "love" medicines that she placed in her vagina to promote her relationships with Masele and Christopher:

> She said the medicine for Masele is intended to make him love her so that even if she makes a mistake he won't beat her or chase her away. She also has medicine to make Christopher love her and forget his family, including his children. . . . She explained, "As you are putting the medicine in [your vagina] you give it instructions, like, 'This man will not hate me or leave me unless I get tired of him.'" [PO-01-I-7-5f]

Tabia also told the researcher about another extramarital relationship that she had had with a fisherman who was a friend of Christopher's. Wives' concurrent relationships seemed to be fairly common and somewhat acceptable in that particular fishing village, in contrast to most non-fishing villages. For example, when Tabia spoke with a girlfriend about another woman's extramarital affair, they laughingly said, "That woman has no problem. Why eat *dagaa* every day? Sometimes you have to eat a little meat, have a little beer!" [PO-01-I-7-5f] As was found for premarital concurrency, extramarital sexual relationships seemed most common for both husbands and wives in the relatively heterogenous and mobile fishing communities.

Polygyny

According to Tanzanian law, a registered traditional marriage can have an unlimited number of wives, while a Muslim marriage can have no more than four, and a Christian or civil marriage can have only one. However, very few marriages of any kind—either monogamous or polgynous—were legally registered in rural Mwanza, and many men who identified themselves as Christian also had multiple wives. Polygynous marriages were common. Forty-one percent of the randomly selected in-depth interview respondents reported that their father was or had been polygynous at some point in their lives. Sixteen reported that their father had had two concurrent wives, eight reported three, one reported four, and one reported five. Eleven said that their mother had lived in a different household from her co-wives, while three said that she had lived with at least one co-wife. The other twelve respondents did not specify such family arrangements.

Similarly, participant observation researchers estimated that about one-third of marriages in study villages were widely perceived as polygynous, with the large majority involving co-wives living in separate households.

This did not include many marriages in which a husband had a semi-public extramarital relationship, but the woman did not seem to be perceived as another wife at that time.

There were several ways in which polygynous marriages formed in rural Mwanza. Sometimes a man who wanted an additional wife due to sexual attraction or a desire for more children simply moved her into his household and identified her as a junior wife, as in case study 2.4. Usually the new wife was younger than the man and his pre-existing wives. Often, she came from a relatively poor family, or she had already been married, had a child, or was considered an *msimbe* for other reasons, so her family did not expect much or any bridewealth. Frequently, marriages to junior wives happened informally, but occasionally a man formally married a junior wife and paid substantial bridewealth for her, particularly if she was young, had only recently left school, and had never been married or had a child.

Polygynous marriages in which the co-wives lived in separate households often came into being after a husband's clandestine extramarital relationship with a woman in a different household evolved into a more openly acknowledged, long-term relationship. Over time, for example, a man might stop providing money or gifts in exchange for specific secretive sexual encounters and instead begin providing general and open support to the woman's household. During that transition, the woman might come to be perceived as one of his wives, at least by some other villagers. This could happen gradually or quickly, as when a mistress became pregnant.

A gradual transition from having one to two wives was illustrated by a Muslim house builder and farmer in his 30s. During a first participant observation visit this man lived with one wife and eight children but he had discreet extramarital sexual relationships. For example, he confided in the researcher that he was anxious after having had a one-time sexual encounter with a woman on New Year's Eve, because the woman "did not have good behavior" and might have infected him with a disease [PO-99-C-2-1m]. During the second participant observation visit one year later, the man took the researcher to visit the household of a woman he referred to as his "second woman," a mother of three in her 20s with whom he had a one-year-old child. The man said that his wife knew about his relationship. Nonetheless,

> because he has a wife, he says he cannot spend the night with the young woman. He said that he has sex with her until late at night, for example 11 pm or midnight, but afterwards he returns home. . . . He has not given any bridewealth for the young woman, but her mother respects him as a son-in-law because he has introduced himself as the father of the baby girl. . . . He has been given land to cultivate by the woman's mother, and he has cultivated cotton there [for her and her daughter]. [PO-01-C-2-1m]

During the third participant observation visit this man explained that his relationship with the young woman had become more widely known in the village, and villagers had begun to see her as his junior wife. He said that his senior wife was initially angry but eventually came to accept the arrangement. At that time he increasingly was involved in his junior wife's household, including sometimes openly spending the night there.

Polygynous men tended to be in their 30s or older. By that age they were more likely than younger men to have had an extramarital sexual relationship that resulted in pregnancy, and they were also more likely to have the income to support multiple households. While few young men had polygynous marriages, many young women were junior wives.

Co-wives in the same household often cooperated with one another, especially if both wives had been aware and willing when entering into the polygynous marriage. For example, one 19-year-old respondent who eloped with a young married man described how she and her senior wife shared their responsibilities within their poor household:

R: The difference [with my premarital life] is that I lived pretty well then. . . . Now it is just rough. . . . At present I have neither clothes nor soap. Not even kerosene. . . . I sold my goat and bought the clothes I am wearing, and my other set I bought when we sold some maize.

I: What about your co-wife, who buys for her?

R: She also only has two dresses, until we harvest more crops. . . . We work in shifts, every three days.

I: Where does your husband sleep during those three days?

R: With the other wife.

I: Have you had sex with him since you gave birth [two months earlier]?

R: We haven't, [but] he still sleeps with me when it is my turn. [II-02-C-309]

Co-wives in the same household typically spent more time together than with their husband, as they shared many domestic and farming responsibilities. Some co-wives seemed to like one another and get along well, while others struggled with resentment and anger for one another, as in the polygynous marriage described in case study 2.4. For example, during one participant observation visit within a polygynous host household, a researcher witnessed a junior wife becoming jealous and refusing to speak for an entire day after her husband bought a dress for his senior wife. In multiple villages there were also accounts of a co-wife using a traditional medicine to win a husband's devotion, as noted in chapter 6. In one participant observation village, for example, a pregnant 25-year-old woman with two children returned to live in her parents' home, reportedly because her husband's new wife had used charms to make him hate her and throw her out of the house.

Co-wives who lived in separate households often had little or no contact with one another. If a man gradually and informally took on support of a second household, his first wife sometimes felt betrayed by his lack of fidelity, or resentful and angry about loss of income. However, if she did not want to divorce her husband she usually resigned herself to another wife. The potential tension between co-wives is illustrated in the following example from participant observation:

[The second wife] said she and her co-wife do not greet each other at all, because the first wife is very jealous and doesn't like her. . . . The second wife used to greet the first wife, but the first wife would never respond, so she has now stopped greeting her too. . . . The first wife has given the second wife the [derogatory] nickname, "the one with big breasts." The first wife's son said that . . . his mother forbids him to greet the second wife . . . because his mother is extremely jealous. [PO-02-C-2-6f]

This family was conflicted about concurrency in other ways. The son mentioned above was 22 years old and had just finished primary school. He had concurrent premarital sexual relationships and expressed solidarity with his father's polygyny, stating, "Has my father done something wrong? No— I will be polygynous too" [PO-02-C-2-6f]. Notably, however, his father disapproved: "When [the father] drinks beer these days, he says that his children have become very promiscuous, and that even his son . . . is disreputable and can make people's daughters pregnant" [PO-02-C-2-5f]. Commenting on this, two women in their 20s said: "But isn't [the father] also promiscuous?" and "Children imitate. Their father doesn't sleep at home every day. Does he think they can't do the same?" [PO-02-C-2-5f]

The typically informal nature of polygynous marriage formation in rural Mwanza meant that it was sometimes difficult to determine whether a woman was a mistress or a junior wife, and opinions could differ about the same woman. In one participant observation household, for example, a wife and her children referred to a woman maintained in a separate household as their husband/father's mistress, but other villagers referred to the same woman as the man's junior wife.

In this study it was sometimes also difficult to determine whether a woman was still married to a man if he mainly lived elsewhere. Some first wives had difficult relationships with their husbands and ran their households independently, rarely seeing their husbands and mainly having contact with them through their children. However, a first wife generally was seen as married if the couple had not separated decisively, if they had children together, if the man still occasionally contributed to the household materially or stayed overnight there, and/or if she did not take on a new sexual partner openly.

Marital Separation or Divorce

Separation and divorce were not unusual in rural Mwanza, including amongst young married couples. In all participant observation villages there were accounts of couples who ran away together, were considered married, and then ended the relationship within a few days, weeks, or months. For example:

> They were talking about a girl who had eloped. They said that what surprises them is that the boy who eloped with her has already returned to the village and is continuing with his fishing work, without saying anything about having eloped with her. She said that nowadays it is common for a girl to elope and then be deserted within a short time, especially when she has gone with a fisherman. [PO-01-I-7-5f]

Another example is provided by Juma and Nyanjige, the couple described earlier that eloped after Nyanjige's father discovered them having sex. They eventually returned to the village as a married couple, but the marriage did not last:

> Juma did not follow up to know the required amount of [elopement fine]. After some time Nyanjige became pregnant and went back to her parent's home and the matter dissolved like that. Her father did not follow-up with Juma. Nyanjige gave birth to a child, but the child died soon afterwards. I asked Juma why the child died, and he told me that he was not sure, but he thought maybe because the girl's father had beaten her while she was pregnant. [PO-99-C-2-1m]

Like Juma and Nyanjige, some couples hardly knew one another before marrying and quickly separated after they found they did not like or love each other enough to stay married, or that their marriage was unacceptable for some other reason. Marriages were most commonly reported to end because of insufficient economic support (from husbands), infidelity (particularly by wives), difficulty having children, and general disagreements, such as whether to use contraception. For example, a 21-year-old woman who had eloped with her husband explained why she eventually left him:

> R: Early in our marriage life was good, but later it became bad. . . . He was a man that just roamed around. He didn't even look for money. . . . I used to tell him we needed to tend our cotton field, and then when we did he just sold it and I didn't even know where the money went. . . . I was annoyed. I told him, "You brought me from my home and then abandon me here, so I am going back

home." . . . Now I had to tell his uncle [a Village Executive Officer]. We were counseled and counseled. I stayed. They said that if someone wrongs you, you must forgive him. They said, "Just put up with each other, because that is how homes are made." I stayed on. . . . [But] when I saw that the same problems persisted, I just had to leave. [II-02-I-325-f]

Other factors which were reported to cause a divorce included incomplete payment of bridewealth, a spouse's drunkenness, a husband's violence, tensions about a husband's family or co-wife, and geographic separation (as when a husband left for work and never returned). Several of the factors listed above seemed to contribute to the two divorces experienced by the young woman in case study 2.4.

The act of divorcing could be sudden if prompted by a particular crisis, such as infidelity, or gradual and more passive, as when an indefinite separation became permanent. In the following example a 22-year-old woman who had eloped one year earlier described how she left her husband's household because of illness and neglect:

R: I had a headache, dizziness, and diarrhea. . . . My husband bought me aspirin but I finished all of those tablets without getting any relief. [After three months] I decided to go back home. . . . I thought I was just going to die there.

I: Did your mother-in-law give you any treatment?

R: Not at all. . . . That disease attacked me . . . I went on cultivating but I fell seriously ill. One day I returned from the farm and went straight to bed without taking my meal. I stayed like that for about four days. I would have porridge at 2 pm and not have it again until 2 pm the next day. . . . I thought, "These people—these people don't even realize that I'm here!" [So] I decided to go back home. . . . My husband forbade me. . . . He told me to wait until he finished his work. But how could I wait for him without eating? I just left.

I: What did your parents do when you arrived home?

R: They tended to me and began treating me [with traditional medicine]. . . . I know it works, because I experienced relief afterwards. [II-02-I-252-f]

Just as many marriages happened informally, separation and divorce could be similarly informal, usually simply signified by one member of the couple moving out of a shared residence as described above. Most typically a young woman moved back into her parents' or a relative's household, but sometimes she might move into a household with one or more other single women. If bridewealth or an elopement fine had been paid, the couple had not been married for long, and there were no offspring, then the woman's family was expected to repay the man's family.

Many villagers shifted between being unmarried and in a monogamous or polygynous marriage repeatedly over the course of one or two decades, depending on their particular experience of separation, divorce, widowhood, and new marriage. Just as marriage represented a reduction in risk behaviors for some, separation or divorce seemed to involve a shift to higher risk behaviors, as men and women sought new partners for sexual satisfaction, material support, or potential marriage.

DISCUSSION

Many of this study's findings about married young people in rural Mwanza are similar to findings elsewhere in the region and Tanzania, including that half of women married by the age of 18–19 years and half of men by the age of 23–24 years, and that the informal nature of many unions meant some couples were perceived as unmarried by some and married by others (Meekers 1992; Boerma et al. 2002; National Bureau of Statistics and ORC Macro 2005). One important finding of our study was that half of young people married someone who they had only met one to two months earlier, whether they married by elopement or engagement. Similarly, anthropologists working with the Sukuma in the early to mid-twentieth century estimated about one month typically passed between a man meeting a woman, proposing marriage to her father, and the wedding (Tanner 1955a; Varkevisser 1973). At that time, for example, it was not unusual for young Sukumas living in widely dispersed villages and homesteads to marry someone fairly soon after meeting them at a central, celebratory event. Compared to this earlier research, however, we found a much higher proportion of marriages involved elopement with someone largely unfamiliar rather than engagement and formal marriage with parental consent. Even when two individuals had known one another for a longer premarital period, they typically had had very limited opportunities to spend time alone and entered into marriage without great familiarity or emotional intimacy.

Chapter 6 described how many young people entered into premarital sexual relationships spontaneously and opportunistically, and many seemed to use a similar approach when deciding to marry. Usually it did not seem necessary to know a partner well before marrying, but what was critical was for both individuals to be at a point in their lives when they wanted to be married. For many young people in rural Mwanza marriage thus seemed to be a "leap of faith" that involved leaving old sexual relationships and childhood homes behind in the hopes of creating a more satisfactory life with a promising new partner. In a study in Cameroon, Johnson-Hanks (2005) described how young women faced with uncertain futures practiced a similar "judicious opportunism" or "seizing of promising chances" when it came to marriage and reproduction.

Young women in rural Mwanza had few alternatives to marriage to create a respectable and economically secure future, and they seemed to take the greatest risks in the "leap" described above, both socially and sexually. For some young women, marrying involved moving to another village to live within an unfamiliar family and community. Many married substantially older men who were more likely to enter the marriage with sexually transmitted infections, and a larger proportion of husbands than wives seemed to have extramarital relationships and thus were likely to introduce infections to a marriage later. When a marriage did not work out, as was not unusual, women also had the most to lose in terms of economic security and social status, as has been found elsewhere in sub-Saharan Africa (Bingenheimer 2010).

As Varkevisser (1973) found in her research thiry-five years earlier, marriages in our study were typically characterized by gender segregation and often took the form of avoidance relationships. A young wife was expected to obey her husband's wishes. Young married couples spent little time together during the day and evening, and it was rare for them to overtly display their affection. However, it is difficult to draw conclusions about emotional intimacy and attachment in marriage based on an absence of such data. First, as discussed in chapter 6, measuring the quality or intensity of emotions based on observation or report is not straightforward. Second, researchers did not see all interactions between married couples, most notably not being present when couples were alone together at night, when they were perhaps most likely to speak intimately and with emotion. Acknowledging these limitations, there nonetheless was little evidence in our study to suggest that companionate marriages, or marriages in which emotional intimacy was valued above all else, were common amongst young people in rural Mwanza.

Extramarital Relationships

Most young men in our study entered into marriage expecting their wives to be sexually faithful, and some were motivated to marry specifically to reduce their own sexual health risk. Most young women also entered marriage hoping that their husbands would be faithful, although they were generally less confident that this would be the case. Thus, importantly, unlike the two other highly promoted behavioral risk reduction goals of abstinence or condom use, young people often perceived long-term fidelity in marriage as both feasible and desirable.

The qualitative nature of this study, its primary focus on unmarried youth, and the very secretive nature of extramarital sexual activity means that we cannot estimate the exact proportions of young married men and women who engaged in extramarital sexual activity, how often they did so, or their numbers of partners. Publicly, most young married people claimed to be faithful to their spouse(s). It seems likely that the number of partnerships and the frequency of non-marital sexual encounters did in fact reduce immediately after marrying, especially for women, as some others have found elsewhere in sub-Saharan Africa (Hattori and Dodoo 2007; Research to Prevention 2009). However, our findings suggest that within several years of marriage most young husbands had experienced at least one extramarital relationship, and sometimes multiple ones. A smaller proportion of young wives engaged in extramarital relationships with great secrecy. This was most often reported in marriages in which a man travelled for work, as has been found in other research in the region (Vissers et al. 2008). Nonetheless, it was not unusual for young men who did not travel to also have experience of one-off or open-ended extramarital sexual relationships.

We collected more data on young husbands' extramarital relationships than those of young wives, but we cannot conclude from this that marital infidelity was rare for women. In chapter 6 we described how many young women reported premarital partners in in-depth interviews before marriage but strongly denied them in in-depth interviews afterwards, suggesting that any extramarital partners would also be denied or underreported, and raising questions about the validity of married women's self-reported sexual histories in general. The women who did report extramarital relationships rarely seemed to engage in one-off encounters like some men, but rather had secretive partnerships with a familiar man or men involving occasional encounters over a period or many months or years, thus contributing to an extended period of concurrency and its related risk.

In chapter 6 we also discussed how many unmarried young people considered faithfulness to be ideal in a partner but did not expect the same of themselves. Such double standards were also evident within married relationships, especially for men. Nonetheless the ideal of fidelity in marriage means that it may have more potential than abstinence or condom use as a promoted behavior. Critically, any such promotion needs to emphasize that fidelity must be both *mutual* and *long-term* between uninfected partners if it is to be effective in protecting one's *self* as well as one's spouse.

Polygyny

Our study could not assess whether polygynous men had more or less extramarital sexual partners than monogamously married men. On the one hand, many men's relationships with their junior wives began as clandestine, extramarital relationships, as has been found elsewhere in sub-Saharan Africa (Clark 2010). This suggests that such men may have had higher risk behavior than men who were faithful to their wives, whether monogamous or polygynous. On the other hand, men with multiple wives may have been more likely to have a closed sexual network than monogamously married men, because, for example, they might have sex with a second wife while a first wife abstained after delivering a child, rather than seeking out a new, extramarital partner (Vissers et al. 2008).

We found that extramarital relationships were one of the only ways for both polygynous and monogamously married women to obtain supplemental income when needed, as has been found elsewhere in sub-Saharan Africa (Caldwell, Caldwell and Quiggin 1989). Our data suggest that women in polygynous marriages who lived in a separate household from their co-wives may have been more likely to have extramarital partners than other polygynous women or monogamously married women. Such women could face greater economic hardship because their husband's material support was shared between households, and they also had more freedom of move-ment than women who lived with their husbands full-time. These findings are broadly in keeping with studies elsewhere in the region and sub-Saharan Africa (Hattori and Dodoo 2007; Vissers et al. 2008). For example, a study in another part of Mwanza region found that 34 percent of polygynous men and 41 percent of monogamously married men reported having had extramarital sexual partners, compared to 5 percent of women in polygynous marriages and 2 percent in monogamous marriages (Nnko et al. 2004).

Polygynous societies in sub-Saharan Africa are often assumed to be fairly uniform and to have more social controls than other societies, for example, greater prevention of sex before marriage, especially for women (Kretzschmar, White, and Caraël 2010). In many societies this may be true, but in rural Mwanza polygyny was practiced in diverse ways by people of dif-ferent faiths, both formally and informally. More research is needed on the di-verse forms of polygyny before determining the sexual health risk involved in it, both at individual and population levels. One area warranting further study is the nature and scale of sexual health risk in marriages where co-wives live apart, relative to those where co-wives share a household. Another is the rela-tive risk in settings where polygyny may be fairly uniform and follow strong religious and social norms, in contrast to those where it is practiced in more diverse and informal ways.

Marital Separation and Divorce

Separation and divorce were fairly common among young adults in our study. A recent survey in a semirural ward in Mwanza Region similarly found that one-half of ever-married men and one-third of ever-married women had divorced at least once, and remarriage soon after divorce was common (Boerma et al. 2002). The researchers suggested that divorce or separation might be increasing in such areas because the increase in informal marriages and incomplete bridewealth payments meant young married couples received less support from their families than in the past. However, it is difficult to know whether divorces truly are more prevalent today than historically. Older people may claim higher rates of divorce today than in the past, but historical documentation does not always support such statements (Kaler 2001; Thomas and Cole 2009). For example, in his review of Sukuma law and custom in the early twentieth century Cory (1953, 59) observed, "marriage, divorce, and re-marriage are regarded as customary stages in a normal life-cycle." Similarly, in his study with the Nyamwezi, Abrahams (1981) found that 66 percent of 30–39-year-old men and 92 percent of men over 60 years of age had experienced divorce. In her 1965–1967 study Varkevisser (1973) also commented on the relatively high rate of Sukuma divorce in comparison to other patriarchal societies, and highlighted that 31 of the 34 divorces officially registered in one court had been initiated by wives. We similarly found that many young women in our study refused to endure negligent or abusive marriages and took the initiative to end them, often with the support of their parents.

Many factors which contributed to divorce in our study have been found in other studies in the region, such as infidelity, infertility, and conflict with a spouse's family (Adeokun and Nalwadda 1997; Twa-Twa, Nakanaabi, and Sekimpi 1997; Boerma et al. 2002). One factor that we have not seen highlighted previously is partners having little familiarity with one another before marrying—whether the marriage was family approved or not—and ultimately being disappointed as they came to know their spouse and new living circumstances better. In our study marrying someone largely unfamiliar was common and some couples seemed to be satisfied with their choices long-term, but others were clearly dissatisfied, which often led to separation and divorce.

CONCLUSION

In this chapter we considered how young people's lives and sexual relationships changed with marriage and, sometimes, divorce. Having children was a central aspect of married life that we have only briefly addressed here. In the next chapter we will thus examine beliefs and practices related to reproduction in depth, for both married and unmarried young people.

Chapter Ten

Contraception, Abortion, and Fertility[1]

Historically, fertility has been valued very highly in sub-Saharan Africa. An individual's ability to conceive and have children has been perceived as both economically and socially important, and reproduction played a central role in many African religions (Caldwell, Caldwell and Quiggin 1989). Early and universal marriage for girls, an emphasis on immediate conception, and extremely low rates of effective contraception have all contributed to women initiating childbearing fairly early and giving birth to an average of six or seven children in their lifetimes (Caldwell and Caldwell 1987; Cohen 1998). In the 2004–2005 Tanzanian Demographic and Health Survey, for example, 20 percent of 15–19-year-old women had already had a child, and another 7 percent were pregnant with their first child (National Bureau of Statistics and ORC Macro 2005). However, fertility in sub-Saharan Africa has declined somewhat in recent decades, particularly in urban areas, due to greater use of modern contraception, older ages at first marriage, and HIV and other sexually transmitted infection epidemics (Kirk and Pillet 1998; Cohen 1998; Harwood-Lejeune 2000; Hinde and Mturi 2000; Terceira et al. 2003; Dyer 2008a; Pellati et al. 2008).

CONTRACEPTION

The meaning and importance of contraception and fertility can vary considerably at different stages in an individual's life in sub-Saharan Africa as elsewhere in the world. Contraceptive desires and practices before marriage or childbearing can vary markedly from those afterwards. As discussed in chapter 6, a large proportion of unmarried youth may be sexually active for several years prior to independent adulthood and/or marriage. Some studies have focused on understanding unmarried adolescents' attitudes and practices related to condoms, but few have examined their broader contraceptive and fertility-related beliefs and practices in depth (Castle 2003a; Williamson et al. 2009). Most research with adolescents has evaluated modern contraceptive use through surveys of urban youth and/or secondary school students, which may have only limited validity and representativeness for the broader population, as noted earlier in the book. A recent review of qualitative studies of young women's modern contraceptive use in developing countries only identified six studies of high standard in sub-Saharan Africa, most of which were conducted in urban or semi-urban settings and did not discuss use of traditional methods in detail (Williamson et al. 2009).

The HIV epidemic has led to intensive research on condom use in sub-Saharan Africa because condoms are the only contraceptive method that also prevents sexually transmitted infection (Davis and Weller 1999). Unlike hormonal contraceptives which women take orally or by injection, a male condom is protective against infection because it consists of a sheath of thin rubber or latex that is rolled down over an erect penis, preventing an exchange of fluids during intercourse. Critically, to be most effective condom use needs to be consistent and correct, that is, condoms need to be used properly for every act of intercourse. A review of 62 condom promotion evaluations in Asian and African countries found some positive intervention effects on reported condom use, especially amongst commercial sex workers and their clients (Foss 2007). Generally, however, reported condom use—and particularly consistent condom use—has not been high in sub-Saharan Africa, even in casual relationships and even after participation in condom promotion interventions (Ferguson et al. 2004; Katz 2006; Sayles et al. 2006; Tassiopoulos et al. 2006; Bankole et al. 2007; Foss et al. 2007; Izugbara and Modo 2007; MacPhail et al. 2007; Rutherford 2008).

Problems with condom distribution and access have contributed to low rates of consistent condom use in sub-Saharan Africa (Bosmans et al. 2006; Sambisa and Stokes 2006), but beliefs and attitudes about condoms play a part as well. Negative beliefs about condoms are widespread, including that they reduce sexual pleasure, indicate infidelity or a lack of trust in a partner, are inherently dangerous, become lodged in the woman's vagina, and are associated with sexually transmitted infections, casual sex, or prostitution (Taylor 1990; Lamptey and Goodridge 1991; Lindan et al. 1991; Karim et al. 1992; Mehryar 1995; Mnyika, Kvåle, and Klepp 1995; Hart et al. 1999; Maharaj 2001; Kaler 2004b; Marandu and Chamme 2004; Thomsen, Stalker, and Toroitich-Ruto 2004; Amuyunzu-Nyamongo et al. 2005; Lees et al. 2009; Harrison and O'Sullivan 2010). Other factors that may discourage condom use include embarrassment and shyness; a lack of perceived personal risk of infection; male socioeconomic control of sexual decision-making; and the importance of male potency, male and female fertility, or the exchange of bodily fluids during sexual intercourse (Taylor 1990; Lamptey and Goodridge 1991; Lindan et al. 1991; Karim et al. 1992; Bond and Dover 1997; Hart et al. 1999; Kinsman et al. 2001; MacPhail and Campbell 2001; Luke 2003; Macintyre et al. 2004; Thomsen, Stalker, and Toroitich-Ruto 2004; Coast 2007; van den Borne 2007; Selikow et al. 2009).

Until 1994, contraceptive counselling and services in Tanzania were only officially allowed for child-spacing purposes. After that time, revision of the National Policy Guidelines and Standards for Family Planning allowed adolescents access to contraceptives, irrespective of marital status or childbearing history (Silberschmidt and Rasch 2001). By the 2004–2005 Tanzanian Demographic and Health Survey, 12 percent of 15–19-year-old women reported having ever used a contraceptive method, mainly condoms (7 percent), traditional methods (4 percent), oral contraceptives (3 percent), and injectables (2 percent), compared to 45 percent of 20–24-year-olds and 59 percent of 25–29-year-olds (National Bureau of Statistics and ORC Macro 2005). Over one-third of the 15–19 years olds who had used a contraceptive only did so after having a child (National Bureau of Statistics and ORC Macro 2005). Adolescent and adult modern contraceptive users were disproportionately urban, in part because rural areas commonly faced shortages of family planning providers and contraceptives (Chen and Guilkey 2003).

ABORTION

In most countries of sub-Saharan Africa, induced abortion is illegal unless the woman's life is in danger (Silberschmidt and Rasch 2001). In Tanzania, abortion for almost any other reason is punishable by fourteen years of imprisonment for the person administering the abortion, seven years for the woman, and three years for anyone who knowingly supplied abortifacients, that is, materials used to induce abortion (United Nations 2002). Despite these deterrents, abortion is believed to be practiced widely in Tanzania and elsewhere in sub-Saharan Africa (United Nations 2002). For example, the World Health Organization recently estimated that 3 percent of East African women aged 15–44 years had undergone unsafe abortions, and 60 percent of unsafe abortions in Africa involved women younger than 25 (WHO 2004).

Such estimates are only "best guess" calculations, however, based largely on hospital admission records for women with complications resulting from incomplete abortions, such as hemorrhage or sepsis (Mpangile, Leshabari, and Kihwele 1993; Benson et al.1996; Rasch et al. 2004; Grimes et al. 2006;

Grady 2009). Abortions that lead to serious health consequences, for which women access and pay for hospital treatment in urban areas, are not likely to be representative of the majority of abortion attempts (Barreto et al. 1992). Less recognized and understood are the experiences of women who attempt abortions but have no complications, minor complications, or major ones—such as infertility, fistula, and other chronic illnesses—for which they do not seek or receive medical care in hospitals (Castle, Likwa, and Whittaker 1990; Barreto et al. 1992; Benson et al. 1996; Grimes et al. 2006; Singh 2006). Similarly, only limited research has been conducted concerning the broader social, cultural, and economic influences on abortion in sub-Saharan Africa (Barreto et al. 1992; Benson et al. 1996), particularly on men's roles as partners, providers, and decision makers; the experiences of adolescent girls; and the psychological and emotional circumstances leading to and resulting from abortion (Benson et al. 1996; Mundigo 1999; Silberschmidt and Rasch 2001; Rasch and Lyaruu 2005; Hess 2007).

Studying abortion in non-hospital settings in sub-Saharan Africa is challenging. Survey participants may underreport abortion because they fear cultural disapproval and legal or religious sanctions (Barreto et al. 1992). For example, although Marchant and colleagues (2004) found that abortion was one of the most important and consistent themes in group discussions of family planning in rural Tanzania, they believed it to be too sensitive a topic to include in a subsequent survey questionnaire. Similarly, in the 2004–2005 Tanzanian Demographic and Health Survey, respondents were asked detailed questions about fertility, contraception, and maternal health, but no questions were asked about abortion (National Bureau of Statistics and ORC Macro 2005). Anthropological research can be more effective than surveys in investigating this highly sensitive topic because it involves building long-term, trusting relationships with informants and allows direct observation of events (Bleek 1978; Castle, Likwa, and Whittaker 1990; Erasmus 1998; Allen 2002; Mundigo 2003; Stambach 2003). For example, in rural Ghana, Bleek (1987) found that six women interviewed by female nurses "lied lavishly," underreporting experiences of birth control, pregnancy, and abortion already discussed with him in-depth during his anthropological research.

FERTILITY PROTECTION AND PROMOTION

In addition to trying to prevent or terminate pregnancies, young women's attempts to control their reproduction can focus on maximizing their fertility in the present or future. Women may be anxious to protect or promote their long-term fertility from an early age, even when they do not want to become pregnant in the short term (Castle 2003a). If they perceive themselves to be infertile, they may attribute this to either a supernatural or a biomedical cause, although understanding of the latter is often very limited (Dyer 2008b). Considerable effort can be expended seeking infertility treatment, but effective methods are often very difficult to access (Nachtigall 2006; Dyer 2008b).

In the 2004–2005 Tanzanian Demographic and Health Survey, only 2 percent of women in their late 40s had never given birth, suggesting a very low rate of primary sterility (National Bureau of Statistics and ORC Macro 2005). However, this statistic does not include a much larger proportion of women who delivered one or more children but were then unable to have more when they wanted to do so later. A study of 3,708 20–44-year-old Tanzanian women found that 16 percent reported having experienced such secondary infertility (Larsen 2000). In a different study, Mwanza Region had a secondary infertility rate of 18 percent, which was significantly higher than 18 of the 21 Tanzanian regions studied (Larsen 2003).

This chapter primarily draws on data collected from *MEMA kwa Vijana* control communities to describe young people's beliefs and practices related to contraception, induced abortion, pregnancy suspension, and fertility promotion in rural Mwanza. Special attention is given to condom beliefs, attitudes and use because of their dual potential in contraception and disease prevention. Abortion decision-making, frequency, methods, and outcomes will also be described in depth, as these topics rarely have been examined in a rural African context.

FINDINGS

Contraception

In rural Mwanza, having children—especially many children—was almost universally viewed as a source of pride, accomplishment, and security in one's old age. Many men and some women considered pregnancy to be "God's will" and desirable in any circumstances, because children would assist and support their family as they grew older. Nonetheless there were many accounts of unmarried adolescent girls and young women who did not want to become pregnant for fear of the stigma, punishment, and hardship sometimes associated with out-of-wedlock pregnancies. Some did not try to prevent pregnancy because they did not know how to do so, or they believed that they could not become pregnant (e.g., due to young age) or that contraception was alien or harmful. However, many school girls and childless young women used traditional contraceptive methods that were unlikely to be effective. Very few boys or men reported trying to prevent pregnancy by using a condom or by helping their partner to obtain a different contraceptive method. Those men were usually in highly secretive sexual relationships that would result in very negative consequences if they became known, such as a married man who was involved with a school pupil.

Young mothers, whether married or not, generally had much more access to modern contraceptives than childless young women, because they attended health services for prenatal checkups and their children's health care, and health facility staff specifically targeted them with contraceptive advice. However, only a minority of young mothers used modern contraception consistently, and often their sexual partners were unaware of this.

Traditional Pregnancy Prevention

Most girls and women learned about traditional contraceptive methods from older same-sex siblings and cousins, but sometimes also from other female friends, mothers, grandmothers, older women familiar with traditional methods, and traditional healers. Most did not inform their partners that they were attempting to prevent pregnancy, as they believed their partners might oppose it, even within clandestine relationships. As one participant in a female group discussion reported: "If you don't want to have a child, seek any means, and keep it your secret. . . . You do not tell that young man" [GD-00-C-10-2f].

Traditional contraception usually fell into two categories: charms that were worn, and solutions of leaves, roots, or wood ashes that were ingested. Many women reported having drunk ash solutions to prevent pregnancy, particularly as young adolescent girls, because they were free, easy to access, and could be prepared and taken without anyone else's knowledge. For example, a 17-year-old married woman who had never gone to school:

> She said she used to drink ashes mixed with water before sexual intercourse to prevent getting pregnant. She said the ashes are effective because she never got pregnant [while single]. She also showed me some plants, which she said are used by boiling the roots, and then drinking the contents. She said that it is very bitter, but combined with ashes it is very effective. [PO-00-C-3-2f]

Opinions varied about the effectiveness of ashes in pregnancy prevention, possible side effects, what ashes could be mixed with (e.g., local herbs or sodium bicarbonate), and whether to take them before and/or after intercourse. A few respondents reported that strong concentrations could cause infertility. A few male group discussion participants reported that, if a man drank an ash solution, it made his sperm temporarily ineffective, and one reported having used this method himself.

Protective charms or talismans were also widely used for pregnancy prevention. These usually were prepared by a traditional healer or an older female family member or acquaintance who claimed knowledge of traditional medicine. Some were worn by a woman for a short time before being buried or hidden (e.g., under a roof) until she wanted to conceive, at which time they were uncovered or removed. Others were worn by the woman until she wished to conceive. A contraceptive **lupigi** consisting of one or two pieces of roots or wood with a hole born through it and herbal medicine sealed inside was worn on a string or beads around a woman's neck, arm, or (most typically) waist. Another form of contraceptive amulet called a *hirizi* consisted of plant materials sewn between two small pieces of animal hide, to also be worn around the waist. Examples from interviews with group discussion participants:

R: I have seen a certain person who proves that a [**lupigi**] works. My aunt, who used to stay at our home, she is the one who had it. . . . She herself stayed for about fifteen years without having a baby, although she was going [having sex] with men. [GDII-00-C-12-4m]

R: One woman from here wears a [*hirizi*] on her waist beads. . . . She told me she uses it to not become pregnant. . . . I also saw one neighbor, after having two children she vowed not to give birth again. . . . She went to a female traditional healer to have that medicine [**lupigi**] made for her. Yes, that stopped her from getting pregnant. [GDII-00-C-11-5f]

Participant observation researchers often observed unmarried young women wearing protective charms, and their use was so common as to be an "open secret." However, they usually were worn discreetly out of sight, and if asked directly, a girl or woman could claim to wear the charm for other reasons than contraception, such as to treat an illness.

In multiple villages young people reported that pregnancy could be prevented by drinking teas made from the roots, stem, leaves or other parts of certain plants, such as the *mwarobaini* tree (*Azadirechta indica*, the neem tree), which has been found to have contraceptive and abortifacient potential in biomedical studies (Sharma et al. 1996; Talwar et al. 1997). Less commonly reported practices believed to have long-term contraceptive effects included placing traditional medicine in an incision made in a woman's skin, or mixing and burying certain substances (e.g., herbs and ashes, a woman's menstrual blood, or her child's feces) in the earth. The following example was provided by a nurse in her 30s:

She talked about one woman who uses special slivers of wood, which she dips in her menstrual blood on the first day of her menses. She said that after doing this, you bury them without being seen by anyone. Then, if you later want to conceive, you unearth them. [She said] after seeing them, if you have sex you will definitely get pregnant. [PO-02-C-3-3m]

Occasionally respondents voiced doubt about the safety of contraception, for example, that if a waist string bearing a charm broke accidentally, or a woman forgot where she had buried a charm, she might become permanently infertile. Most respondents believed that such methods were effective. As one male group discussion participant commented, "With that [charm], no matter how many times you do it, no matter how long you have sex, there will be no pregnancy" [GD-00-C-12-2m]. However, some questioned their effectiveness, particularly if they knew someone who became pregnant while using them. For example:

> *P:* They once tied the *lupigi* that they talk about on [my waist] . . . I was surprised to become pregnant while wearing it. . . . So I told the traditional healer, "Healer, you completely tricked me, you!"
>
> *F:* And what did he/ she say? . . .
>
> *P:* [He/she said], "You probably dropped [the *lupigi*]." I said, "No, you deceived me and, lo! Now I'm pregnant. . . . You have brought problems to me." So I had to give birth. [GD-00-C-10-3f]

Female-Controlled Modern Contraception

Few young people in our study reported having used modern contraceptives themselves: in all methods, most reports about them were third-person observations and opinions rather than personal experience. Reports of school girls using modern contraception were extremely rare. Judgment about adolescent contraceptive use could be harsh, as evidenced by a comment from a 20-year-old unmarried woman: "Birth control pills are only used by adults, particularly those who are married. When a girl uses contraceptive pills, she must be a prostitute" [PO-02-I-4-5f]. Even if school girls were aware that such options were available at health facilities, they were very unlikely to seek them out, because of distance to facilities and, most importantly, fear that health workers would judge them and discuss their visit with other villagers.

The simulated patient exercises in five of the ten *MEMA kwa Vijana* control communities found health workers engaged with adolescents in a responsive and nonjudgmental way and also provided them with adequate, basic information. In the remaining five communities, health workers were ranked as moderately to extremely judgmental in their comments and provided little or none of the appropriate information. In one example, a girl requested birth control from a health worker who responded abruptly and rudely, interrogating her about her parents' names and village, and stating that the girl was "most primitive" and "never went to school" when she did not take her shoes off prior to getting on the examination table. The health worker ultimately asked her if she wanted injectable or oral contraceptives but did not explain them to her. The girl requested oral contraceptives, which the health worker gave her after a brief physical examination. However, the health worker's criticism continued:

HW: Who taught you about it?

SP: About what?

HW: That you should go for family planning pills?

SP: I heard about it in the streets.

HW: So, if you hear that people are stealing, you also go and steal?

SP: No!

HW: A young person like you, why do you hate having babies? Hmm, we provide [contraceptives], yes, that's fine. But you haven't—haven't even had a baby. [It would be acceptable] if a baby is disturbing you, or your husband doesn't care about you. . . . But a young person like you, you have just begun hating having babies." [SP-00-C-24-10f]

Villagers and health workers consistently reported that the only women who used modern contraceptives were a limited number of single or married mothers who mainly used Depo Provera, or, to a lesser extent, oral contraceptives. Depo Provera was popular because it is a hormonal contraceptive that only requires injection into a woman's muscle once every three months. It typically was perceived as more convenient and less detectable by others than oral hormonal contraceptives, which needed to be swallowed once per day. For example, a 22-year-old single mother who had children by different fathers reported that she used Depo Provera injections, but she hid this from her mother because her mother would disapprove of her continued sexual activity. In another example:

[A male health officer] told me about a woman who, after [secretly] using the [Depo Provera] injection method, did not get pregnant. Her husband took her to a traditional healer to get medicine to help her get pregnant. [She] was given a traditional medicine, but didn't take it. Instead, she emptied it slowly over time, pouring out the amount she had been told to drink every day. [PO-01-C-3-3m]

Very few women reported use of oral contraceptives, and those who did tended to have more formal education than most villagers. For example, during a participant observation interview a village health officer reported that his wife used oral contraceptives, and showed the researcher her pills. Many respondents voiced wariness of hormonal methods, and particularly oral contraceptives, because they were widely reported to have negative side effects, such as weight loss or gain, continuous or sporadic menstrual bleeding, reproductive cancer, and infertility. For example, a mother of nine who was relying on a traditional contraceptive at the time of the research:

> She said she once used injections [Depo Provera] for a year. She said that few women use such methods because they believe the medicines are dangerous and cause cancer . . . and some are said to have a rotting uterus after using contraceptive pills or injections for a long time. [PO-01-C-2-5f]

One of the most commonly cited concerns about both traditional and modern contraception, and especially oral contraceptives, was that they could harm a woman's long-term fertility. The following example was provided by a 25-year-old unmarried mother of two:

> She told me that parents would prefer their daughter to get pregnant before getting married rather than use contraceptives that will completely damage their reproductive system. She gave me an example of a Year 7 girl whose younger sister showed their mother her contraceptives. That mother became very angry, and beat the girl severely, as she thought she was intending to destroy her reproductive system. [PO-02-I-4-5f]

Such beliefs mainly were reported in informal village discussions, but the simulated patient exercises suggest that the information patients received in health facilities might have sometimes also perpetuated misunderstandings about modern contraceptives. In each of the following exchanges a girl requested a birth control method and the health workers responded by encouraging her to use condoms. In the process, they provided her with incorrect information about other contraceptive methods. In the first example, the health worker suggested that both oral and injectable contraceptives were poor alternatives to condoms because they might damage the girl's short-term or long-term fertility, while in the second example, the health worker told her she was too young to use oral contraceptives:

> *HW:* This [condom] is really good, because it protects your health and it prevents conception. . . . Try this rather than oral contraceptives, which can mess up your [future] child bearing.
>
> *SP:* Right.
>
> *HW:* They [condoms] are just as good as pills [at preventing pregnancy]. The injection can delay child-bearing, in case you desperately need to have babies

after [discontinuing]. However, these [condoms] are good, because when you want to have babies. . . you just don't put it on.

SP: Then you conceive [immediately]?

HW: Yes. [SP-00-I-21-7f]

HW: Why shouldn't a man [your boyfriend] use condoms? You see, you're too young to start using oral contraceptives. . . . Now, what if people at your home realize [you are taking them]? You know, some parents do not like to see their children use these pills. Suppose they see them at your home?

SP: Mm! They won't know about it.

HW: Some parents are not—are not educated enough to understand that . . . it's a disadvantage if a girl becomes pregnant. You're insisting on using those pills, but suppose they see them? You're not looking on both sides of the coin, you're just looking at one side of it only. [SP-00-C-12-7f]

Occasionally individuals mentioned other contraceptive methods such as Norplant, the female condom, vaginal microbicides, withdrawal, the calendar method, and sterilization, but it was rare for any to report personal experience of them.

Condom Use

Many villagers in *MEMA kwa Vijana* control communities had heard of condoms through radio, public meetings, or informal discussions. People who had some familiarity with condoms usually referred to them by the brand name *Salama*, which literally means "safety," or slang terms, such as "sock," "equipment," "load/burden," "dose," "passport," "jersey," "rubber," "General Tyre," "Scud" (as in Scud missile), "police," "soldier," and "traveler," the latter term being associated with a local bus of the name "Safe Traveler." Sex without condoms was similarly referred to using metaphors such as "barefooted" and "flesh-to-flesh."

People generally associated condoms with the prevention of sexually transmitted infection, not contraception. Condoms were available for free in government health facilities, and they usually could be purchased in kiosks for Tshs 50 ($0.06) for a pack of three. However, few villagers had seen a condom outside of its packet or had a clear understanding of how one was used, let alone had used one during intercourse.

A small minority of adult villagers had favorable comments to make about condoms and disease prevention, but most were government officials and health workers who did not discuss their own sexual activity. Generally, condoms were perceived negatively. The vast majority of respondents reported many reasons why they would not use condoms, including: a belief that condoms reduce sexual pleasure; not being "used to" condoms (particularly men); not having a say in the decision to use condoms (particularly women); not wanting to prevent conception; willingness to leave exposure to chance or God's will; perceiving no personal risk of acquiring HIV/AIDS or other sexually transmitted infections; trust in a partner; fear of stigma, rejection, or punishment; and suspicion that new condoms might have holes or contain HIV.

For many men a reduction in pleasure seemed to be the main reason they perceived condom use as unacceptable, even if their other concerns about condoms were resolved. A bicycle taxi driver, for example, said that he did not use condoms when having sex with his main girlfriend or with his other sexual partners because of this reason. He explained, "I would rather completely stop having sex than use condoms" [PO-99-I-6-1m], but he did not seriously consider abstaining. Men used numerous metaphors to describe how they believed condoms must dull sexual sensation, defeating the purpose of the sexual encounter, including "eating a sweet or chewing gum in its wrapper," "eating delicious, spicy meat in a paper bag," "staying at home and sleeping," and "farming with your hoe in a sack."

In addition to the belief that condoms reduce physical pleasure, some male informants reported that, if sex is to be satisfying and meaningful, it is important to ejaculate inside of a partner without a barrier. For example, a young carpenter: "If I have sex with a woman, I must spill my semen into her, so that she walks about with it" [PO-01-I-1-3m]. A few mentioned the belief that when sperm is ejaculated into a woman's body, it has the desirable effect of causing her to gain weight and become beautiful.

In several villages women reported that they would not consider condom use because they believed a condom might fall off during intercourse and remain lodged in the vagina. However, the overwhelming determinant in whether a woman would use a condom was whether her partner wanted to do so. For example, when a 23-year-old woman was asked whether she would use a condom if her husband requested it: "You will have to accept it. He is your husband, isn't he? You just accept it if he wants it that way" [II-02-I-252-f]. Outside of marriage men also generally felt entitled to set the terms of sexual encounters after providing a woman with a gift or money, and most considered condom use to be poor value for their money. For example:

[A 29-year-old cassava seller] said that when the man refuses to use condoms, the woman doesn't have any say. The other youths present said that very few women tell their men to use condoms, and [if they do] the men refuse and demand to be paid their money back. They said women can't do that, and eventually the couple agrees to make love without using condoms. [PO-01-I-1-3m]

Many villagers reported that they did not use condoms because they were not at risk of acquiring a sexually transmitted infection or AIDS. The most common circumstance in which men reported that they might use a condom was if they suspected a partner of having many other partners, or of having a sexually transmitted infection. However, even in such circumstances few men used condoms. For example, a 36-year-old woman who was widely perceived as a prostitute in one participant observation village:

> She said that she stays with a man for 2–3 days and then she gets another one. . . . She likes to tell her lovers to use condoms and she always keeps some, but not one of her lovers in that village have ever used them. . . . They refuse, saying that they won't get any happiness [pleasure] if they use condoms, as they prefer spilling/scattering their sperm into a woman's vagina. [PO-00-C-9-3m]

The association of promiscuity with condoms may have contributed to a fear of stigma among some potential condom users, particularly women. Broaching the issue of condoms also raised uncomfortable questions about a partner's infidelity, or one's own, potentially offending and alienating a partner. For instance, when a group of married women were asked why they had thrown away free condoms that they had been given at a health facility, they replied, "Why take them home? To be beaten by our husbands? To be told that we have become prostitutes?" [PO-01-C-3-3m] Similarly, a young man in his late teens reported:

> If you put on a condom, a girl will be afraid of you and think that you have encountered sexually transmitted infections before, and therefore she will tell other girls that you used a condom. She might also see you as a *mhuni*, or believe that you don't trust her. [PO-99-C-9-1m]

One of the most common reasons given for not using condoms was trust of a prospective or current sexual partner. For example, a single woman who was pregnant with her second child reported that she had never used condoms because she and her lover trusted each other. For those rare couples who began a sexual relationship using condoms, a period of one or two weeks, or a couple of sexual encounters, seemed sufficient for them to feel that they had established mutual trust and no longer needed to use condoms.

Those villagers who said they might consider condom use were sometimes concerned that if they tried to obtain condoms from local kiosks or health facilities it would not remain confidential. Health workers and kiosk staff said that their customers usually were embarrassed to request condoms and would not make eye contact, or would use slang terms to conceal what they were purchasing from other customers. Some condom providers contributed to customer or patient discomfort by asking personal questions or making inappropriate comments, as shown in a girl's interaction with a shopkeeper in case study 2.1. The following exchange between a male simulated patient and a health worker provided another example:

HW: What's your problem?

SP: I have come to request condoms.

HW: Condoms? . . . A young boy like you, you put on a condom! Who has sent you here for them?

SP: I just came on my own.

HW: You want to use them yourself?

SP: Yes.

HW: A youth like you! Whose son are you?

SP: . . . William's.

HW: My God! A young boy like that, you want to do those things, young like that?

HW: . . . Which class are you in?

SP: Year 6.

HW: . . . [Later] Now, just stay here and let me find some for you. . . . You should not get accustomed to these things; you're still a young person. My God! The day it bursts, you might even acquire diseases. . . . [Later] But if you are so desperately in need of sexual intercourse, as a natural desire of the human body, it is better that you use them than not, isn't it so?

SP: Yes! [SP-00-C-20-9m]

Shopkeepers reported that they sold condoms mainly to men in their twenties and thirties. In one large fishing village two shopkeepers independently estimated that they sold three to five packs of three condoms on a normal day, and as many as eight packs per day on market or video show days. Reports of condom sales were substantially lower in other villages. Cost rarely was mentioned when people discussed reasons why they did not use condoms, and a number of young men specifically noted that the cost of condoms was not a problem. Some respondents knew that condoms were available in health facilities but were uncertain whether they were free. In addition, the typical three to ten kilometer walk required to visit a health facility made it inconvenient to obtain them.

A small minority of villagers reported that they had used condoms. Usually, this involved having used them once or twice out of many prior sexual encounters. Consistent condom use with any or all partners over an extended period was very rare. Men whose work and income facilitated concurrent partnerships—such as shop owners or bicycle taxi drivers—and some women engaged in commercial sex work reported that they occasionally used condoms, or their sexual partners reported this. For example, a 16-year-old school girl who twice had sex with a shop owner in the district capital:

> *R:* He began telling me, "I want to marry you." . . . I told him, "I will never get married while still in school." He told me, "Let us have sex." . . . So we did, in his room in [the district capital], before he got married. . . . We use condoms. He wears it. [II-99-I-57-f]

Men sometimes were motivated to use condoms if they had personal experience of a sexually transmitted infection and/or if they considered their partners to be high risk. For example, a 20-year-old carpenter "said that he personally started using condoms [three years ago], after contracting a sexually transmitted infection. He said that he has continued using them until now, particularly when he is with a lover from outside, but that he doesn't use them when just with his wife" [PO-01-I-1-3m]. Similarly, a 25-year-old, married church choirmaster:

> He said that he uses condoms with lovers who he doesn't trust—those he fears have sexually transmitted infections or AIDS. He said usually he gets condoms from a heath worker he knows at the health facility, who gives them away for free. He also said that, whenever he brings some, those few other youth who also use them come to him to get condoms if they don't have them and want to have sex. He said he gives them away if he has them, for those youth also give him condoms when he needs them. [PO-00-C-3-3m]

Some men reported that they used condoms with a partner specifically because they had heard she had a sexually transmitted infection. An example from a male group discussion:

> *R:* The first time [I used a condom] it was normal, but when I ejaculated I found that it is useless. I didn't continue to have [unprotected] sex because I had doubts about the girl. I used to hear she had syphilis. I had only one condom, so when I finished I escaped, I didn't even say goodbye. . . . The second time I used a condom, when I put it on my penis, it took a while before I entered her [vagina] and the condom became dry. I mean when I touched it, it sounded like paper. I tried to have sex with the girl but I failed, so I had to take it off, throw it out, and then penetrate her without any protection. . . . I decided that it will be bad luck if she has a disease, and that will be my burden, but thank God she did not have any, and we had sex until morning. [GD-02-I-1-36m]

Women who had used condoms typically reported that they used them at their partner's initiative. For example, a 19-year-old single mother and kiosk worker:

> She said she is a bit confused on the issue of using a condom, because they were told . . . in church that condoms are used to prevent sexually transmitted infections, but not AIDS, because the virus can pass through a condom . . . She said she has never bought a condom on her own, as her boyfriend comes with it . . . and she has never felt unusual when having sex with a condom. [PO-99-C-5-2f]

Church and mosque leaders rarely opposed hormonal contraception in rural Mwanza, but their attitudes and advice about condom use were quite variable, ranging from leaders who voiced adamant opposition to it, to some who discreetly endorsed it, for example, by hosting an AIDS awareness workshop.

Rarely, school girls reported having used condoms for one or two sexual encounters after learning about them in their school lessons or due to unusually great fear of pregnancy, such as a girl who did not want to lose a hard-won place in secondary school. Girls who were "hard-to-get" and insistent on condoms were more successful in negotiating their use. For example, the girl in case study 1.4 ended a first sexual liaison with a man prior to intercourse because he did not have condoms, which ensured that he brought condoms to the next liaison.

Most women who had used condoms said that it did not feel very different from unprotected intercourse. In contrast, men who had used condoms sometimes reported that a condom use negatively delayed the onset of intercourse, changed friction, reduced sensation, and (most commonly) delayed ejaculation. As noted in chapter 8, achievement of multiple ejaculations within one sexual rendezvous was considered ideal for young men. They may thus have viewed prolonged intercourse with a condom negatively if they felt it reduced their total number of ejaculations within a given rendezvous.

Abortion

Abortion Frequency and Methods

Induced abortion in rural Mwanza was highly stigmatized, hidden, and infrequent, but nonetheless there were plausible first-hand reports of abortion attempts across the study area. Several participants in the female discussion group based in the largest village reported their own or a close acquaintance's abortion attempt. Female researchers heard a few first-person accounts of abortion attempts in each participant observation village, but male researchers did not. In most participant observation villages, female researchers also heard widespread rumors about one or more women who were believed to have recently terminated a pregnancy with dramatic consequences, and several relatively discreet and plausibly detailed stories about a friend's or relative's abortion attempt.

The most widely and frequently reported abortion method was ingestion of particular materials, mainly wood ashes in solution, high doses of chloroquine, and/or a solution of "Blue," a brand of laundry detergent sold in tablet form. Reports of the appropriate dosage, pregnancy timing, and effectiveness of these abortion methods varied. Most informants believed that too high of a dose of Blue could harm the woman and even kill her, but many also acknowledged that, because of the illicit nature of abortion attempts, women often did not know how much would be effective or dangerous. Many additionally reported that certain plants, such as *mwarobaini*, were abortifacients. Less frequently, informants reported that other brands of laundry detergent or high doses of aspirin or antibiotics were abortifacients. Most of the substances reported to be abortifacients could be obtained discreetly in rural areas at low cost, for example, Tshs 10–30 ($0.01–0.04) per chloroquine pill, or Tshs 50 ($0.06) per "Blue" tablet.

Many informants were also aware that abortions could be performed manually. A few reported that a woman could terminate her pregnancy using a twig; in two districts, cassava stems were specified. A few believed that certain villagers (usually older women) were experienced at performing manual abortions, using unknown instruments in their own homes. However, most young people who talked about manual abortions described them as being performed by health facility staff, typically costing Tshs 10,000–15,000 ($12–18) per procedure. These were mentioned most often in the larger villages and villages close to a health facility.

Opposition to Abortion

The vast majority of informants opposed abortion as illegal, dangerous for the woman, morally wrong, and particularly unacceptable if the man who caused the pregnancy did not consent. They often cited examples of specific women who they believed had experienced serious health problems as a result of abortions. For instance, an 18-year-old mother: "She said that abortion is bad and can lead to infertility. She gave an example of one woman who cannot give birth now, after having had several abortions when she was a girl" [PO-01-I-1-2f].

In each of the four study districts informants reported that ancestral spirits in some Sukuma clans opposed abortion and would kill any female members, and particularly the sexual partners of any male members, who attempted it. This is illustrated by the following three excerpts:

She said that a girl can only abort successfully if the man responsible for the pregnancy comes from a clan that allows abortion. If not, she will die in the course of the abortion. She gave the example of [a certain woman], who died while trying to abort against the wishes of the man who had impregnated her. [PO-00-C-3-2f]

P1: In our clan we are not allowed to abort.

F: For both girls and boys?

P1: Yes. . . . Once you're pregnant, you're not allowed to abort, but you just leave [the fetus] to grow, and then you give birth.

F: And if you abort?

P1: You will die in the course of aborting it.

P2: Perhaps that is so if you don't go to a doctor, but if you go to a doctor, the abortion will be successful.

P1: No, we are strictly forbidden to abort. So whether you go to the doctor or anywhere else, you're going to die. [GD-00-C-10-f]

R: There are very strong spiritual ancestors in our clan who do not allow abortions. If a girl attempts to abort a pregnancy that I caused, she will die. . . . I will tell her, "If you want to abort, you must ask me, you see!"

I: And how about the women from that clan, for instance your sisters, . . . if they have abortions, are they also affected?

R: It is only for the men [in the clan]. [GDII-00-C-12-4m]

Closely related to this clan taboo was the belief that abortion was particularly unacceptable if the man responsible for the pregnancy did not consent to it. Men were perceived as entitled to their potential offspring, and some male respondents expressed outrage that this right might be undermined. Two young men in their twenties gave the following examples:

R: If [my lover] aborts and I know that I made her pregnant, I would take her to court, because she has destroyed my property, she has killed my child. [GDII-00-C-12-5m]

He said that he decided to separate from [his wife of ten months], because she did things without his permission, [like] using birth control pills. He said that after discovering this, he hid the pills, so she became pregnant. He said what annoyed him enough to separate from her is that she then aborted without consulting him. . . . After taking her back to her parents' home, he told her parents [that] he would like her to stay there to reform and correct herself. [PO-00-C-3-3m]

Less frequently reported reasons why people opposed abortion were that it was illegal, immoral, disrespectful (for example, insulting to infertile individuals), or unwise (for example, reducing the number of children who could care for a woman in her old age).

Toleration or Acceptance of Abortion

Although most informants said they were opposed to abortion, some were also sympathetic, acknowledging that women usually terminated a pregnancy because of difficult life circumstances. A minority of informants did not condemn the act of abortion when the topic came up. These tended to be women who had attempted to end a pregnancy themselves, or who had friends who had done so. This group ranged in age from young to middle-aged, and included women of different social status, for example, women who were single and considered somewhat disreputable, single and socially respected women, and married women. Informants commonly reported inter-related reasons why a girl or woman might terminate a pregnancy, including being in school and living with parents, being unmarried and unsupported by the baby's father, experiencing financial hardship, being afraid to jeopardize marriage prospects, and/or wanting longer intervals between children. Generally, school girls and single women were considered the people most likely to have an abortion.

Abortion Decision-Making

Some young women faced with unwanted pregnancies were advised to have an abortion by those close to them, but they chose not to do so for fear of potential health problems. The following example was provided by a mother in her 20s:

> *R:* When I became pregnant, I didn't think of aborting it, but my father [a district hospital nurse] called me and counseled me, [saying], "My daughter, come here to abort, so you may continue with your studies. . . ." But I refused. . . . The idea is not good at all, because you may die from the abortion, so it is meaningless. [GDII-00-C-10-3f]

A small number of women reported feeling desperate to end an unwanted pregnancy. In the following example, a young guest in a female researcher's household confided that she had come there from a smaller village because she needed postabortion care at a health facility. The researcher recorded the woman's account in her field notes:

> Her lover promised to marry her, and went to his [distant] home village to tell his family. However, they forbade him to marry her, and he was told to become engaged to someone at home. . . . [Eventually] he admitted [to her]

that he was engaged to another, but he stopped her from terminating her pregnancy. . . . She waited for him to travel, and then [one month ago] she aborted the pregnancy by drinking a solution of "Blue." She bled profusely and experienced severe pain. . . . Today she paid Tshs 5,000 ($6) for a dilation and curettage procedure. She asked me to escort her because she was told that the anesthetic would put her into a heavy sleep. . . . I left her when she went into the room for the procedure. [Afterward] she told me that she was treated without any problems. [PO-01-I-7-5f]

Outcomes of Abortion Attempts

A number of women reported secret abortion attempts which failed, from which they had no apparent consequences. These women carried their pregnancies to term. The following two examples were reported by adult women who had attempted abortion when they were school girls:

R: I looked for any medicine to drink, so that I could have an abortion and continue in school. My best friend [a classmate] advised me to drink "Blue." I drank that . . . but I didn't abort. . . . I changed the medicine and drank ashes [recommended by the same friend]. I still didn't abort. . . . One woman told me, "If you are looking for medicine to drink to abort, then you should go to a traditional healer." Of course, I went there . . . [and the traditional healer] gave me medicine [for Tshs 3,000 ($4), to be paid afterward]. . . . It was just crushed, dried, and ground roots. . . . [The healer] told me, "You must eat until you are full, and then . . . you drink it and go to bed. When you wake the next morning, your pregnancy will have come out. If you bleed profusely, you shouldn't worry much; that is how it is with this medicine." Of course, I drank that medicine, but I didn't bleed, not even a drop. . . . So I just had to carry that pregnancy until I gave birth. [GDII-00-C-11-5f]

[The first time she had sex], she was in Year 7 . . . She agreed to make love with [a married man] because he offered to buy her shoes to wear when singing in the choir. [During intercourse], her lower vagina ruptured, and she couldn't stand the pain, so she had to tell her mother, who told her to massage herself with hot water. It was on that day that she conceived. . . . She tried to abort by using traditional medicine, "Blue," and chloroquine, but she failed. . . . After four months, she quit school, because she was forbidden to have a [different kind of] abortion. Eventually, she gave birth and married the man who made her pregnant. [PO-01-I-7-5f]

Of the women who reported having terminated a pregnancy, most said they had at least short-term negative health consequences (for example, severe pain and bleeding for days or weeks), but none mentioned regretting the decision later. In the following account, a woman revealed how she ultimately saw her abortion as beneficial in her life:

During the meal, Grace said, "Kulwa, truly, if I hadn't done that, I would have nothing now." Kulwa said, "If you hadn't done what?" Grace said, "What I did that time when I was pregnant." Kulwa exclaimed, "Aha! Ee! If you hadn't done that, you would have many worries." I asked Grace what she had done, but she only laughed and said, "These are just our personal issues." [Later] Kulwa told me that Grace became pregnant before marriage, while living at [her parents'] home. . . . She said that Grace had had an abortion. Three days later she began feeling stomach pain. She went to the dispensary and they found unclean detritus in her stomach. She was injected with anesthetics, and the material was removed. [PO-01-I-7-5f]

The negative consequences women experienced from induced abortion included opposition from their sexual partners, sexual exploitation by practitioners, health problems, social ostracism, and quasi-legal sanctions. Both first- and third-person abortion reports commonly mentioned postabortion health problems that eventually led women to visit a health facility (usually for curettage) some days or weeks after the initial procedure. Two examples follow.

She mentioned that her cousin tried to end her pregnancy with her aunt's assistance, but when her condition became serious, her aunt rushed her to the district hospital. When her cousin's father heard about this, he strongly condemned his daughter and her aunt and refused to give them any assistance. [PO-01-I-1-2f]

She said that during [her niece's] first abortion, the girl narrowly escaped death and was taken to the hospital, where she received a blood transfusion. She said that [the second time her niece terminated a pregnancy], she managed to do so without any problems. [PO-01-I-1-3m]

In a group discussion, one woman described both the immediate pain of the manual abortion that she experienced and how she was compelled to have sex with the abortion provider to compensate him:

P: I once used the white person's method to abort [had an abortion in a health-care facility], because I became pregnant unexpectedly, when I already had a six-or seven-month-old baby. So I was afraid. . . . I was told [by a health-facility staff person], "Don't tell [anyone]." . . . I told him that I would pretend to be suffering from backache. So he agreed, [saying,] "Those people at home will ask to take you to the hospital, and you will say, 'No. I will just buy some medicine, and I will recover.'"

F: You paid a lot of money [for the abortion]?

P: Ah, that man used to know me. We agreed that once the abortion was successful, we would talk it over again. . . . I just paid him with my body [had sex

with him later]. . . . He conducted the abortion without anesthesia. He asked me
to just tolerate it. I said okay. . . . In fact, I felt pain, because you know those
modern methods, using scissors and what not . . . He harassed it inside there. . . .
[Afterwards] I took nearly 15 [painkiller] pills. I recovered. . . . I had to keep it a
secret, so those people at home did not know anything about it. [GD-00-C-10-f]

Some women experienced social ostracism after an abortion, or when
others thought that they had had one. Single women who gained weight,
appeared pregnant without acknowledging it, and then suddenly lost weight
were sometimes believed to have induced an abortion. One researcher observed how a young woman experiencing debilitating symptoms was rumored to have had an abortion. Excerpts from two months of the researcher's
fieldwork follow:

Day 6: Helena was suffering from a stomachache. . . . She said that she took
some herbs [traditional medicine] and felt okay.

Day 21: Helena was still suffering from a stomachache. She said she has pain,
especially when she menstruates. She said she now has a fever, a backache, and
a lack of appetite.

Day 27: Helena's stomach condition has become critical. She said that she has
taken almost every type of traditional medicine, but she hasn't experienced any
relief. . . . After two months [of symptoms] . . . she began taking aspirin and ace-
tominophen . . . but they gave her no relief. Helena's mother said that she will
take her to the hospital for treatment today. . . . [After returning from the hospi-
tal] Helena said she was given a dose of five injections and some yellow pills.

Day 32: Helena told me that she thanked God for being able to walk upright,
because during the last two days she could only walk bending forward over her
belly, because of the acute pain in her stomach. Her friend interrupted her, saying that, in the hot sun, Helena had been walking like an expectant mother who
was about to deliver.

Day 37: After greeting Helena, a male kiosk owner told her that she has done
something very bad if she really has had an abortion. The kiosk owner went on
to say that many people struggle day and night to have children, without success, but Helena [wastefully] aborted. Helena replied that those who say [she
had an abortion] are fools, because their accusations are baseless. The kiosk
owner looked at Helena and said, 'How have you become very long and thin? It
is true that you aborted.' Helena became annoyed. . . . While heading home, she
said that the whole village believes that she has aborted a pregnancy, but only
God knows if she really did. [PO-00-I-4-4f]

Although researchers heard multiple reports of specific women who had
terminated their pregnancies recently, they saw no evidence of formal le-

gal proceedings and only one case in which quasi-legal proceedings took place. In that village, a man in his mid-20s was charged large fines because he paid a health worker Tshs 15,000 ($18) for his girlfriend (who was also the mother of his two children) to end a pregnancy caused by another man. Both the woman and the father of her children were participant observation informants and openly discussed their relationship and other sexual partners with researchers, but neither mentioned an abortion. Details of the incident only became widely known when the man who had caused the pregnancy brought charges against the first man at a *sungusungu* meeting. The first man confessed and, as punishment, his family paid the *sungusungu* Tshs 28,000 ($35) and the village Tshs 200,000 ($240) and one cow. They were threatened with formal ostracism if they did not pay the fine, for example, other villagers would not have been allowed to visit the family's home, even in the event of a funeral. Soon afterward, the young woman married another man and moved to another village. The abortion practitioner appeared to continue his practice without consequence.

Pregnancy Suspension: "Moving It to the Back"

Some people, such as the young woman described in case study 2.3, referred to a practice of using traditional medicine to move a woman's pregnancy indefinitely to her back (*kupindya nda ku ngongo*). This practice was believed to suspend fetal development for months or years until traditional medicines were used to return the pregnancy to its original position, after which growth resumed. This belief was reported independently in five participant observation villages, and in response to questions in each of the villages where group discussions were held. The following example was reported by a health officer who was married to a traditional healer: "He said that some women use magic with their [unmarried] daughters and can shift a pregnancy to the daughter's back so that it will not be seen, especially if the girl is still young. The girl then gives birth at the time her parents choose" [PO-00-C-3-2f].

Although pregnancy suspension was widely believed to be possible, it was considered rare, and no woman reported that she had used it herself. However, a male traditional healer and a male fisherman in different districts reported having made such medicines for women who successfully suspended their pregnancies, and a few other respondents reported that they knew someone who had suspended a pregnancy in this way. For example:

P: When my cousin was in Year 6 . . . she became pregnant by a boy whose grandmother is a traditional healer . . . and the grandmother made some medicine for her. They usually say in Sukuma that they take it to the back, here [gesturing], so that it can't be seen. That girl stayed like that for two years. She completed school and stayed for another year, and then it was returned to her womb and she gave birth. [GD-00-C-10-m]

P: I, too, heard about this from my classmate, when I was in Year 7. . . . The teachers took her to be examined [and she was found to be pregnant]. . . . Her mother gave her some medicines and told her to go back to school. . . . The teachers took her to be re-examined, and she was not pregnant. The pregnancy had moved into her back. . . . [After completing school] she continued being pregnant just as before. People were surprised. [GD-00-C-12-f]

Most people believed that the woman and fetus did not suffer any symptoms in this condition and that no signs of the pregnancy could be detected, even upon medical examination. Generally, people reported that girls or women moved their pregnancies to their backs for the same reasons that a woman might seek abortion, for example, because they were in school and not married. Often, however, these stories involved a woman who became pregnant by one man but wanted to attribute the pregnancy to another man at a later date, ideally a future husband. As one young woman explained:

R: If that pregnancy was, let's say, three months old, a woman will suspend growth until after staying with a [new] man for three months. Then it is returned to the womb again and it is released to grow. So the man will think that that pregnancy is his, but, in fact, it belongs to another man. [GDII-00-C-10-3f]

Frequently, pregnancy suspension accounts described a girl's mother or grandmother as having a key role in this process. Few informants seemed to condemn girls who they believed used it, and it was not considered as shameful or stigmatized as abortion. An example from a primary school teacher: "She said that people even move pregnancies to the back in her [distant] home village. She said it is done more often there [than here], because abortion is not accepted there at all and is condemned by many people" [PO-01-C-3-3m].

Although suspending a pregnancy generally was reported as a woman's choice, a couple of informants said that it might also be performed against a woman's will through bewitchment. For example, a traditional healer reported that a pregnancy could be moved to the back by malicious sorcery (*kabugume*):

[For *kabugume*] he said that usually the medicine is prepared by using soil from a place where the woman urinated. . . . [He said] the woman experiences a lot of back pain, and can be treated by a traditional healer. . . . He said that there are some who request this traditional medicine for themselves, but in such a case, the pregnancy would be hidden for just a few months, [whereas for *kabugume*] the pregnancy is hidden for a long time. [PO-01-C-2-1m]

Only a few participants stated that they did not believe that a pregnancy could be suspended, and most of them had attained an unusually high level of formal education, such as completing some secondary school.

Beliefs about Fertility Protection and Promotion

Protection and promotion of future fertility was paramount for young, unmarried women in rural Mwanza even if they did not want to become pregnant in the near future. Thus if girls believed that contraception or an induced abortion might affect their long-term fertility, they would generally rather risk immediate pregnancy and childbearing than later infertility. For example, a Year 7 girl who was the daughter of a Pentacostal preacher feared being thrown out of her home if she became pregnant, but she declined another girl's offer to make her a traditional contraceptive: "She fears being infertile in the future. She said that people say traditional contraceptives are only good [safe] for people who have given birth, not girls [who have never been pregnant]" [PO-01-I-1-2f]. When the researcher returned to that village one year later this young woman was pregnant and had left the village after being thrown out of her father's house.

Once a woman married her priority quickly shifted to becoming pregnant. Infertility and miscarriage were widely attributed to physical causes (such as sexually transmitted infections, contraception, or abortion history for females; "cold" sperm or one testicle for males) as well as supernatural causes (such as God's will, witchcraft, or ancestral punishment). For example, a 17-year-old woman who recently had completed Year 7:

> She said she doesn't use any contraceptives because she knows she can't get pregnant. She said she has *michango*, which cause her a lot of pain during her monthly period. . . . She was told that the moment she takes traditional medicine to cure the problem, she will conceive. [PO-00-C-3-2f]

Mchango (pl. *michango*) literally means "intestinal worm," but in rural Mwanza was often used interchangeably with the term **nzoka** (literally "snake"), to mean a broad range of illnesses which might have supernatural causes and require traditional treatment. For example: "The informant said that *michango* could pierce a woman's womb and cause her to have a miscarriage. . . . He gave the example of [a certain woman], who . . . had several miscarriages and had to take traditional medicines, [after which] she had her current child" [PO-01-C-2-1m]. An infertility-related *mchango* or **nzoka** was often characterized by severe menstrual cramping and bleeding.

If a married couple did not conceive within one or two years, the woman was almost always assumed to have fertility problems. Typically, a man was only considered to be infertile if he had had multiple long-term sexual relationships with women who did not conceive, particularly if the women were known to have conceived children with other men. In most study villages, people reported that wives of infertile men might seek secret extramarital partners specifically to become pregnant. This was a rare instance when discreet female infidelity was considered understandable and even warranted.

There was very little opportunity for biomedical treatment of infertility in rural Mwanza, with the exception of treatment of sexually transmitted infections, which indirectly could protect or promote fertility. Active attempts to treat infertility were almost always traditional in nature. Traditional medicines used to treat infertility caused by sexually transmitted infections or *michango* usually consisted of specific plant roots that were prepared for the woman to ingest, although there were also reports of medicines being placed in a woman's vagina, marked on her body, or left at a crossroads to be stepped on so that the condition would be taken away by another woman. An example provided by a 27-year-old man:

> He told me that [his partner's] condition had become worse and that she had been taken to the hospital. She had been taking some local plants [to become pregnant] which she was given by a certain man who . . . had been taught about it by his late grandmother. He said that the traditional medicine had affected her, because she had been given a large dose and hence it had burnt her abdomen. [PO-99-C-2-1m]

If pregnancy did occur, most beliefs about carrying a healthy pregnancy to term related to the woman getting adequate nutrition and rest and not over-exerting herself. One participant observation researcher noted that this seemed more difficult to achieve for young women who were pregnant out-of-wedlock. He commented:

> Those women who get pregnant within marriage receive early services; sometimes their husbands even take them to the health facility and do [extra] domestic chores. In the household where I am staying, [an unmarried girl] is pregnant. I see that there isn't any relief for her, relief that is normally given to those who are pregnant when doing different domestic work. . . . I feel this situation is causing her to be weak, which she shows most of the time. [PO-01-I-1-3m]

Across the study area problematic pregnancies frequently were explained in terms of supernatural forces, but the interpretation often differed depending on whether it was first-person or third-person accounts. Speaking about themselves, women usually explained their problematic pregnancies in terms of other people's maliciousness and witchcraft. For example, a 42-year-old widow with eight children described the negative outcome of her sixth pregnancy:

[In her ninth month of pregnancy], one day she felt something protruding from her private parts . . . she found someone with a bicycle to take her to the hospital. . . . she said that [her child was stillborn] because of the mischief [witchcraft] of people of that village. . . . She said people who don't have children are not happy when they see other women deliver without problems. [PO-00-I-4-4f]

In contrast, when respondents explained another woman's problematic pregnancy or delivery in supernatural terms, the problems were sometimes explained as punishment for her immoral behavior. For example, many respondents reported that, if a pregnant woman had sex with a man other than the one who impregnated her, she would encounter certain dangers during delivery (*lwikilo*). In fact, difficult deliveries were sometimes taken as evidence of a woman's infidelity in pregnancy. This belief was reported in each study district, with many accounts involving parents-in-law discovering a daughter-in-law's infidelity. No respondents reported that they had experienced *lwikilo* themselves. *Lwikilo* related to a belief that, after conception, a sexual partner's sperm or blood influenced fetal development. While fluids from the child's father were believed to help the fetus grow, fluids from another man were believed to confuse it, and to make it move upwards towards the woman's chest, possibly harming her and the fetus. In two districts the fetus was reported to try to emerge from her mouth during delivery. A 25-year-old man provided one example: "He said that if a woman becomes pregnant and continues to have sex with different men, then . . . the child would want to burst through his/her mother's liver and ribs and might come out of the mouth." [PO-02-I-4-1m] *Lwikilo* reportedly could be treated during delivery if the woman swallowed traditional medicines and named her lovers. A mother of seven provided an example:

She reported if the woman takes traditional medicines, she will vomit, and she will have to mention the names of any sex partners she has had other than the man who caused the pregnancy. . . . She said [a certain man's daughter-in-law] was in the hospital when she had that problem, but she was given those [traditional] medicines and then delivered her child safely. [PO-01-C-2-6f]

DISCUSSION

Contraception

Our study found that many school girls in rural Mwanza were sexually active and highly motivated to prevent pregnancy but relied on traditional contraceptive methods which were similar to practices documented by Tanner (1955b) in the mid-twentieth century and were unlikely to be effective. Young, single

mothers in our study had better access to modern contraceptives than adolescents who had not borne children, but many chose not to use them. This
may reflect external pressures related to their fertility, ambivalent personal
desires, and a general openness to chance, as has been found elsewhere in
sub-Saharan Africa (Johnson-Hanks 2005; Harrison and O'Sullivan 2010). It
may also result from contradictory information they received about possible
side effects from family planning providers and informal village discussions.

Concerns about potential contraceptive side effects, particularly of oral
contraceptives and condoms, were very similar to those documented in other
studies in the region (Mgalla and Boerma 2001; Allen 2002) and elsewhere
in sub-Saharan Africa (Rutenberg and Watkins 1997; Castle 2003a; Westhoff
2003; Wood and Jewkes 2006; Williamson et al. 2009). Many of the reported
side effects of hormonal contraceptives are known possibilities in the short-
term (e.g., menstrual or weight change) and the long-term (e.g., delayed
return to fertility once an injectable contraceptive is discontinued) (Castle
2003a; Westhoff 2003). However, some widely reported side effects had
no scientific basis, such as permanent infertility. It may be that information
about possible negative health effects provided during family planning counseling sessions (such as possible associations of hormonal contraceptives and
specific cancers) may be misstated by health workers and/or misunderstood
or exaggerated by patients afterwards. As Mgalla and Boerma (2001) found
in their study of infertility in another rural Mwanza district, the limited health
education available in school or health facility settings may sometimes be
integrated with existing incorrect beliefs, reinforcing them by making them
appear more scientific and credible.

Finally, there were widespread misconceptions and negativity towards
condoms in our study population. A number of factors contributed to this, including: the dynamics of gender and power; cultural values concerning meaningful, decent, or natural sex and reproduction; the alien nature of condoms;
the association of condoms with infection, promiscuity, and reduced sexual
pleasure; and the difficulty of accessing condoms due to embarrassment or
distance. The single, strong belief that condoms reduce sexual pleasure—particularly for men—was widely reported by study participants. Indeed, many
of the other reported concerns about condoms (for example, that they might
be contaminated, old, ineffective, or prohibited) may have been secondary
rationalizations fueled by this fundamental male concern.

Fertility Protection

In our study, young women's concern that contraceptives may reduce their
later ability to have children underlines the fundamental importance of future

fertility for them, and their potential anxiety related to it. As Castle (2003a) found in her study of young people in Mali, unmarried women's contraceptive decision making was often not driven by a current need to limit fertility (or current issues such as accessibility, availability, and cost of methods), but rather by a future need to maximize it, in order to raise their status through childbearing in their marital households. Similarly, in her ethnographic research on maternal health in a Sukuma village, Allen (2002) found that many women were concerned from an early age about both physical and spiritual factors that may affect their ability to conceive or give birth in the future.

Single young women's concern to protect and promote their future fertility may represent an opportunity for condom social marketing campaigns. Unlike hormonal contraceptives, condoms were not rumored to affect long-term fertility. To the contrary, condoms could be promoted as a means of pregnancy prevention in the present that also actively protect future fertility, specifically because they reduce the possibility of contracting sexually transmitted infections which may cause infertility. With greater education about the links between sexually transmitted infection and male infertility (Pellati et al. 2008), such an approach could also be employed with boys and men. While these findings suggest promising new approaches to condom promotion in sub-Saharan Africa, it is important to recognize that other barriers to condom use remain high, including multiple misconceptions, reduced sensation during intercourse, and the male decision-making role, so new and/or intensified strategies are necessary to address them as well.

Abortion

We found plausible evidence that induced abortion was a widespread but infrequent practice in rural Mwanza. Abortion was highly secretive, dangerous, and stigmatized, but nonetheless a small minority of women had attempted it at some point in the past and managed to keep this a secret whether or not the abortion was successful. Abortion attempts involved a range of potentially unsafe methods with variable results. Some women ingested dangerously high doses of medications or products not intended for human consumption; some trusted people with little or no training or resources to perform manual abortions; some were financially or sexually exploited in their desperation; and some suffered serious health consequences and social ostracism afterward.

Most of the voiced opposition to abortion in rural Mwanza was not based on the concept of the sanctity of human life, as it is in Western, and particularly Christian, arguments, although the majority of villagers identified themselves as Christian, and approximately one-third as Catholic. This belief may be so fundamental as to be assumed and, therefore, was not stated explicitly. Instead, opposition to abortion usually was expressed in practical terms, such as concern about it causing physical harm to the woman, which was a serious possibility in this setting. When moral concerns were raised, they usually related to the violation of the authority of ancestors, or to the undermining of the reproductive entitlement of the man who caused the pregnancy. These two issues frequently were linked in people's statements and usually included descriptions of extreme retribution such as severe illness or death that the man's ancestors would visit upon a woman who aborted a pregnancy he had caused.

As discussed in chapter 3, Sukuma men traditionally secured primary entitlement to any offspring upon payment of bridewealth (Cory 1953; Varke-visser 1973; Wijsen and Tanner 2002). If a wife was found to have induced an abortion, her husband was entitled to divorce her (Cory 1953). Although payment of bridewealth is less common today than in the past, our findings suggest that even in the absence of legal, religious, or traditional marriage agreements, some men aggressively prevented their partners from aborting specifically because they felt entitled to any potential offspring. Notably, while such an entitlement was suggested in both men's and women's reports, only male informants voiced outrage that a woman might end a pregnancy against her sexual partner's wishes. Previous research on abortion in sub-Saharan Africa has identified a gap in understanding about the role that women's sexual partners play in abortion decision making (Benson et al. 1996; Mundigo 1999; Silberschmidt and Rasch 2001; Rasch and Lyaruu 2005). Our study suggests that, while some men were informed and supported their partners in obtaining an abortion, others' strong opposition led women to seek even more clandestine abortion methods.

Despite powerful social norms and highly restrictive laws opposing abortion, most rural informants' reactions to girls and women who attempted it seemed to be ambivalent and pragmatic. Parents who encouraged or assisted their daughters to terminate a pregnancy might have voiced opposition to abortion in a general discussion, but chose to support it when their family faced potential stigma, and their daughters faced a difficult future as school drop-outs or single mothers. Similarly, when strong public evidence existed that abortions had taken place, the women generally were stigmatized and ostracized, but none faced formal prosecution or imprisonment, and medical staff who were rumored to perform abortions appeared to continue their practice without challenge. Only one case of abortion led to quasi-legal proceedings, and it involved exceptional circumstances: a man arranged for his lover to terminate a pregnancy caused by another man. The first man's role in "usurping" the reproductive entitlement of the other man was particularly unacceptable to the community, and he was forced to pay a large fine. These findings are in keeping with Stroeken's (2001) observation that Sukumas generally feel ambivalent towards breeches of community norms and would rather heavily fine someone guilty than moralize and reprimand.

Of the limited range of manufactured products available in rural Mwanza at the time of the study, certain of them taken in high doses were believed to be abortifacients throughout the study area and beyond, for example, chloroquine and, earlier, quinine (Bleek 1978; Bledsoe and Goubaud 1988; Etkin 1992; Allen 2002; Marchant et al. 2004; Grimes et al. 2006). The laundry detergent "Blue," for example, was identified by villagers as an extremely dangerous abortifacient in Ghana in the early 1970s (Bleek 1978). This finding is in keeping with studies in different low income countries which have found products designed and distributed for a specific purpose may sometimes be widely used in a different way than recommended (Bledsoe and Goubaud 1988; Etkin 1992).

Prior research on abortion in Tanzania has suggested that adolescents are more likely than older women to attempt abortion by unsafe means and to experience harsh physical consequences (Rwebangire 1994; Silberschmidt and Rasch 2001; Allen 2002; Stambach 2003; Rasch et al. 2004). Similarly, in our study most of the detailed and plausible accounts of abortion involved young, single women who were desperate to end an unintended pregnancy. Adolescents were most likely to ingest harmful substances rather than seek an illegal abortion at a health facility, because such substances were widely discussed as abortifacients and were cheap and easy to obtain secretly. We found little evidence of women who were in their late twenties or older attempting to induce abortion, possibly because older and married women had less incentive to terminate pregnancies, but possibly also because the study specifically focused on young people.

Misclassification can be a problem in any study of abortion (Rasch et al. 2000). For example, clinical records of abortion attempts may be falsified intentionally in settings where the procedure is illegal (Grimes et al. 2006), as was demonstrated in a study of hospitals in Dar es Salaam, Tanzania, where on-site, safe abortions were routinely recorded as incomplete or septic off-site abortions requiring follow-up dilation and curettage (Rwebangire 1994). Another possible source of misclassification is honest but inaccurate reports, for example, from informants who believe that they aborted although they were not pregnant, or community members who reported that a woman moved her pregnancy to her back when, in fact, she experienced a miscarriage or induced abortion. In this study, however, many first-person and third-person accounts of abortion attempts were highly detailed and plausible, which argues for their validity.

Pregnancy Suspension

Our findings on stigma related to abortion may help explain the widespread belief that a woman's pregnancy can be moved to her back, indefinitely suspending growth and delaying childbirth. The belief that herbal medicine can be used to extend a pregnancy well beyond nine months is not unique to this part of Africa, as reports of pregnancies being made to "sleep" or "lie down" have also been documented in Nigeria (Kleiner-Bossaller 1993; Renne 1997). In Tanzania, Varkevisser (1973) and Allen (2002) found this belief to be widespread in their anthropological studies conducted in Mwanza Region (1965–67) and in neighboring Shinyanga Region (1992–94), although their interpretations of the belief differed. In Allen's (2002) study, virtually all 154 women surveyed had heard of moving a pregnancy to the back and believed that this was the result of malicious sorcery, requiring diagnosis and treatment by a traditional healer. Nine of the women interviewed reported first-person experience of this, and the author noted that some may have been attempting to account for infertility in a society in which a woman's ability to bear children is highly valued. In contrast, Varkevisser's (1973) informants from Mwanza, like those in our study sample, reported that women intentionally ingested materials believed to move inopportune pregnancies to their backs. Whether any of Varkevisser's informants reported first-hand experience of this is unclear.

In our study, the lack of first-person reports of this practice may result from the broadly different interpretation of the practice in the two regions. In Shinyanga the belief that a woman has been victimized and her pregnancy involuntarily suspended by witchcraft may make infertility more acceptable, both socially and personally. In Mwanza, however, where the condition generally is believed to result from a woman's secret attempt to postpone an unintended pregnancy, those who have attempted it may be much more reluctant to reveal it. Alternatively, it may be that few if any women attempted to suspend their pregnancies in Mwanza, but third-person reports about it persisted as people tried to explain the reproductive anomalies of others.

Fertility Promotion

Our findings that newly married women rarely attempted traditional or modern contraception were in keeping with traditional Sukuma beliefs that adults were not "whole" or "complete" (***mhola***) until they had had children (Brandström 1999), and that they must prove their fertility with a first child before considering birth control for child spacing purposes (Varkevisser 1973). In this study, many of the symptoms which were believed to indicate an infertility-related *mchango* may have related to conditions like endometriosis, but biomedical diagnosis and treatment was rarely possible. The dearth of clinical infertility services, other limitations of biomedical care, and traditional health and illness beliefs meant that individuals instead mainly sought traditional methods to promote their fertility. Similar findings have been found elsewhere in sub-Saharan Africa and the developing world (Sundby, Mboge and Sonko 1998; Nachtigall 2006; Folkvord, Odegaard, and Sundby 2005). We found that some of those traditional treatments—such as those for perceived infertility, or for certain kinds of difficult labor—may have been at best ineffective and at worst emotionally and physically harmful.

In this study, reports that certain problematic deliveries were attributed to a woman's promiscuity (*lwikilo*)—and that such problems could be avoided by naming the men involved—are similar to those of other studies in Mwanza Region, neighboring Shinyanga Region, and elsewhere in sub-Saharan Africa (Caldwell, Caldwell, and Quiggin 1989). Varkevisser (1973) also described beliefs about *lwikilo* as a condition in which a child tried to emerge from a mother's mouth, for which the mother must divulge her sexual partners' names and receive traditional treatment to be cured (Varkevisser 1973). More recently Allen (2002) witnessed a prolonged, stalled labor at which the birth attendant, a traditional healer who specialized in pregnancy and delivery, treated the woman with herbal medicine because she believed the child was moving towards the woman's chest as a result of the woman's promiscuity during pregnancy. After 24 hours the woman was moved to a hospital where staff noted that her full bladder probably had impeded her child's descent. Her child died soon after delivery there.

CONCLUSION

Since the time of our study, reproductive health services in rural Mwanza have not changed dramatically. For example, in the 2004–2005 Demographic and Health Survey in Mwanza Region, 9 percent of currently married women were using modern contraceptives and 47 percent of live births took place in a health facility, while in the 2009–2010 survey the figures were 12 percent and 46 percent, respectively (National Bureau of Statistics and ORC Macro 2005; National Bureau of Statistics and ICF Macro 2010). There remains a critical need for improved reproductive health education and services in rural Mwanza as in many other parts of sub-Saharan Africa, including interventions to address widespread misconceptions about hormonal contraceptives and condoms, increased access to modern contraception for sexually active young people who have not borne children, improved fertility services for women who have difficulty conceiving, and better medical care for pregnant and delivering young women. Condom promotion campaigns may be more successful if they emphasize both the contraceptive value of condoms, and that condoms may protect future fertility through sexually transmitted infection prevention.

Increasing the practice of effective contraception is likely to prevent some unsafe abortions, but it is unlikely to eliminate them completely, because unwanted pregnancies will occur when couples do not use contraceptives and when contraceptives fail (Bongaarts and Westoff 2000). Many sub-Saharan African countries have increased women's access to legal abortion since 1995, and advocacy for legal access has increased in several others (Grimes et al. 2006). Globally, increased legal access to abortion has not increased the demand for abortions appreciably, but it has greatly improved their safety, resulting in significant improvements in sexual and reproductive health (Grimes et al. 2006). For example, after abortion became legal upon request in South Africa, abortion-related deaths dropped 91 percent from 1994 to 1998–2001 (Jewkes et al. 2005). The Tanzanian government has expressed concern about maternal morbidity and mortality related to the estimated high incidence of illegal abortions (United Nations 2002). Our findings that women in Mwanza persisted in obtaining unsafe abortions despite strong disincentives suggests that, in addition to improving reproductive health education and services, legal access to safe abortion should also be considered in Tanzania.

We will now move to another critical sexual health issue in sub-Saharan Africa: HIV/AIDS and other sexually transmitted infections. The next chapter will focus on beliefs about these infections in rural Mwanza, and traditional and biomedical treatment practices related to them.

NOTE

1. Some material in this chapter was adapted from: (a) Plummer, Mary L., Daniel Wight, Joyce Wamoyi, Gerry Mshana, Richard J. Hayes, and David A. Ross. 2006. Farming with your hoe in a sack: Condom attitudes, access, and use in rural Tanzania. *Studies in Family Planning* 37(1):29–40. (b) Plummer, Mary L., Joyce Wamoyi, Kija Nyalali, Gerry Mshana, Zachayo S. Shigongo, David A. Ross, and Daniel Wight. 2008. Aborting and suspending pregnancy in rural Tanzania: An ethnography of young people's beliefs and practices. *Studies in Family Planning* 39(4):281–92. (c) Plummer, Mary L., Joyce Wamoyi, Zachayo S. Shigongo, Gerry Mshana, Angela I. N. Obasi, David A. Ross, and Daniel Wight. 2010. "Seek any means, and keep it your secret": Young women's attempts to control their reproduction through contraceptive and fertility practices in rural Tanzania. *Tanzania Journal of Health Research* (12)3:178–93.

Chapter Eleven

HIV/AIDS and Other Sexually Transmitted Infections[1]

Sexually transmitted infections are widespread in sub-Saharan Africa, particularly amongst young people (WHO 2001; UNAIDS 2010). During the 1998 *MEMA kwa Vijana* survey, for example, less than 1 percent of males of average age 16 years and 2 percent of females of average age 15 years tested positive for HIV, gonorrhea, or Chlamydia (Todd et al. 2004). However, three years later 14 percent of males tested positive for one or more of five infections tested for males, and 45 percent of females tested positive for one or more of six infections tested for females (Helen Weiss, personal communication).

Some sexually transmitted infections can be cured and the symptoms of others can be treated, but such biomedical care usually requires symptom recognition, a health facility visit, correct treatment, and patient compliance (Grosskurth et al. 1995; Wald and Link 2002; Freeman et al. 2006). At the time of our study only one-quarter of rural sub-Saharan African women with sexually transmitted infections or reproductive tract infections were believed to recognize their symptoms and to attend health facilities for treatment (Hayes et al. 1997). When people did seek such treatment in rural Mwanza, health workers managed sexually transmitted infections syndromically, that is, in the absence of laboratory tests they treated patients for all possible infections that could have caused their symptoms (Grosskurth et al. 1995).

One barrier to appropriate treatment of sexually transmitted infections is the belief that the illness has a different cause. As described in chapter 3, illnesses in sub-Saharan Africa historically have been attributed to a range of possible supernatural and natural causes. In the case of HIV/AIDS and other sexually transmitted infections this has included witchcraft, evil spirits, or a violation of sexual taboos, as well as sexual contact with a person who has an infectious organism (Ingstad 1990; Green 1992a, 1992b; Schoepf 1992b; Yamba 1997; Pool and Washija 2001). Another barrier to biomedical treatment of sexually transmitted infections is that people may prefer to use traditional medicine because of its perceived effectiveness, accessibility, ratio of providers to patients, cost, payment options, and/or confidentiality (Kale 1995; Crabbé et al. 1996; Awusabo-Asare and Anarfi 1997; Mogensen 1997; Yamba 1997; Okonofua et al. 1999; Muela, Mushi, and Ribera 2000; Ndulo et al. 2000; Ashforth 2002; Zachariah et al. 2002; Stadler 2003; Kusimba et al. 2003; Kiapi-Iwa and Hart 2004; Chimwaza and Watkins 2004; Kalichman and Simbaya 2004).

As discussed in chapter 1, historical data on the prevalence of different kinds of sexually transmitted infections in sub-Saharan Africa are very limited. Nonetheless, gonorrhea, and syphilis were common enough amongst the Sukuma in the early twentieth century that there were laws related to them (Cory 1953). For example, if a man was found to have infected a nonmarital partner with gonorrhea or syphilis he was required to pay cattle compensation to her or her father, brother, or husband. Similarly, in her anthropological research in a Sukuma village in the 1960s, Varkevisser (1973, 95) noted that a father who "tranquilly" accepted a daughter's out-of-wedlock pregnancy could become volatile if he learned she had a sexually transmitted infection, specifically because he believed it might make her infertile.

HIV/AIDS

At the time of our study, HIV/AIDS education in rural Mwanza was mainly limited to radio programs and a few small-scale, short-term health promotion interventions. Many villagers did not understand how HIV is contracted or that those infected may appear healthy for many years before developing symptoms of AIDS. Efforts were underway to reduce HIV transmission during medical care, including testing blood before using it for transfusions and ensuring all needles and syringes were sterilized. However, the possibility of transmission via those mechanisms was not completely eliminated. The blood supply was limited, so it was not unusual for family members or friends to provide untested blood when a patient needed a transfusion (Berege and Klokke 1997). In addition, traditional healers or lay people who claimed knowledge of biomedicine sometimes used injections outside of health facilities, and in such practice sterilization was unregulated (Gumodoka, Favot, and Dolmans 1997). Only very limited HIV testing services were available at district or regional hospitals, and villagers rarely knew of or used such services. Antiretroviral therapy was not available, so medical treatment of HIV/AIDS amounted to treatment of opportunistic infections, at best.

Most studies of AIDS treatment-seeking behavior in sub-Saharan Africa have involved HIV-positive patients recruited through major hospitals, and have focussed on their adherence to antiretroviral therapy, that is, the extent to which they accurately follow instructions over time (Weiser et al. 2003; Nachega et al. 2004; Byakika-Tusiime et al. 2005; Mills, Nachega, Buchan, et al. 2006; Bell et al. 2007). Few studies have examined HIV/AIDS treatment-seeking more broadly, considering home care, traditional medicine, and/or biomedical treatment of opportunistic infections, particularly in the many areas where antiretroviral therapy remains largely or entirely unavailable (Setel 1999b; Pool and Washija 2001; Mshana, Wamoyi, et al. 2006; Roura et al. 2009).

MALE CIRCUMCISION

Recently three randomized trials demonstrated that male circumcision—the surgical removal of the foreskin that covers the tip of the penis—reduces the risk of acquiring HIV (Auvert et al. 2005; Gray et al. 2007; Bailey et al. 2007). There is also evidence that circumcision protects against other, ulcerative sexually transmitted infections, such as herpes and syphilis, both of which may increase acquisition and transmission of HIV (Fleming et al. 1999; Weiss et al. 2006; Sobngwi-Tambekou et al. 2009; Tobian et al. 2009). As a result, international and government agencies are now exploring how male circumcision can be promoted amongst ethnic groups which do not traditionally circumcise, and it has become important to understand how circumcision is perceived by such populations (WHO and UNAIDS 2007).

Based on linguistic evidence, Marck (1997) postulated that the Sukuma practiced male circumcision many hundreds of years ago, like other Bantu ethnic groups in the currently non-circumcising region of Africa extending from southern Sudan down to inland southern Africa. However, the Sukuma ethnographies of the early to mid-twentieth century do not mention circumcision, suggesting it was not practiced during that period (Tanner 1955b; Varkevisser 1973).

In the next section we will examine causation, prevention, and treatment beliefs and practices related to HIV/AIDS and other sexually transmitted infections in *MEMA kwa Vijana* control communities. At the end of this chapter we will discuss these findings in light of developments since the end of the study, particularly efforts to introduce and scale-up HIV testing and antiretroviral therapy services in rural Mwanza and across Tanzania.

FINDINGS

Beliefs about the Causes of Sexually Transmitted Infection

When villagers were asked if they could name any sexually transmitted infections (*magonjwa ya zinaa* or **bunyolo**), many named syphilis (*kaswende*) and gonorrhea (*kisonono* or **kasogone**). A minority also incorrectly identified other illnesses as sexually transmitted infections, such as schistosomiasis. A large proportion of informants knew that sexually transmitted infections were contracted during sexual intercourse. Notably, *magonjwa ya zinaa* literally means "illnesses of fornication/adultery," so it suggests the mode of infection. Many informants reported that people who have multiple sexual partners out-of-wedlock are in danger of getting sexually transmitted infections. For example, a 29-year-old woman in a polygynous marriage reported, "Syphilis, Chlamydia, and gonorrhea greatly bother [local] people, especially the youth . . . because sexual intercourse has just become normal to the youth of this era." [PO-00-C-9-5f]

On a few occasions informants mentioned that sexually transmitted infections are caused by organisms. For example, one man diagnosed and treated himself for a sexually transmitted infection after experiencing an unusual penile discharge: "He used sixty co-trimoxazole tablets, and when the symptoms disappeared, he used traditional medicines which made him urinate a lot, in order to clean out the *uchafu* (dirt or filth) and the germs" [PO-01-C-2-5f].

With the exception of HIV/AIDS, which will be discussed below, few informants reported that illnesses which were recognized as *magonjwa ya zinaa* were caused by witchcraft, ancestral spirits, evil spirits, or anything other than sexual contact. However, our data suggest that some villagers had symptoms of sexually transmitted infection which they did not recognize as such. In those cases the illnesses were attributed to nonsexual causes, such as stepping on contaminated material that had been left on a pathway by someone attempting to rid themselves of the same illness. Case study 2.3 provides one example of this.

Beliefs and Practices Related to the Prevention of Sexually Transmitted Infection

We described in the last chapter how many villagers knew condoms were promoted to prevent sexually transmitted infections, but they did not always believe condom use was effective or safe. In addition, several villagers reported that sexually transmitted infections could be prevented through traditional methods. A few young people independently reported that an ash solution could be drunk before or after intercourse to prevent infection. For example, a young man stated:

> *P:* The Sukuma people know well that if one is promiscuous one can sometimes get sexually transmitted infections. So if a person goes to someone they know has sexually transmitted infections, they first protect themselves by stirring those ashes in water and drinking the solution, and then go have sex without any problems. . . . But regarding AIDS, people don't know how to prevent it like they do for other sexually transmitted infections. [GD-02-C-3-43m]

A few respondents also reported that traditional herbal medicines could be taken to prevent initial infection and/or the relapse of an existing sexually transmitted infection. One young woman described how she and her husband both took traditional medicine after experiencing a sexually transmitted infection, and she said she continued to take it to prevent illness reoccurrence:

> She believes that the medicine cured her, because she has conceived another pregnancy since then and some women don't conceive after contracting sexually transmitted infections. However, she said that even after giving birth she will continue using the medicine, because **bunyolo** germs do not die and just hide in the stomach, where they can completely destroy the reproductive organs. [PO-01-C-2-5f]

During the first in-depth interview series, 40 male and 28 female pupils were asked about beliefs and practices related to male circumcision. Those in-depth interviews suggested widespread and consistent respect for male circumcision, whether it was an individual, family, ethnic, or religious decision. Twenty-one male respondents said that there were benefits to being circumcised and only two raised possible negative outcomes. Many referred to uncircumcised penises retaining more *uchafu* or **budogo** (dirt or filth) (n = 10) or being more susceptible to disease (n = 8). For example:

> *I:* You may find one [boy] still has skin on the top of his private part . . . You may find he has plenty of dirt inside of it. Yes, the one who doesn't have [foreskin], he does not have dirt. Someone who has not been circumcised can have a disease . . . any disease which will get him. [Circumcised men] cannot easily get a disease. [II-99-I-49-m]

Five male pupils reported that they had been circumcised, and the ages they reported for this were quite variable (3, 9, 13, 14, and 18 years), as were the costs (Tshs 1,000-5,000, or $1.20–6.00). Three of the circumcised respondents were Muslims, two of whom had ceremonies accompanying their circumcisions. One of the non-Muslim circumcised boys said he decided to do it because a group of girls had mocked him for being uncircumcised, and he felt embarrassed. The other reported that an uncircumcised penis can retain *uchafu*. Four circumcisions took place in health facilities and one was done by a traditional healer. Several respondents also described circumcisions they had witnessed in their village, performed by a traditional healer or a medical person, usually involving circumcision of groups of Muslim boys and men. A circumcised Muslim boy reported:

> *I:* [The man who circumcised me] is a traditional healer who passes here very often. . . . Whenever he comes, all of the [Muslim] young people who are not circumcised are brought to him, as well as others who want to be circumcised. . . . Everyone must bring his own [razor blade or scissors]. . . . He first injects them with anesthetics. And there are some leaves, I don't know what they are. When applied to the wound, the blood clots / stops immediately. . . . But when there is no more numbness, then you can feel pain and cry. [II-99-I-27-m]

There were two uncircumcised Muslims amongst the male respondents, and they said that they planned to get circumcised soon for religious reasons. One said his procedure had been delayed because he could not pay the Tshs 1,000 ($1.20) it would cost. Nine uncircumcised, non-Muslim men said that they planned to be circumcised because of cleanliness and/or disease concerns. One explained:

> *I:* When you get older, you develop shame. . . . You see, we go to bathe in the lake. You'll be laughed at [people may say], "Hey, I didn't know you were dirty!" So now you think that maybe you will get circumcised. . . . [But] the big reason [to get circumcised] is that your private parts otherwise stay dirty between baths. [II-99-I-80-m]

The female pupils showed little knowledge of male circumcision. The majority (21/28) said that they had never heard of male circumcision and/or did not know what it was, even when interviewers used synonyms and descriptions to explain it. Eighteen of these 21 reported having already had sexual intercourse. The remaining seven only had a vague idea of male circumcision, for example, that it involved cutting the private parts, and/or that it might be done to boys of all ages, particularly Muslims. None of those seven reported that their male relatives or sexual partners were circumcised, although two who were sexually active said that they did not know how to tell whether a sexual partner's foreskin had been removed.

Experience and Treatment of Sexually Transmitted Infection

Seven percent of males and 42 percent of females who had been randomly selected for the first and second in-depth interview series tested positive for one of five or six sexually transmitted infections at the end of the *MEMA kwa*

Vijana trial, similar to the proportions for the broader survey population. In addition, however, a few in-depth interview respondents who tested negative for all infections during the *MEMA kwa Vijana* surveys reported in their second interview that they had had a sexually transmitted infection that had been treated at a health facility. Of the female respondents, fewer of those who were married (5/17) than single (9/16) tested positive for an infection in the final survey, but two of the married women had two sexually transmitted infections, whereas none of the unmarried women had more than one.

Most adolescent and adult villagers in our study could describe symptoms of sexually transmitted infections, such as genital sores, unusual genital discharge, and painful urination. Treatment was opportunistic and pluralistic, similar to that of other illnesses in rural Mwanza. However, there was greater stigma associated with sexually transmitted infections, so if people suspected they had one their fear of stigma could delay their treatment-seeking. Almost all reports of treatment initially involved traditional home remedies. For example, a female researcher had the following exchange while at a female bathing area:

> I noticed [a certain woman] scratch her private parts. . . . She was at first uncomfortable talking about it, but later . . . said that she has felt itchy [for three months] and when she scratches, small pimples appear. . . . She said she had been shown medicines/herbs by her mother-in-law . . . And hoped to start using them tonight. [PO-00-C-3-2f]

In a second example, a mother of six reported that she learned how to treat her sexually transmitted infection from a male acquaintance:

> She said that she contracted a sexually transmitted infection while pregnant . . . she had pain in her abdomen, and after she gave birth to her daughter, she developed some small scabs in her vagina. She started using local medicine . . . consisting of certain insects mixed with certain roots, which had been soaked in water and dried in the sun. [PO-00-C-9-5f]

When villagers had persistent symptoms of sexually transmitted infection they often consulted a traditional healer or someone else who was believed to have expertise in traditional medicine. A 41-year-old traditional healer explained that he saw the most people for sexually transmitted infections soon after *ngoma* events in the dry season. He attributed this to increased sexual activity around such events, and especially sex with *ngoma* performers and other travelers who could have many partners in different locations. Another man in his 50s explained how he treated sexually transmitted infections:

> He said that his father taught him the local herbal medicines. . . . He first makes sure a person really has a sexually transmitted infection by asking the patient to urinate on the leaves of a certain tree. If the patient has one, the leaves of that

tree will dry up after one day. Then he treats the patient by using a mixture of water and the roots of three different types of tree for 1–2 weeks until the symptoms disappear. He then gives the patient a different medicine and the patient is cured and can have sex again if he/she wants after one month. [PO-00-C-3-3m]

Treatment of sexually transmitted infection by traditional healers was not limited to solutions which were drunk or applied topically. The young woman in case study 2.3, for example, described how a traditional healer used a razor to cut off growths on her genitals which may have resulted from a sexually transmitted infection, such as genital warts.

Some people with sexually transmitted infections combined both traditional and biomedical treatments. For example, a 20-year-old single mother reported that:

She was diagnosed [and given tablets] by a health worker . . . who told her she had syphilis or gonorrhea. . . . She was also given traditional medicines by her paternal aunt . . . [and was shown others] by a certain man and a 20-year-old single woman who had also suffered from a sexually transmitted infection. [PO-00-C-3-2f]

Officially, syndromic management of sexually transmitted infections was available free-of-charge at government health facilities. In practice some facilities did not have a complete medication stock, and it occasionally was rumored that health workers were involved in illegal reselling of drugs and supplies. Some health facility staff also insisted that patients purchase a treatment book to facilitate their pharmacy purchases and follow-up visits, although the existing protocol did not call for this and the cost was prohibitive for adolescents. In some simulated patient exercises young people who did not have a treatment book were chastised and one was sent away without a consultation for this reason.

Kiosk staff reported that some men but very few women purchased medication to treat sexually transmitted infections from them, but health workers reported that women were much more likely than men to seek such treatment from health facilities. Health workers typically stipulated this was because health facility treatment was free, and because pregnant women and mothers of young children already attended the facilities for prenatal or pediatric care. However, most health workers also reported that women were shyer than men when seeking sexually transmitted infection treatment. For example:

[A health worker] said that men are quick to discover that they have been infected, and when they come to the health facility they immediately say that they have been infected with sexually transmitted infections. He said they use words like, "I have sores on my genitals." He said that, to the contrary, you must follow up more closely with women, who usually say that they are suffering in their stomach, below the navel. [PO-01-C-3-3m]

During both in-depth interviews and participant observation, young people and older adults who had received treatment for sexually transmitted infections at health facilities generally spoke positively about the experience and were very grateful that their symptoms resolved. However, some symptomatic young people—especially girls—feared that they would be verbally abused and that their consultation would not be kept confidential in a health facility, so they did not seek treatment even if their symptoms intensified, as illustrated in case study 1.4. Concern about health worker confidentiality was often warranted, both within a health facility and when health workers socialized with other villagers outside it. For example, while visiting a health facility during participant observation, a female researcher overheard a young man being diagnosed with a sexually transmitted infection in the next room, and then the health worker directly mentioned the man's diagnosis to her when he spoke with her later. Lack of privacy within the clinic setting was a problem observed in almost all simulated patient exercises, as consultations often took place in rooms without doors and with open windows immediately next to the waiting area.

Four of the simulated patient exercises in *MEMA kwa Vijana* control communities involved a sexually transmitted infection concern, and in two of these the provider was fairly responsive and nonjudgmental, and generally provided good information. For example, one control community health worker reassured a young woman as follows:

HW: You have made a good decision [to come here], not a bad one. . . . Because if you stay with a problem [without trying to resolve it], it may cause you trouble in the future. . . . your organs could be damaged, you could suffer a [reproductive] loss. . . .

SP: Mm. Please just tell me the symptoms of sexually transmitted infections, so if I see them one day I will come back for treatment. . . .

HW: Eh, I don't know if it will help . . . first, for a woman, the early symptoms are itching on one's private parts. A second one is showing discharge of fluid or pus from the private parts. A third is the presence of sores on the private parts. Then a fourth is swelling. A fifth is pain in the waist or the private parts. Sixth, you could have a sexually transmitted infection without displaying symptoms. . . . Therefore, if you see that you have—one of those symptoms—you will come back, right?

SP: Yes! [SP-00-C-2-7f]

This health worker also took time to write down the symptoms for the patient, but did not mention condoms at any point during the exchange.

In two of the simulated patient exercises the health workers were very judgmental or disrespectful about the young person's sexually transmitted infection concern, and provided him or her with very little or no information. For example, one control community nurse neither asked the girl about her symptoms nor tried to examine her, but instead asked many questions about her school, class, residency, and the names of her sexual partner, guardians, and parents. Such questions were not unusual, as similar questions were asked during almost all simulated patient visits, sometimes repeatedly throughout a visit, as noted in chapter 10. However, this health worker also insisted that the girl return to the facility with her parents, and instructed her to lie to her sexual partner, so that he would also come to the health facility. Throughout the exchange the health worker loudly berated the girl, drawing the attention of another nurse from a nearby room who then participated in chastising the girl. An excerpt follows:

> *HW:* You are just doing it [having sex] without a condom? . . . Do you want to leave school and die? . . . Why have you decided to have sexual intercourse—to do such immoral acts—while you're in Year 6? . . . Go back home right now. Come with your aunt tomorrow. . . . If your parents refuse to come, I will not give you treatment. [In that case] I will write you a letter, so that you can go to the police. The police should give me permission to do what . . .?
>
> *SP:* To follow up with me.
>
> *HW:* Yes . . . Now, you're—dying of AIDS when you're—still young. [SP-00-C-27-7f]

Beliefs about HIV/AIDS Causation

The common term for AIDS in Tanzania is the Swahili acronym, *UKIMWI*. At the time of our study many people in rural Mwanza who knew the acronym did not know its full meaning, that is, lack of protection for the body (*Ukosefu wa Kinga ya Mwili*). Colloquially AIDS was also referred to as "our illness" in several villages, an expression that suggests the community was burdened with the illness rather than that the speaker or someone in their immediate family had AIDS. In addition, individuals were heard to refer to AIDS as "slim," "the new illness," "two hundred," "submarine," "wire" and "the four corners illness." "Two hundred" may here refer to an amount of Tanzanian shillings that a man or boy might give a girl for a sexual encounter. "Submarine" is a slang term for a sexually "loose" woman that was popularized in a national musician's song about AIDS, and ultimately came to be used as a slang term for AIDS itself. "Wire" was also a national slang term often used to describe HIV infection and AIDS through metaphors such as "stepping on a wire" or "being short circuited." A 22-year-old single mother explained her use of "four corners": "If one gets AIDS it definitely leads to the grave, which in all cases has four corners" [PO-99-C-5-2f]. In Swahili, the expression for HIV (*virusi vya UKIMWI*) literally means "the AIDS virus."

The majority of villagers in our study had heard about AIDS from the radio, public meetings, fellow villagers, or school. In all villages, many people reported hearing about someone in the village having AIDS, although some said they had never heard this. A small proportion of villagers said that AIDS, like many other illnesses, is simply a result of chance or bad luck. This is illustrated in the following account by a divorced 35-year-old man who had several concurrent partners: "He said AIDS is like any other disease and if it gets him, let it come. What he cannot do is to stop having girlfriends. . . . He said if he gets AIDS it will be bad luck, but if he doesn't, it will be his [good] luck" [PO-99-C-5-2f].

Some villagers believed that AIDS is unavoidable. A 31-year-old female farmer explained: "Some people say that to die of AIDS is like an accident at work, and sometimes accidents can't be avoided" [PO-01-I-1-2f]. In several villages informants said that dying of AIDS may be inevitable, so most or all villagers would eventually die of it. For example, one 16-year-old school girl stated, "Even if a person does not get AIDS through a blood transfusion, the fact remains that we are all going to be finished by this illness of ours [AIDS]" [PO-01-C-2-5f]. Similarly, after the death of a young man from what was believed to be AIDS, a female researcher noted:

> It is said that he used to have sex with many people, a situation that makes people in the village become very worried. People say this is due to the situation that young people and adults have sexual interaction, and it is possible that people in the whole village have been affected and may die to the last person in the family. [PO-02-I-4-5f]

In our study population, the main causes attributed to AIDS were natural (biological) and witchcraft, both of which will be described in the following sections.

Natural Causes

Most informants reported that AIDS is contracted through sexual intercourse, a blood transfusion, or contact with a sharp, infected object (such as razors).

People especially associated AIDS with sex. For example, a conversation that took place between three teenage boys:

> They talked about a teacher who had died of AIDS, [and] they became very sad. . . . They said that AIDS is very dangerous, especially if one person with AIDS participates in *kuliwa susa*. One informant said his grandfather told him, "AIDS has come to the wrong place. Had it been [transmitted through] food, people wouldn't be dying." They all laughed. [PO-01-I-4-5f]

Many informants said that **wasimbe**, *wahuni*, and/or *malaya* spread AIDS in the villages through their sexual activity.

Few informants specifically knew that HIV causes AIDS, and those who did usually did not understand the term "virus" or its relationship to immune deficiency and opportunistic infections. Some villagers knew that a person could be infected and infectious but not yet show signs of AIDS, but many did not fully understand or believe this. For example, a female kiosk owner and tax collector was widely believed to have AIDS when her husband was diagnosed with it, and then he and her co-wife died. Nonetheless, by her own account she did not have difficulty finding sexual partners:

> She said people became afraid of her, especially men, that they would be infected if they agreed to have sex with her. Later on, she managed to get two sexual partners. . . . Before having sex with a third man, he explained the prevailing rumors to her, that all of the people know that she has AIDS, and that he also had information that she has AIDS. He did not care and once they had sex, she conceived and gave birth to her child. [PO-00-I-4-4f]

Importantly, even villagers who knew that there is an asymptomatic period prior to the onset of AIDS were confused about the length of that period and the diverse illnesses that a person with AIDS might eventually have. For example, a male laborer dismissed the possibility that someone's rapid, fatal illness could have been AIDS, saying: "This is just witchcraft, [when] a person is sick for seven days or a month and dies. But with this situation we hear about [AIDS], the person's illness takes years" [PO-99-C-5-2f].

Finally, a few informants believed that AIDS is spread through natural means which in fact do not transmit HIV, such as touching or sharing food with a person with AIDS. Individuals in several villages reported that AIDS was created by white people with the intent to kill Africans, and/or that it was transmitted sexually through new condoms. For example, a Village Executive Officer said, "Using condoms and trusting white people is a disgrace to our culture, as [new] condoms have been infected with HIV" [PO-01-C-2-5f]. However, such comments mainly seemed to occur during general discussions about why villagers did not use condoms, and these beliefs did not seem to be a great or immediate concern for the individuals who said them.

Witchcraft

In this study there were no reported beliefs of AIDS having been caused by ancestral spirits, and only one report that it could be caused by evil spirits. However, many people in all participant observation villages reported that individuals rumored to have had AIDS may in fact have had an AIDS-like illness that was caused by witchcraft. These informants typically reported belief in both a "real" (natural) AIDS, which leads to certain death, and a similar illness caused by witchcraft, which could be cured by traditional medicine. A ferry owner in his 40s described this:

> He said that if a man decides to chase away his wife, the woman often may decide to kill him. . . . Nowadays they bewitch such men with an illness having the symptoms of AIDS. If you are quick to go to a traditional healer, he/she will treat you and you will be cured, but at the hospital this illness can't be cured. [PO-01-I-7-5f]

Numerous accounts of people who initially were thought to have died of AIDS, but who later were believed to have died of another illness, were attributed to witchcraft. A 38-year-old male farmer provided one such report:

> He said that before the man died last year, he was bedridden for a long time and had a rash all over his body. He said that that man's widow now has sex with any young man who goes to her. He said that the men who have sex with her believe her husband died of witchcraft, not AIDS, because this widow is so healthy and so are their children. [PO-01-I-1-2f]

Similarly, in another village, a 50–60-year-old female farmer and a 38-year-old male teacher voiced their belief that witchcraft can be mistaken for AIDS:

> They said that the sickness of a certain woman's daughter was not exactly AIDS, for she had been bewitched and caught an illness similar to AIDS. Other sick people were brought as patients to the village, so it is possible that they too had already been bewitched, because their spouses are still alive and they are not sick with AIDS. [PO-02-C-2-6f]

A third example was reported immediately after the death of a man rumored to have had AIDS:

> She told me that the man had had sex with a woman who came to this village from a district capital . . . When that woman left the village, they heard that she was critically ill and afterwards they learned that she had died. People said that the woman had just been bewitched, and they continued having sex with that man. After some while, his wife died, so people said that she also had been bewitched, as her husband's condition was just fine. [PO-02-I-4-5f]

The presentation of "real" AIDS and AIDS-like bewitchment was reported to be very similar and sometimes indistinguishable. One traditional healer, for example, reported that "real" AIDS had only slightly different symptoms than "false" AIDS, such as certain skin problems and unusually red lips. He said that witches bewitch people with an AIDS-like illness because they want the victims to despair and believe there is no cure, ultimately dying for lack of traditional treatment.

In two villages 150 kilometers apart, informants reported that people who have committed an offence such as theft could be bewitched to become ill with a prolonged traditional illness, *lusumbo*, which involves symptoms similar to those of AIDS. Three young male farmers explained:

> They said that nobody had died with AIDS in their village. But they said there are people who have died with diseases with similar symptoms to AIDS, but people say it is *lusumbo*, a certain spell cast on them because they stole other people's maize or vegetables from their farms. [PO-99-C-9-1m]

Several explanations were given for why someone might be bewitched with AIDS-like illness, including envy, punishment for an offence, and a desire for revenge on someone in authority. One bicycle taxi man described an example of the latter as follows:

> He said that the man said to have AIDS could have been bewitched, for he was an Assistant Ward Executive Officer and was not on good terms with people, and this was cause to be bewitched. He said that if one is an authority figure but doesn't respect others, one is bewitched. [PO-01-I-1-2f]

In our study there were no definite reports of punishment of a witch accused of causing AIDS. However, there were occasional reports of traditional healers declaring revenge upon a witch who caused the death of a patient. In addition, researchers learned of two violent incidents which occurred just before participant observation visits, each of which may have involved an AIDS-related death. In the first a woman was accused of bewitching and killing a baby, and men of the baby's family reportedly attacked her with machetes. In the second incident a woman was stabbed to death, and her sister-in-law was arrested for her murder. The Village Chairman reported that the sister-in-law had earlier accused the woman of using witchcraft to kill her three children.

Only a minority of villagers in our study doubted whether witchcraft can cause an AIDS-like illness. One villager to question this was a 50-year-old male nursing assistant, who illegally practiced both western and traditional medicine out of his home. After identifying three plausible cases of AIDS in his village, this man stressed the need for discretion:

> He said that all the examples of people he had mentioned as having died from AIDS are confidential. He told us if the relatives of the deceased know about this, they may feel hurt . . . because they lack education and because they believe what traditional healers tell them, that their deceased relatives were bewitched. [PO-01-I-1-2f]

This statement reflects other findings that "false" AIDS was less stigmatized than "real" AIDS.

Finally, a number of the accounts about witchcraft and AIDS involved people who had tested positive for HIV, or who had been diagnosed with AIDS at a medical facility, but who reportedly did not let that be known publicly. For example, the brother of a deceased woman said:

> "Many people feel there is no AIDS, because they feel there are not many incidents of death by AIDS, so they say it is just witchcraft. Like our sister, they said she was just bewitched over there [in the capital] by those witches. But we knew the truth, because they tested her at the [national referral] hospital." [PO-02-I-1-2f]

This example demonstrates how people diagnosed with AIDS and their relatives were among those most aware of "real" AIDS in rural areas during the study period. Nonetheless, there also were numerous reports that those with AIDS and their relatives were the most likely to claim an illness was due to witchcraft rather than AIDS. For example, a Village Executive Officer commented that, "Most people, especially the patient's relatives, allege that he/she has been bewitched with a disease resembling AIDS" [PO-01-I-4-5f].

Becoming Infected with HIV

In-depth interviews were conducted with twenty-nine young people who had had a preliminary HIV-positive test result in a *MEMA kwa Vijana* survey. As described in chapter 2, results from more rigorous tests after the trial determined that thirteen of those individuals were truly HIV-positive. Like all trial participants, they had been offered the opportunity to learn their HIV status at each survey. If they agreed, they participated in voluntary counseling and testing following the national protocol at the time. Those who declined this within the trial surveys were unlikely to know their HIV status from being tested elsewhere, since no HIV testing took place in health centers or dispensaries at that time, and very little took place in district and regional hospitals.

There was little in the in-depth interviews with HIV-positive young people that clarified how they had become infected with HIV, or that otherwise distinguished them from interviews with randomly selected young people. All of the HIV-positive respondents reported that they had never received a blood transfusion. A few reported having had medical injections within a health facility in the past, but none reported experiencing this outside of a health care setting. All denied having ever shared a razor. Most of the respondents who first tested HIV-positive at the beginning of the trial (two male, five female) and those who first tested HIV-positive later in the trial (one male, five female) described sexual histories typical for young people in rural Mwanza, or of even lower risk. Of those who reported sexual experience, almost all said that they had had only one or two sexual partners and denied having ever had concurrent partners. Importantly, some contradicted themselves in ways that suggested they did not report all of their sexual partners, but such inconsistencies were also common amongst randomly selected individuals, particularly females, as described in chapter 6.

It seems likely that some of the seven in-depth interview respondents who were HIV-positive at the start of the trial were long-term survivors of mother-to-child HIV transmission; the young man in case study 3.1 is one example. Three of these respondents' mothers had died of unspecified illnesses, and a fourth had not heard news of her mother since early childhood, but her father's current wife was seriously ill at the time of the interview. Four of these seven respondents had polygynous parents, two had parents in monogamous marriages, and the seventh did not know what her parents' marital status had been. Six respondents said that they had already had sex and described their first sexual relationship. Three of these specifically said they had had no other sexual partners, while the other three did not clarify whether they had had other partners.

In contrast, it seems likely that most or all of the six respondents who became HIV-positive in the course of the trial contracted HIV sexually, including the young woman in case study 3.2. The one young man in this group, a 20-year-old farmer, estimated that in the three years prior to the interview he had had eleven sexual partners. He said that he had never had concurrent sexual relationships, but that once a relationship ended he usually began a new one within one week. The remaining five female respondents in this group did not report unusually high numbers of partners or experience of concurrent partnerships. Two said that they had never had sex. The interviews with the remaining three suggested their HIV risk may have been unusually high because they had a partner who was likely to have had many partners, such as a truck driver or a cotton ginnery operator, and/or they had lived in Mwanza City, a district capital, or large villages on major truck routes, settings where HIV prevalence was likely to be high. For example, one 21-year-old divorced woman said that she temporarily left school when she was 16 years old in order to work in domestic service in a district capital. She explained: "You take a [female] friend with whom you are on very good terms. You just go and look for work and start working. I stayed there for five months . . . cooking and washing dishes and clothes." [II-02-I-325-f]

Living with HIV/AIDS

Some of the HIV-positive in-depth interview respondents reported having had common health problems such as fever, headaches, stomachaches or coughs. Many randomly selected respondents also reported these symptoms, although they may have been more persistent and recurrent amongst HIV-positive respondents. Such symptoms typically were treated with aspirin, acetaminophen, and/or homemade traditional medicines. Several of the HIV-positive respondents also reported more serious health problems which had been treated by medical professionals or traditional healers, some of which were commonly associated with AIDS in rural Mwanza at the time, such as chronic shingles and oral thrush (Todd and Barongo 1997). For example, a 20-year-old married woman reported:

> *R:* I am suffering from a stomachache and a headache. When I was finishing Year 7 I lived with a traditional healer [for treatment]. I just left that place to take my Year 7 examination at the end of the school year. . . . Now my health is okay, but sometimes it worsens. . . . The traditional healer told me, "You are suffering from [throat] ulcers. And you also suffer from schistosomiasis." So he/she gave me medicines, and now in fact I have recovered from the schistosomiasis. . . . But as far as the ulcers are concerned, no, they just recur. And my head aches a lot. [II-02-I-293-f]

In participant observation villages, a few individuals were widely rumored to have AIDS, particularly if they were known to have had an AIDS diagnosis from a health facility, or if they or their sexual partners were very thin and had common health problems with an unusual frequency and severity, such as diarrhea, fevers, skin rashes, or chest infections. One such woman described how she had struggled with schistosomiasis, hook worms, malaria, high blood pressure, chest infections, skin infections, frequent fevers, and extreme thinness for seven years. When faced with such persistent illnesses many people repeatedly consulted traditional healers and/or health facilities for treatment. For example, at the funeral of a man in his 20s, who was rumored to have had AIDS:

> They said he was suffering from a stomach illness and . . . a skin infection. . . . he had a stomach operation [at the hospital]. . . . After a short while he started

ailing again. He was treated by traditional healers, but . . . continued being sick until he was taken to [the local health facility] last week. [PO-02-I-4-1m]

Some people living with HIV/AIDS seemed to pursue traditional treatments for longer than biomedical treatment because they offered more hope of a cure. For example, a 30-year-old, widowed food kiosk worker, who was rumored to have AIDS

appeared emaciated and weak. She walked slowly and talked softly. . . . She said the first and second time [she went to a health facility] she had pain all over her body, especially in her head . . . [and] a third time, she had a rash all over her body. . . . She did not have the Tshs 5,000 ($6) to have the blood tests done [to determine the problem] and thus just came back home. [PO-01-I-1-2f]

A week after the above interaction, the same woman optimistically reported that she had raised Tshs 5,500 ($6.60) for treatment by a traditional healer. She reported:

She was sick yesterday and drank and bathed in traditional medicines she had been given by traditional healers. She said that traditional medicines like the ones she is using are quite effective. She said that after the traditional healer tested her by use of magic, he told her she had been bewitched by her deceased husband's relatives, because they feel she abandoned him when he was quite ill, and she only came back when he had died. [PO-01-I-1-2f]

Some traditional healers claimed that they could cure people who had "false" AIDS, that is, an AIDS-like illness caused by maliciousness, such as witchcraft. A traditional healer and Sub-Village Chairman's account follows:

He said that there are two main types of AIDS. . . . He gave me an example of a certain man who had come . . . believing he had the real AIDS. . . . The man had received treatment for a long time from a modern hospital, but in vain. . . . He said [the man was ill because] his wife had given give him a drug so that he would die. . . . He gave [the man] some medicines to stop the diarrhea and vomiting . . . and increase/recover his lost energy. He said that the man was cured. [PO-99-C-2-1m]

In contrast, the account of a traditional healer and Village Chairman:

He said he has healed many people of illnesses such as paralysis, worms, leg diseases and many others, but not AIDS. He said that traditional healers who advertize themselves as being able to cure AIDS are liars, for there is no medicine [cure] for AIDS. . . . At the most he used to give [his AIDS patients] medicines to calm them and give them more time to live. [PO-01-C-2-6f]

Some people who suspected that they had "real" AIDS may have become hopeless, as did their families. For example, one man reported that when his sister tested positive for HIV, his eldest brother told the family not to take her for treatment as her condition was fatal. Hopelessness and despair may have been more of an issue for professionals who had received HIV/AIDS education as they were more likely to comprehend both the severity of their condition and the lack of options available to them. For example, one health worker was rumored to have attempted suicide by overdosing on chloroquine tablets because he had AIDS. A similar despair was shown by an AIDS education teacher whose husband, two co-wives, and four step-children had died:

> She said her only male child was killed due to the hatred [witchcraft] of the people of [that village]. . . . She said even she herself sometimes falls into a critical state, a situation which makes her fail to work. She was almost weeping whenever she talked. [PO-00-I-4-4f]

DISCUSSION

Sexually Transmitted Infections

In rural Mwanza, as elsewhere in sub-Saharan Africa, self diagnosis and treatment was typically the first response to illness, including sexually transmitted infections, increasing the chance of inappropriate medication and dosage and the development of drug resistance (van der Geest 1987; Msiska et al. 1997; Geissler et al. 2000). We found that, if symptoms did not resolve, villagers often sought treatment from a health facility and/or a traditional healer. The 2001–2002 *MEMA kwa Vijana* survey similarly found that, for those males who reported experiencing an unusual genital discharge in the last twelve months, 22 percent saw a traditional healer for treatment, while 36 percent saw a medical provider (Larke et al. 2010). The figures were 13 percent and 28 percent respectively for females. Some people sought treatment not only for the relief of symptoms but also because they feared a sexually transmitted infection might affect their fertility, as Varkevisser (1973) also found in her anthropological study in the 1960s.

In our study several patterns emerged specifically related to biomedical treatment of sexually transmitted infections. Women were more likely to make use of free health facility services, while men were more likely to self-diagnose and treat themselves using medicine obtained at kiosks. Stigma was powerful and people sometimes did not seek treatment unless their symptoms became severe, particularly adolescent girls. Young people typically were greatly concerned about health worker's judgment and lack of confidentiality, and the simulated patient visits found such concerns were warranted. However, those villagers who did receive treatment for sexually transmitted infections from health facilities seemed satisfied and very grateful for the services, suggesting that syndromic management of infections was often effective.

Some villagers trusted traditional healers more than medical providers to treat sexually transmitted infections. As Green, Jurg, and Djedje (1993) found in a study in Mozambique, traditional healers and their patients may have had faith in their treatments because: symptoms go into latent stages; simultaneous use of different therapies blurs which treatment is successful; some traditional medicines may indeed be biomedically effective; and biomedical treatment may be ineffective, for example, if the full course of treatment is not completed. It is possible that some traditional treatments for sexually transmitted infections in rural Mwanza were beneficial and helped to relieve symptoms. However, our study suggests that some were harmful. The description of a traditional healer cutting off a young woman's genital growths in case study 2.3 is particularly concerning, as the harshness of this treatment may have only worsened her condition.

Finally, although only a minority of boys in our study were circumcised, we found that most young men had positive perceptions of male circumcision, as also found among other non-circumcising populations in southern and eastern Africa (Westercamp and Bailey 2007). This suggests that cultural factors would not prevent the promotion of male circumcision to reduce sexually transmitted infections amongst the Sukuma. Indeed, recent studies indicate that male circumcision is becoming more common among the Sukuma (Nnko et al. 2001; Boerma et al. 2002). In the 2001–2002 *MEMA kwa Vijana* survey, for example, 17 percent of young men were found to be circumcised upon clinical examination, only 62 percent of whom were Muslim and thus were likely to have done this as part of their religious practice (Weiss et al. 2008). When a follow-up survey was conducted with the older trial population in 2007–2008, 40 percent of male respondents were found to be circumcised on clinical examination (Doyle et al. 2010).

"Real" (Biological) AIDS

In rural Mwanza, we found that symptomatic sexually transmitted infections usually were attributed to natural causes, that is, sexual infection with an organism. In contrast, explanatory models of AIDS at the time of the study often included both natural and supernatural causes, and beliefs about natural causes were sometimes erroneous. For example, reports that white people intentionally introduced HIV/AIDS in condoms in order to kill Africans were widespread in our study population. This belief was similar to other tales of white people trying to harm Africans through medicines and consumer products, and reflected a general distrust of people who were perceived as former colonizers. There have been similar findings elsewhere in sub-Saharan Africa (Ashforth 2002; Castle 2003b; Kaler 2004a; Thomsen, Stalker, and Toroitich-Ruto 2004) and the world (Farmer 1992; Bogart and Thorburn 2005; Van Dyk 2008). However, in rural Mwanza discussions about this topic seemed to be rare, and tended to involve a somewhat detached conjecture about AIDS, condoms, and white people in general.

At the time of our study, many Mwanza villagers believed "real" AIDS to be sexually transmitted, but they often also believed that a separate, AIDS-mimicking illness was caused by witchcraft. Only a minority of the villagers who understood that HIV/AIDS could be contracted through sexual intercourse seemed to also understand that there is typically a very long period in which someone may be infectious but look and feel healthy. Other studies in Tanzania and elsewhere in sub-Saharan Africa have also found that such a fundamental misunderstandings has persisted well into the third decade of the HIV epidemic (Uiso et al. 2006; Steinberg 2009; Robins 2009). For example, a 2006 study found that young Tanzanians commonly believed they could assess people's HIV status from their appearance, and they were thus concerned that healthy-appearing antiretroviral therapy users might undermine their ability to avoid HIV infection (Ezekiel et al. 2009).

Such beliefs are reinforced by the fact that the majority of sub-Saharan Africans who are infected with HIV still have neither been tested for HIV nor received an AIDS diagnosis (UNAIDS 2008; Somi et al. 2009; UNAIDS and WHO 2009). For example, Demographic and Health Surveys conducted between 2003 and 2005 in Kenya and Malawi found that 80 percent of HIV-positive participants were unaware that they were infected (Anand et al. 2009). The limited available HIV testing services have tended to target adults, while HIV-positive adolescents have been least likely to be tested, whether they are long-term survivors of mother-to-child transmission or became infected through sexual activity (Ferrand et al. 2009).

In the first decade of the HIV epidemic it was generally believed that HIV-infected people in sub-Saharan Africa only lived a few years before developing AIDS and dying (Colebunders et al. 1991; Anzala et al. 1995). As the epidemic has progressed there has been increasing evidence that, in the absence of antiretroviral therapy, sub-Saharan Africans typically live 10–12 years after infection, and a minority live well beyond that (Morgan et al. 2002; Isingo et al. 2007). Similarly, at the time of our study it was widely assumed that very few or no children who received HIV from their mothers in utero, during childbirth, or via breastfeeding survived into adolescence in sub-Saharan Africa. However, recent modeling and epidemiological research suggests that a small minority have indeed survived into their teen years despite never having received antiretroviral therapy (Marston et al. 2005; Bagenda et al. 2006; Walker et al. 2006; Ferrand et al. 2007; Ferrand et al. 2009). In our study, in-depth interviews with the few adolescents who were HIV-positive at the start of the *MEMA kwa Vijana* trial in 1998 also suggest that some were long-term survivors of mother-to-child transmission.

"False" (Bewitchment) AIDS

Our study found a widespread belief that some people who seemed to have AIDS instead had been bewitched with a non-infectious, curable "false" AIDS. This "false" AIDS shared several attributes with other illnesses often reported to be caused by witchcraft. First, it was fatal, which Varkevisser (1973) found in the 1960s characterized illnesses particularly likely to be attributed to witchcraft; second, many AIDS-related opportunistic infections could be perceived as "normal" illnesses that had an abnormal frequency or intensity; third, powerful people seemed to be particularly targeted; and fourth, affected people sometimes emigrated to try to escape the spell's power (Fortson 2008; Msisha et al. 2009). Such ideas may have been reinforced by a belief that "false" AIDS was in fact *lusumbo*, a witchcraft-induced illness that reportedly preceded the HIV epidemic. Similar associations of AIDS with pre-AIDS traditional illnesses have been found elsewhere in sub-Saharan Africa (Schoepf 1992b; Green, Jurg and Djedje 1993; Mogensen 1997; Chimwaza and Watkins 2004; Uiso et al. 2006). In rural Mwanza there did not seem to be a common focus of AIDS discourse, although reports were found over a wide geographic area. While villagers often expressed uncertainty about whether a person had been afflicted by "real" (biological) or "false" (bewitchment) AIDS, we found little evidence that people believed that they had "real" AIDS *because of* bewitchment, unlike some other studies (Farmer 1992; Ashforth 2002).

HIV/AIDS causation beliefs in rural Mwanza may differ from those for other sexually transmitted infections because of the extraordinary characteristics of AIDS. The gap between infection with HIV and the onset of AIDS is very long, making it difficult for people to perceive the connection between the two. In addition, unlike most other sexually transmitted infections, symptoms of AIDS-related opportunistic infections are highly variable and their symptoms may not involve the genitals. Many people nonetheless understood that HIV/AIDS transmission is often sexual, and AIDS was thus stigmatized in a way similar to other sexually transmitted infections. However, its fatal severity placed it in another, more frightening category. "False" AIDS had less stigma and more hope associated with it than "real" AIDS, because it was not linked to sexual behavior, the potential to infect others, or a perception of certain death. Yamba (1997, 203–4) came to a similar conclusion in his study of HIV/AIDS witchcraft beliefs in a Zambian village:

> The rising death toll, due to HIV/AIDS, among the young and middle-aged adults, the nature of the disease itself as a latent long-drawn-out killer, the stress resulting from the breakdown of society, all fit well into local notions of witch-craft affliction. Witchfinders offer hope and are perceived as the sole resource not only for obtaining a "cure" for the disease . . . but also for vengeance against those who are believed to have caused the disease, namely witches.

In Yamba's 1994–1995 study, witchcraft accusations resulted in an intense period of violence, when sixteen people who were accused of witchcraft were killed during a four-month period. In our study in rural Mwanza, reports of "false" AIDS did not seem to lead to similar violence, possibly because witches were rarely named and/or the afflicted family secretly knew that the illness was truly AIDS. In ethnographic research with the first people diagnosed with AIDS in a rural Haitian village in the late-1980s, Farmer (1992) similarly found that no physical harm came to people accused of sending AIDS via sorcery.

Nonetheless, there remains a potential for retaliation against people who are accused of bewitching others with "false" AIDS in rural Mwanza (Mesaki 1994; Ashforth 2002). As discussed in chapter 3, there seems to have been an increase in witchcraft accusations amongst the Sukuma over the last century (Varkevisser 1973). From 1970 to 1984, the Tanzanian government documented 3,693 killings of people who had been accused of being witches, 61 percent of whom (377 men, 1,869 women) were killed in Mwanza and neighboring Shinyanga Region (Wijsen and Tanner 2002). More recently, Miguel (2005) conducted group interviews in 67 Shinyanga villages to assess the extent of such killings from 1992–2002. He found evidence of 138 attacks on people accused of witchcraft, 65 of which were fatal. Victims were nearly all women (96 percent) who had relatives in the village (98 percent) and/or were ethnically Sukuma (96 percent); they had a median and mean age of 50 years (Miguel 2005). That study found that the killing of people accused of witchcraft happened twice as often in years of insufficient or excessive rainfall, as those conditions caused droughts or floods, which in turn resulted in poor harvests and near-famine conditions.

As Stroeken (2001, 296) noted in his discussion of witchcraft amongst the Sukuma, many political, social, and economic factors may influence witchcraft accusations, but personal experience is ultimately critical: "the core of the matter remains that when people fall seriously ill—and they will continue to do so—they usually attribute the cause to someone bewitching them."

The unique characteristics of the HIV epidemic and its potentially profound impact on income and welfare in villages (Ngalula et al. 2002) may thus contribute to witchcraft accusations and harsh repercussions.

The Role of Traditional Healers

Our study found that traditional healers played an important role in perpetuating or refuting beliefs about AIDS and witchcraft. Some traditional healers did not understand the nature of AIDS and claimed that they could cure it, sometimes reinforcing beliefs about "false" AIDS and bewitchment, as has also been found in other settings in sub-Saharan Africa (Chirwa and Sivile 1989–1990; Awusabo-Asare and Anarfi 1997; Ashforth 2002; Robins 2009). Rather than see this as a limitation in the fight against HIV/AIDS, it could also be viewed as an opportunity. Traditional methods of prevention and treatment are often a first line of defense against illness in rural Africa, so HIV/AIDS interventions which educate and enlist the support of traditional healers may be very important. Indeed, some studies have shown that, once educated about HIV/AIDS themselves, many traditional healers used their health care and leadership positions to better educate, treat, and appropriately refer people (Green 1997; UNAIDS 2000; UNAIDS 2002; Homsy et al. 2004).

Given traditional healers are based in the communities they serve—and many have established practices providing long-term care in their own homes or patient's homes—they could play a valuable role in home-based care programs for people with AIDS after training on relevant topics, such as nursing care, hygiene, prevention of cross infection, medication adherence, health and social service referrals, and the provision of emotional support (UNAIDS 2002). However, the development of culturally-specific and safe traditional healer interventions is challenging. Any such efforts must be monitored closely to ensure they do not reinforce incorrect understandings or inappropriate treatments for HIV/AIDS (Neumann and Lauro 1982; Green 1988; Bodeker et al. 2000; Dickinson 2008).

Implications for Antiretroviral Therapy Programs

Possibly the greatest factor contributing to beliefs in a curable "false" AIDS at the time of our study was villagers' hopelessness and despair in the face of "real" AIDS. The recent introduction and scale-up of HIV testing and antiretroviral therapy in Tanzania has had a great impact on this issue, dramatically improving the quality of life and aspirations of many people living with HIV/AIDS (Somi et al. 2009).

At the time of our study in 2000, the cost of first-line antiretroviral therapy on world markets was between $10,000 and $12,000 per person per year, but by 2004 that cost had dropped to $300. Nonetheless, at that time only 3,000 (1 percent) of the estimated 440,000 HIV-positive Tanzanians who needed antiretroviral therapy actually received it, because regional and district hospital staff still lacked training in antiretroviral therapy management, laboratory facilities were inadequate, medications were insufficient, and outpatient monitoring was very limited (Hardon et al. 2006; Landman et al. 2006; Mapunjo and Urassa 2007; UNAIDS 2008; Somi et al. 2009). Antiretroviral therapy services have improved since then: for example, between 2004 and 2007 over 70,000 people—14 percent of all of those estimated to be living with AIDS in Tanzania—were started on antiretroviral therapy (Somi et al. 2009). Despite this progress, HIV testing and antiretroviral therapy services remain very limited in Tanzania and elsewhere in sub-Saharan Africa today, particularly in rural areas (Mmbaga et al. 2009; Waako et al. 2009; Gatell 2010).

Adherence to treatment is critical for antiretroviral therapy to be successful, and patients must achieve at least 95 percent adherence to avoid treatment failure and the risk of developing drug-resistant strains of the virus (Hardon et al. 2006). The findings presented here suggest that it may be possible to attain genuinely high, long-term adherence to antiretroviral therapy in rural Tanzania, because villagers demonstrated initiative and commitment in their general treatment-seeking behavior, and they were accustomed to preparing and managing their own medicines carefully. Nonetheless, this research also highlights potential challenges, including the powerful nature of AIDS-related stigma and how it may inhibit treatment-seeking, and the pluralistic nature of treatment-seeking, which may make it difficult for people to distinguish between effective and ineffective treatments. Three great concerns for both HIV prevention and antiretroviral therapy programs are that many villagers in our study still did not understand the long period of asymptomatic HIV infection prior to the onset of AIDS; many believed in a "false" AIDS that was non-infectious and curable with traditional medicines; and many believed that illnesses were cured once symptoms resolved. Each of these misunderstandings could contribute to a false sense of safety when engaging in unprotected sexual intercourse, as well as poor adherence to antiretroviral therapy over time, resulting in reduced treatment effectiveness and increased drug resistance.

Other recent research has raised similar concerns. For example, a study of HIV-positive individuals receiving HIV counseling and antiretroviral therapy in two Tanzanian cities found that, despite participants generally having good knowledge of HIV and AIDS, belief in AIDS-related bewitchment was also common and inhibited adherence to treatment (Hardon et al.

2006). Furthermore, two studies conducted with HIV-positive individuals elsewhere in Mwanza Region found that, in addition to programmatic and structural barriers, stigma was a formidable obstacle to uptake and long-term adherence to antiretroviral therapy (Mshana, Wamoyi, et al. 2006; Roura et al. 2009). Roura and colleagues (2009) concluded that antiretroviral therapy programs should contain a community level component that pro-actively engages patients' social networks, including increased education and sensitization of family members by home-based AIDS care providers.

CONCLUSION

At the start of the twenty-first century, villagers in Mwanza were more aware of, and concerned about, other kinds of sexually transmitted infections than HIV/AIDS. Yet few grasped how prevalent such infections were in their community, particularly as some were asymptomatic and others did not recognize the symptoms. Young people who did recognize they had symptoms of a sexually transmitted infection often did not seek treatment at a health facility for fear of punishment or stigma, while others tried to treat their illnesses using traditional methods, some of which were harmful. However, those villagers who did receive treatment for sexually transmitted infections at health facilities were typically very appreciative after their symptoms resolved.

During our study, most people with AIDS in rural Mwanza lived with little understanding of their disease and grossly inadequate services. As such individuals experienced painful, drawn out illnesses, they attempted to make sense of them in terms of both natural and supernatural causes, seeking out both biomedical and traditional treatments, as is still common in sub-Saharan Africa today (Chimwaza and Watkins 2004; Hatchett et al. 2004; Kapata 2004; Anand et al. 2009). Despite three decades having passed since HIV was first identified, there remains an urgent need for improved HIV testing and antiretroviral therapy services in rural Africa, as well as culturally appropriate interventions which convey clear and accurate information about HIV/AIDS and address widespread traditional beliefs and practices related to illness causation and treatment.

The next section of this book provides the final case study series, an in-depth description of the lives of two HIV-positive teenagers in our study. In the concluding chapter we will then review our findings on the social, economic, and cultural context of young people's sexual behavior in order to consider factors which may be barriers to, or facilitators of, sexual risk reduction.

NOTE

1. Some material in this chapter was adapted from: (a) Mshana, Gerry, Mary L. Plummer, Joyce Wamoyi, Zachayo S. Shigongo, David A. Ross, and Daniel Wight. 2006. "She was bewitched and caught an illness similar to AIDS": AIDS and sexually transmitted infection causation beliefs in rural northern Tanzania. *Culture, Health and Sexuality* 8(1):45–58. (b) Plummer, Mary L., Gerry Mshana, Joyce Wamoyi, Zachayo S. Shigongo, Richard J. Hayes, David A. Ross, and Daniel Wight. 2006. "The man who believed he had AIDS was cured": AIDS and sexually transmitted infection treatment-seeking behaviour in rural Mwanza, Tanzania. *AIDS Care* 18(5):460–66. (c) Weiss, Helen A., Mary L. Plummer, John Changalucha, Gerry Mshana, Zachayo S. Shigongo, Jim Todd, Daniel Wight, Richard J. Hayes, and David A. Ross. 2008. Circumcision among adolescent boys in rural northwestern Tanzania. *Tropical Medicine and International Health* 13(8):1054–61.

Case Study Series 3

"The Fever Went Away but Always Returned"

HIV-Positive Young People's Lives and Sexual Relationships

This case study series describes the lives of two young HIV-positive individuals, including their family and school backgrounds, socioeconomic activities, sexual relationship histories, and experiences of illness and health care. Case study 3.1 describes Shabani, a boy in his mid-teens who was HIV-positive when he was first interviewed at the start of the *MEMA kwa Vijana* trial in 1999. Shabani was most likely a long-term survivor of mother-to-child transmission during pregnancy, childbirth, or infancy. He became seriously ill during the trial, and his family sought medical treatment for him in multiple facilities before he died. Case study 3.2 describes Paulina, a young woman who most likely was infected with HIV sexually, because she tested negative for HIV in 1998 and again in 2000, and only tested positive for it at the end of the trial in 2002. Paulina reported that she had only had two sexual partners in her life, both within her village, one of whom was a migrant truck driver.

Like all trial participants, these two young people were offered the opportunity to learn their HIV status at each survey through counseling and testing services that followed the national protocol at the time, but neither took that option. The interviews suggest that both of them had experience of HIV-related illnesses, but it is not clear whether either was ever tested for HIV elsewhere or was diagnosed with AIDS by the medical providers they saw when they were ill. The HALIRA interviewers did not know that Shabani and Paulina had been selected for interviews because of preliminary HIV-positive test results. As discussed in chapter 2, over half of the trial participants who had a preliminary HIV-positive result during a survey did not in fact have HIV. Shabani and Paulina were only confirmed to be truly HIV-positive after more rigorous laboratory testing of their survey specimens was completed approximately one year after the fieldwork ended.

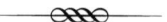

3.1. SHABANI: A TEENAGE BOY WHO PROBABLY WAS A LONG-TERM SURVIVOR OF MOTHER-TO-CHILD HIV TRANSMISSION

Shabani was 15 years old and in Year 7 when the researcher interviewed him. About one year later Shabani became seriously ill, and he died several months after that. Two and one half years after the first interview, the same researcher interviewed Shabani's father.

During his interview Shabani explained that he was the third of seven children that his parents had had together. Shabani's mother had also had two other children from two prior marriages, one to a man in the capital of a neighboring district, and another to a man in a different village. Shabani's father was polygynous and also had 15 other children. Shabani's mother was the third of his father's four wives. Two of her co-wives lived in the same village, while the first wife lived in the district capital. Shabani's father rotated between households by spending two nights at a time with each wife in Shabani's village, and then one week with his wife in the district capital. Shabani's village lay on a main rural thoroughfare between two district capitals.

Shabani's family was Sukuma and Muslim. They seemed to be comfortable financially. Shabani lived with his parents and siblings in a four-roomed cement brick house with a roof of galvanized iron sheets. His father was a welder and had a metal-working shop where he mainly repaired bicycles. He also owned several houses that he rented out. Shabani's mother farmed rice, maize, cassava, peanuts, and beans. Shabani described sometimes eating meat and fish at home, suggesting that he and his family had an unusually good diet for rural Mwanza. Shabani said that he farmed in his parents' agricultural plots, but he did not work for money as his father provided for all of his material needs. Shabani described a contented home life and good friendships with neighborhood youth with whom he studied and shared farming chores.

Shabani was enthusiastic about school, saying he greatly valued learning to read and write. He said he enjoyed his lessons a lot, and when asked for an example he named his *MEMA kwa Vijana* intervention lessons. He explained: "It helps me very much. . . . It helps me to protect myself . . . knowing not to have sex while you are still under age, to wait until you are a fully grown person and old enough to marry" [II-99-I-47-m]. Like most pupils, the only thing Shabani disliked at school was being hit by teachers or prefects for minor issues, such as forgetting to bring building supplies to contribute to school construction. Shabani said he wanted to go to secondary school and ultimately to become a teacher or a driver with a salaried position. He hoped to marry around the age of 25, to have one wife, and then to have no more than five children. He was emphatic about having only one wife, repeatedly stating "she will be the only one," even if it turned out she was unable to have the five children he wanted.

Shabani was very familiar with the sexual activity of his peers, and could describe how they typically negotiated and arranged to have sex. He said he himself had only had sexual intercourse once, when he was in Year 3 and about 10–11 years old. He said the girl had been the same age but in Year 2. Shabani said that he liked that girl a lot and considered her a friend long before their sexual encounter. He explained how their spontaneous sexual encounter occurred:

> *S:* We just started playing. There were also other children there. First we all played games like "bride and bridegroom." Then I told her, "Let us go have sex." She agreed. . . . We waited until everybody had dispersed. . . . We agreed that she should go in the house first, and then I followed. [II-99-I-47-m]

Shabani said that they had vaginal intercourse in an empty house, and he did not give her anything in exchange for it. He said the only reason the relationship ended was that she told others that they had had sex, and he had wanted to keep it a secret.

When asked why he had abstained after initiating sexual activity, Shabani said that after participating in the *MEMA kwa Vijana* intervention he became concerned about possibly getting a sexually transmitted infection. His knowledge of sexual health seemed extraordinarily good. For example, unlike most villagers he referred to HIV rather than simply AIDS:

> *S:* I have heard of HIV, and how a person contracts it. HIV is a virus that enters into a person's body during sexual intercourse. . . . It is found in blood in the veins and also in vaginal fluids and in semen. It is also transmitted by using sharp instruments which were already used by a person with AIDS. [II-99-I-47-m]

Shabani knew that condoms were used for both contraception and prevention of sexually transmitted infection, and he knew they could be obtained from shops and health facilities. He described a condom as follows:

> *S:* It is made of rubber. It is like . . . like a sock. The difference is that it is elastic. . . . It is wrapped in something that looks like a rind. You carefully tear off the wrapper, [because if not] you many accidentally tear the condom, rendering it useless. If you put on [a torn condom] like that and then have sex with a person with AIDS, you will definitely contract AIDS. Next you take off your underwear, then you put the condom on your penis. It has an opening at its top, and you push the penis through that opening. . . .
>
> *I:* In the future, if you agree to have sex with a girl but she tells you to use a condom, how will you feel?
>
> *S:* I will just feel fine. I will think that she wants to use condoms so that she does not get diseases. [II-99-I-47-m]

The only thing Shabani said he would like to learn more from his *MEMA kwa Vijana* participation was how to care for a person with AIDS. This was an unusual comment in interviews, and one that seemed to be made mainly by youths who were close to someone with AIDS, suggesting that this was the case for Shabani.

When the researcher interviewed Shabani's father Hamisi two and one half years later, his father said that Shabani had completed Year 7 soon after his interview and had then begun working in his father's metal-working shop:

> *H:* It was only after he completed school that I became very close to him. I told him, "Since you haven't had luck passing your examination, since you don't even want to repeat school, it will be good if you join me at work, if you're interested. Because this work that I'm doing is what supports our life." . . . So we would spend the whole day together at work. In the evening we would separate, and perhaps he would go watch a video trailer or go to mosque, and then he would return home. Shabani was not a person who would be out for long, no, because he liked/loved his religion so much. When he was out, most of the time he would be in the mosque, praying and whatnot. [II-02-I-247-m]

Hamisi said that Shabani had only occasionally had mild illnesses such as fevers or nose bleeds in childhood, and nothing serious that kept him out of school for more than a couple of days. When Shabani first became ill at the age of 16, he had a fever which they thought was caused by malaria and treated at home with acetaminophen tablets. But the fever kept returning, so Shabani's parents took him to a local private dispensary where he was diagnosed and given medications for malaria and typhoid. Shabani tried to resume normal life:

> *H:* He got some relief, but that relief confused us. The fever went away, but always returned. . . . He would wake up in the morning and say, "Father, let's just go to work." We would stay at work together and when it reached a certain hour you would see he had become weak, or he had fallen asleep. I would tell him to go home if he felt feverish. [II-02-I-247-m]

Shabani's parents decided to take him to the district hospital, where he was re-tested for malaria and typhoid and further treated for both. He was admitted to the hospital for 18 days until his health seemed to improve and he returned home. Some time soon afterwards, however, he became very ill again. His father described how they took care of him at home: "His mother and I, and the entire family that stays here—his sisters and his brothers—all of us had a timetable for attending him while he was here at home. If I went out, his mother would stay with him" [II-02-I-247-m].

Shabani's parents soon took him to a different district hospital in a neighboring district to see if he would be treated more successfully there. The health workers there also tested and diagnosed him as having typhoid, but additionally said that he was anemic and speculated that he might have sickle cell anemia. Shabani was then given a series of blood transfusions, first from blood donated by his father and then purchased from a blood bank every 3–4 days. Shabani was in great discomfort and pain during this period, often feverish and sometimes delirious. His father reported that Shabani also had very little appetite, and experienced weight loss, physical weakness, nausea, vomiting, muscle pain, and very yellow skin, eyes, and urine. For example:

H: He would say, "I feel so weak." . . . Sometimes he used to tell me that he felt very cold. He would just say, "Father, cover me with a bed sheet, I feel very cold." Then I would cover him. . . . Towards the end, he would only eat when forced. You would threaten him a little bit, maybe say, "They're going to feed you intravenously unless you eat." You would call the nurses and arrange with them to rebuke him in order to convince him to eat. But he didn't like to eat. He didn't like to eat." [II-02-I-247-m]

After twelve days in the second hospital, Hamisi was arranging for Shabani's fourth blood transfusion when Shabani died. His father explained: "He was talking until the time of his death. I was with him there on the bed. He told me, 'Father, my condition has become worse, I think I am going to die.' He said those words to me, 'Eee, I think I'm dying, father.' Then he never spoke again" [II-02-I-247-m].

Shabani had not seen a traditional healer during his illness. His father said that he had not seen anything to suggest that the illness was caused by witchcraft, although he added that he might not recognize witchcraft as he did not have expertise in such matters.

Shabani's mother died of unspecified causes soon after Shabani died. At the time of Hamisi's interview, Hamisi reported that his senior wife had also recently developed symptoms similar to those Shabani had had. There is no way to be certain how Shabani became infected with HIV, but the interviews and the timing of his ill health suggest that he may have been a long-term survivor of mother-to-child HIV transmission. Shabani's mother could have been exposed to HIV in one of her three marriages, particularly as her third marriage involved a long-term, concurrent sexual network of at least five people based in large villages and towns, where sexually transmitted infection rates were relatively high.

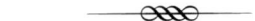

3.2. PAULINA: A YOUNG WOMAN WHO PROBABLY CONTRACTED HIV SEXUALLY

Paulina was 15 years old in Year 7 when she participated in the first *MEMA kwa Vijana* survey. She tested negative for pregnancy and sexually transmitted infections at that time. At the second survey 18 months later she tested positive for Chlamydia and gonorrhea, and at the third survey another 18 months later she tested positive for HIV, herpes and Trichomonas. Paulina's in-depth interview took place several months after that final survey. At that time she was living with her father and two aunts in two rented rooms in the center of a large village in a remote rural area. Paulina and her family were Sukuma and Catholic. She typically spent her days engaged in domestic tasks, farming, working in her aunt's kiosk in the village center, and, on Sundays, attending church. She said she did not attend video shows or discos, but she sometimes went to *ngoma* events. She explained that her father and aunt forbade her to go to video shows, because "There are bad/evil things there. You find people might just dance freely, and men may seduce those who go" [II-02-I-333-f].

Paulina had participated in the *MEMA kwa Vijana* intervention during her last year in school, and remembered some of the information she learned then. She described sexually transmitted infections as follows:

> *P:* They taught us the symptoms are to have pain in the stomach and to emit abnormal fluid from the private parts. Then you have some irritation and . . . some scabs appear. If you see that, then you have to go to the hospital immediately. We were taught that at school by the teachers and those who came from [the government health facility]. [II-02-I-333-f]

Similarly, Paulina was able to explain how HIV/AIDS was transmitted:

> *P:* Say for example a person comes here to this village. You don't even know where he . . . where he comes from. On that same day he seduces you and you have sex with him without condoms. Maybe he has diseases and then you, as the girl, you make love with another man without using a condom. Definitely you will spread the disease. . . .
>
> *I:* Do you think that you can also get AIDS?
>
> *P:* Of course I can, if I have sex with a man without using a condom. [II-02-I-333-f]

During her interview Paulina reported having had two sexual partners and she seemed to speak fairly openly about them, but the dates she reported were sometimes inconsistent and it was difficult to determine the exact sequence of events related to her sexual health. She told the researcher that she had had a one-year relationship with a schoolboy from a neighboring village, and more recently a two-month relationship with a migrant truck driver, which she considered to still be ongoing. Paulina met her first boyfriend at an inter-school sports tournament when she was 15 years old, but she said they did not have sex for almost a year:

> *P:* At the school he told me, "I like/love you . . . you must come to my house." . . . We kept conversing like that until a year went by and we had completed school. I refused when I was still at school because they would have found out about it at my home. Sometimes he would bring me money and tell me to go to buy something, but I refused. [II-02-I-333-f]

Paulina described her first sexual encounter with this boy:

> *P:* Our intermediary brought me shoes from him. My family was there, so the intermediary said she was giving me the shoes because they were too small for her. . . .

Later he and I went to the intermediary's house to have sex. It was during the day. We didn't take long, just a short while, just one hour. I felt some pain, and afterwards I felt exhausted down there [gesturing to her genitals]. The pain went away that same day. [II-02-I-333-f]

Paulina and this young man continued having sex about once a month for over a year. She broke off the relationship because people told her he had other girlfriends, but she said he was still the boyfriend she had liked/loved the most.

Sometime during or after that relationship, Paulina migrated to Mwanza City where she worked in domestic service for one to two months. She said she did not stay there for long because she missed her home. At some point in this period Paulina also developed *mkanda wa jeshi* (literally "soldier's belt"), a form of shingles strongly associated with HIV in rural Mwanza (Todd and Barongo 1997). She described it as follows:

P: *Mkande wa jeshi* is very painful, it is painfully prickly. It is piercing and just very painful. It was right here [gesturing to her arm]. I went to the government health facility where they injected me with medicine and gave me pills and solution to apply. I continued to improve until it was cured. [II-02-I-333-f]

At the time of her interview Paulina explained that her current boyfriend was a truck driver who transported grains between district capitals and the country's commercial capital. She said an intermediary arranged for them to meet: "He just sent a woman who came here at home to look for me" [II-02-I-333-f]. It is unclear whether Paulina's boyfriend had seen her already and requested to meet her specifically when he sent the intermediary, or he had simply asked the intermediary to find a sexual partner for him. However, the matter-of-fact way Paulina described this experience suggested it might not have been an unusual practice for male travelers in the village center where she lived and worked. Paulina and this man had sex in his room in the evening a few times over a two month period before he left on a work assignment. She considered the relationship to still be ongoing because he said that he would return to the village. Paulina said one of her girlfriends and her same-aged aunt knew about this relationship, but she hid it from her father and her older aunt because they would scold and hit her if they found out.

Paulina told the interviewer that she had never had symptoms of a sexually transmitted infection. However, she said she had once cut herself with a razor blade while she was shaving her pubic hair, and afterwards she developed a genital rash. The rash resolved, and since that incident she said she had only trimmed her pubic hair with scissors.

During her interview Paulina repeatedly said that she had used condoms every time she had had sex and that she would continue to do so in the future. She explained: "Definitely I will continue using them with him [her current partner], because he is away at present, and I just don't know what he is doing while he's away. Because there are many diseases these days—sexually transmitted infections and AIDS" [II-02-I-333-f]. Paulina said that her partners had always brought condoms to their sexual encounters and she could not imagine obtaining them herself. She explained:

> *P:* I can't buy them; he goes to buy them himself. No, I can't. . . . What will they say when you go there? [Laughter] Maybe you go to a shop here in the village where they know you. I mean, from then on that person will always make fun of you, saying, "Why did you buy condoms? You must have gone with a man!" Mm, he may even tell other people. [II-02-I-333-f]

Despite Paulina's assertions of consistent condom use, when the interviewer asked her if she had any questions at the end of the interview Paulina revealed uncertainty about whether it was necessary to use a condom after an initial sexual encounter with a partner:

> *P:* I have only one question, that . . . if perhaps you have had sex with a man . . . now, if you are seduced by that man again, is it important that you take a condom with you, or can you just have sex with him like that, without using a condom? . . .
>
> *I:* Like you said, condoms prevent many diseases . . . so it is important to take and use a condom. Because even if you know the person . . . when you look at him, you can't know what he is suffering from, right?
>
> *P:* Definitely not. . . . No, you just can't know.
>
> *I:* Therefore it is important to use . . . to use condoms. [II-02-I-333-f]

Given Paulina was found to have contracted five sexually transmitted infections over a three year period it seems unlikely that her report of consistent condom use was accurate. From her interview it is not possible to determine who exposed her to HIV and other sexually transmitted infections. However, several possibilities are evident, including: her first boyfriend who reportedly had multiple partners; unacknowledged partners she might have had in the village or in Mwanza City (where HIV prevalence was higher than in rural areas); or her recent partner who was a migrant truck driver and thus likely to be high risk.

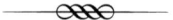

CONCLUSION

Shabani's and Paulina's interviews were very similar to other interviews with HIV-positive young people in our study. Experiences such as theirs may still be common in many parts of sub-Saharan Africa today, despite the recent scale-up of HIV testing and antiretroviral therapy services, and the good progress made in preventing mother-to-child HIV transmission. These two individuals' reported sexual behavior and illness histories were also not very different from those reported by randomly selected young people, at least before Shabani became seriously ill. Notably, both Shabani and Paulina reported that they tried to reduce their sexual risk behavior after participating in the *MEMA kwa Vijana* intervention. While it is not possible to know the extent to which they succeeded in this, their sexual histories nonetheless highlight the importance of HIV prevention education for both HIV-positive and HIV-negative individuals.

Chapter Twelve

Barriers and Facilitators of Sexual Risk Reduction

Our findings on young people's sexual culture, relationships, and activities in rural Mwanza have revealed their exposure to sexual coercion, unwanted pregnancy, and sexually transmitted infections, in particular HIV. In this final chapter we will review our findings on the social, economic, and cultural context of young people's sexual behavior by first discussing those factors which make it difficult for them to avoid risk behaviors, and then identifying those which might facilitate sexual behavior change and risk reduction. Understanding such barriers and facilitators is critical to developing effective behavior change interventions, which is the focus of the companion volume to this book (Plummer, forthcoming).

CONTEXTUAL BARRIERS TO SEXUAL RISK REDUCTION

In the following discussion we will distinguish between economic and cultural barriers to sexual risk reduction, but in practice these dimensions are deeply intertwined. Determining whether economic or cultural barriers are more important in inhibiting risk reduction is a macro-level, theoretical debate that is beyond the scope of this book. Our findings do show, however, that like economics culture operates at a structural level, that is, as a fundamental pattern of social systems that is very difficult for individuals to resist, whatever their ability for independent action. Both economics and culture should thus be regarded as profound underlying drivers of sexual health or ill-health.

Economic Factors

Women's Lower Status and Economic Dependence on Men

We found that women's subordinate status and very limited economic opportunities were fundamental barriers to sexual risk reduction. Girls were socialized to accept male superiority, deferring to male decisions and seeing their role as serving men. Girls' education was valued far less than that of boys. For example, of the minority of young women who passed their Primary School Leaving Examination, many did not go to secondary school because their parents said they could not afford it. However, it was not unusual for families to pay for young men who failed the same examination to reenter primary school under assumed names, in order to resit the examination and get another chance at secondary school. Girls grew up expecting early motherhood, married life within their husband's home and village, and economic dependence on their husbands. The very small minority of young women who had different aspirations tended to have both extraordinary parental support and high academic achievement.

Sex as an Important Economic Resource for Women

Young women had far fewer economic opportunities than young men, so for many—perhaps the vast majority—sex was a critical resource to help them meet their requirements, as shown in chapter 7. In their teens, girls frequently were expected to provide for their basic needs, such as soap and underwear, and they often also went without a daytime meal unless they bought themselves a snack at school. However, girls had very few ways to earn cash and these were not lucrative. In stark contrast, throughout their teens girls often were offered money, food, or other products in exchange for sex, and female peer pressure only reinforced this option. Unmarried young women in their late teens and early twenties had more small business opportunities than younger teenagers, but they still earned relatively little from such activities compared to what they could acquire from sexual encounters. Furthermore they often had greater expenses than teenage girls, particularly if they had children.

Despite the findings above, transactional sex in rural Mwanza should not be seen simply as "survival sex" among the poorest females, for it was embedded in the culture at all income levels. A young woman's respectability and self-worth were closely linked to the compensation she received for sex; this was also found in a more recent study in Mwanza (van Reeuwijk 2010). Material exchange for sex could be regarded as an extension of the established institution of bridewealth, within which men paid for sexual and other rights over women.

Poor Quality of Health Services

At a broader level Tanzania's poverty meant that both education and health services were underfunded and of extremely poor quality, particularly in remote rural areas. Self diagnosis and treatment with traditional medicines and/or medications bought at kiosks was typically the first response to illness and an ongoing strategy, increasing the chance of inappropriate medication and dosage and the development of drug resistance (van der Geest 1987; Msiska et al. 1997; Geissler et al. 2000). If symptoms did not resolve, villagers often sought treatment from a traditional healer before biomedical services. Some traditional treatments may have been beneficial and helped relieve symptoms, but some were likely to have been harmful, as described in chapters 10 and 11. Biomedical health care was limited by widely dispersed facilities, inadequate staff training, chronic understaffing, poor facilities, very basic technology, and drug and equipment shortages. Even if young people walked the typical three to ten kilometers to their local health facility, their consultation was unlikely to be confidential and the health worker's advice might be inappropriate.

Poor Quality of Formal Education

Many primary school teachers in rural Mwanza had little training beyond primary school themselves, and pupils had very low literacy, very little knowledge of mathematics or biology, and received few opportunities and little encouragement to think critically. In high income countries most young people have had sufficient education in these areas to readily grasp key concepts about HIV and AIDS, for example, that a person can be HIV-infected but appear healthy for many years. In such settings acquiring adequate knowledge is thus often seen as the most straightforward step towards reducing sexual risk behaviors. However, two decades into the HIV epidemic we found that basic understanding of HIV and AIDS was very poor amongst both adolescents and adults in rural Mwanza. Other recent studies in eastern and southern Africa have also found this continues to be a fundamental problem, particularly in rural areas (Uiso et al. 2006; Steinberg 2009; Ezekiel et al. 2009; Robins 2009).

Problematic teacher–pupil relationships also posed great challenges within rural Mwanza schools and limited the potential role teachers might play in adolescent sexual health promotion. As described in chapter 4, teaching was highly authoritarian and was characterized by recitation and corporal punishment, which fundamentally differ with the trust-building and participatory methods that are generally promoted in sexual health programs (Kuhn, Steinberg, and Mathews 1994; World Health Organization 1997). In addition, several official and unofficial school practices had serious implications for teacher–pupil relationships. Mandatory pregnancy examinations raise ethical concerns about pupil privacy and teachers' motivations, and sometimes led to pupils leaving school, being beaten and fined. Instead of reducing pupil sexual activity, forced pregnancy examinations and corporal punishment may have contributed to pupils' secretiveness about it.

Sexual abuse of school girls by teachers is a very serious issue that has been found in many countries in sub-Saharan Africa (World Health Organization 1997; Mlemya, Justine, and Mgalla 1997; Kinsman et al. 1999; Jewkes et al. 2002; O-saki and Agu 2002; Panos Institute 2003). Punishing such offences by transferring the guilty party simply moves the problem to another school. In such contexts, close supervision and appropriate responses are crucial and there is a broader need for national policies and norms that better prevent, monitor, and correct such abuses (World Health Organization 1997; Panos Institute 2003).

Finally, while some teachers in our study seemed to have fairly positive and respectful relationships with villagers, in some villages substantial tensions existed between the two, which could affect the acceptability of teacher-led sexual health programs. Preexisting problems, such as teachers' alcohol abuse or sexual abuse of pupils, could create or reinforce controversy and stigma associated with a sexual health program in a community.

Cultural Factors

Contradictory Sexual Norms and Secrecy

In chapter 5 we analyzed how contradictory norms both encouraged and discouraged young people's sexual activity, which led youth to conceal their sexual relationships and parents not to acknowledge them. Such concealment of unmarried relationships is also common elsewhere in Tanzania (Setel 1999) and sub-Saharan Africa (Nzioka 2001; Helle-Valle 2004). In our study, young people often believed that maintaining discretion was more important than strictly adhering to moral norms. From an early age they learned to present themselves differently in different social contexts, and, as Helle-Valle (2004) found in his study in Botswana, this principle particularly applied to sexual relationships. In rural Mwanza this was one of the most important barriers to monogamy, as was also found among adult men in Uganda (Parikh 2007). Unmarried sexual relationships were not reinforced through the acknowledgement and endorsement of families and peers, which could possibly promote longer, more exclusive, and more familiar relationships. Being socialized into a sexual culture of clandestine unmarried relationships facilitated rapid partner change and concurrency, as shown in chapter 6. This probably also profoundly influenced marital infidelity later in life, and particularly men's common expectation that their wives should be faithful but they need not be, as described in chapter 9. Furthermore, it is likely that widespread secrecy affected perceived susceptibility to sexual risk. Ignorance about a sexual partner's past and concurrent partners was probably an important barrier to realistic risk perception.

The hidden character of young people's sexual relationships was also connected to most parents' inability to communicate with their children about sexual issues, since discussion of such topics was deemed improper and shameful. Similar inhibitions have been documented by others in Mwanza (van Reeuwijk 2010) and elsewhere in Tanzania (Mbonile and Kayombo 2008; Bastien 2009a; Namisi et al. 2009), as well as elsewhere in sub-Saharan Africa (Boileau et al. 2008; Phetla et al. 2008; Biddlecom, Awusabo-Asare, and Bankole 2009). This meant that parents rarely discussed with their children the sexual risks they might face, even in a depersonalized way, and parents had little opportunity to endorse and reinforce more protective values and beliefs. Parent-child communication was further hampered by many parents having a very poor understanding of sexual health risk themselves. However, international research on parent-child relationships suggests that a lack of communication about sex is probably of less importance for children's sexual risk behavior than the expression of parental affection or connection (WHO 2007), which was also typically limited in rural Mwanza, or parental monitoring of children's behavior (Biddlecom, Awusabo-Asare, and Bankole 2009), which was widely attempted, at least for girls.

Sexuality and Masculinity

Being sexually active was central to young men's identity, as discussed in chapter 5, and the ability to seduce the most desirable women was greatly admired by other young men. Limited alternative ways to affirm masculine identity—such as through sports, employment, entrepreneurship, active fathering roles, or becoming a patriarchal head of household—may have contributed to this emphasis on sexual prowess (DeVisser and Smith 2007; Steinberg 2009). This resulted in persistent male pressure on young women to have sex, particularly directed at girls who were considered to be "virtuous." Such pressure was often effective, even with girls who initially were determined to resist, as seen in case study 1.4. Young people's behavior is unlikely to change without modifications to such gender roles and values.

A Belief in the Inevitability of Sex Once Started

We found that young men were primarily motivated to have sex because of physical desire, and most believed it was not possible to abstain from intercourse once they had already experienced it. As noted in chapter 8, masturbation was probably practiced by many young men, especially adolescent boys, but negative attitudes and misunderstandings about it were widespread, such as the belief that it might reduce a man's virility or fertility. Masturbation was rarely perceived as a safe, alternative to unprotected vaginal intercourse; to the contrary, some youth believed it was a more harmful way to satisfy their sexual desire.

The widely held belief that it is too difficult to abstain from intercourse after sexual debut supports the internationally promoted idea that sexual health interventions should start at young ages prior to sexual experimentation (WHO 1997; Gallant and Maticka-Tyndale 2004; Dixon-Mueller 2009). In rural Mwanza targeting adolescents at an early age would be logistically challenging, however, as pupils typically ranged in age from 12—18 years in each of the last three years of primary school, yet programs should preferably be tailored for specific ages (Van Dyk 2008). In addition, the younger the target group, the greater resistance to sexual education there is likely to be from parents and education officials, so more community education and advocacy may be required to achieve community support.

Misconceptions and Ambivalence about Contraception

As shown in chapter 10, many girls and young women were misinformed and/or ambivalent about pregnancy prevention. Most hoped to avoid premarital pregnancy because it would lead to parental punishment and an end to schooling for school girls. However, many sexually active young women believed that pregnancy prevention was beyond their control, and that only God or chance could determine whether they conceived. Most expected to marry and bear children very soon after leaving school, and some regarded out-of-wedlock pregnancies positively as a demonstration of their fertility. For those young women who did wish to prevent pregnancy, misinformation about contraception was widespread. Many used ineffective traditional methods, while those with access to hormonal contraception—usually young mothers—often mistrusted it, believing it might make them infertile.

Very few villagers in our study had experience with condoms, and among those who had, most had only used them once or twice. Condoms were rarely used because of beliefs that they prevented meaningful, decent, natural, or satisfying sex. The most widely expressed belief was that condoms reduce men's sexual pleasure, but they were also thought of as alien, unnatural, and associated with promiscuity and infection, and some thought them ineffective or even dangerous. Many of the reported concerns about condoms seemed to be secondary rationalizations fueled by the fundamental male concern about physical pleasure, and men typically determined whether condoms would be used in sexual encounters. Furthermore, adults were opposed to the discussion of condom use with young people because this acknowledged youth sexual activity and could be interpreted as promoting it. Even for those rare young people who may have considered using condoms, access to them was very limited.

Low Salience of, and Perceived Susceptibility to, HIV/AIDS

Several factors contributed to the low prominence of HIV/AIDS in day-to-day life in rural Mwanza. At the most general level daily concerns with subsistence were more pressing than worry about such a long-term and seemingly invisible threat. Most rural young people, but especially the poorest, had difficulty developing concrete future plans because of immediate material insecurity and the need to focus on routine domestic and agricultural tasks, getting food and water, finding soap, and maintaining their parents' approval and peers' respect. This was probably particularly the case for young people who lacked specific long-term education, business, farming, or family goals. For those who understood it, the long duration between HIV infection and symptoms also dissipated immediate concern: many other misfortunes might afflict them before the possibility of developing AIDS.

Another factor contributing to the low salience of HIV/AIDS in village life was that people typically distanced themselves from those they perceived to be vulnerable to HIV/AIDS, reducing their sense of personal risk. Many villagers thought the disease only affected those living in towns and cities, particularly those with "immoral" sexual practices, and adults rather than young people. Relatively low HIV prevalence, very limited HIV testing, poor health services, stigma, and secrecy made the disease largely invisible in rural areas. Few of those infected were ever clinically diagnosed, and those who were did not necessarily inform others. Thus although deaths due to AIDS occurred, they were often attributed to the specific opportunistic infections, related symptoms, and/or witchcraft. When close relatives or friends did know the root cause, AIDS was rarely openly acknowledged, although it might be discussed in rumors. Therefore HIV/AIDS had little visibility in rural Mwanza, making it difficult for some people to take the immediate threat seriously.

Finally, limited knowledge about the biology of HIV also reduced people's sense of susceptibility to the disease, as discussed in chapter 11. An enduring misunderstanding was that healthy looking people could not be infectious, so many villagers were only concerned about sexual transmission from those with visible symptoms. Even when someone *had* visible AIDS-related symptoms they often were not seen as potentially infectious because their condition was not recognized as AIDS, as described above. Belief in the supernatural origins of many illnesses meant that people could be equally or more concerned about avoiding witchcraft than they were about having unprotected intercourse.

Excessive Alcohol Use

Our study did not set out to investigate alcohol use, but it was such an important part of village life that we collected extensive data on it. In chapter 3 we described how every village had venues where alcohol was brewed, distilled, and/or sold, and a small minority of villagers drank alcohol frequently and excessively and were often seen drunk in public places at any time of day. In all villages a sizeable proportion of adult men and a small minority of women drank alcohol socially in the evening or when traveling, leading to varying degrees of drunkenness, and this was especially common around special events. The patterns of harmful alcohol use were thus similar to those reported elsewhere in rural and urban sub-Saharan Africa, namely becoming intoxicated in public spaces, heavy drinking during cultural festivals, and drinking outside of mealtimes (Chersich et al. 2009).

In rural Mwanza alcohol use promoted sexual risk behaviors in a number of ways. A small number of women were responsible for making alcohol and thus had relatively easy access to it, but other young women who drank homemade or bottled alcohol were likely to obtain it in exchange for sex. Most commonly, intoxication impaired decision making for both men and women, so that some had sexual encounters that they would not otherwise have had, such as sex with a casual partner, with multiple partners, or against a woman's will, as described in chapter 7. Similar findings have been documented elsewhere in sub-Saharan Africa (Zablotska et al. 2006; Parkes et al. 2007; Akarro 2009; Chersich et al. 2009; Page and Hall 2009).

Decision-Making and Fatalism

Our study found that many young people made important, long-term decisions quickly and almost arbitrarily, such as the fairly common practices of young men migrating to another area on short notice because of a tip about a possible job, or youth of either sex marrying people they had only met recently because they felt ready to marry. Often such decisions did not seem to involve much reflection or consideration of possible negative long-term consequences, despite, for example, the fairly common nature of divorce. As noted in chapter 9, the practice of marrying someone largely unfamiliar had historical and cultural precedence amongst the Sukuma (Tanner 1955a; Varkevisser 1973), as did the practice of striking out on one's own to pursue new opportunities (Wijsen and Tanner 2002). In our study population such practices may have also reflected limited aspirations and/or youthful adventurousness. Such rapid decision making could also be seen in sexual behavior, when many young people focused on the immediate advantages of sex, rather than possible unwanted pregnancy or infection later, even when those possible consequences were well known to them. This short-term orientation of sexual decision making was also found in a more recent anthropological study with children in Mwanza (van Reeuwijk 2010).

Importantly, adults also sometimes made similarly fast, life-changing decisions, either for themselves or their children. For example, there were many accounts of parents allowing a man who was essentially a stranger to marry their daughter if he formally proposed marriage and paid bridewealth. However, parents may have felt they had adequately considered the long-term consequences if the man seemed to be financially secure and/or came from a known family, believing that issues such as emotional intimacy and compatibility were unimportant or would develop after marriage.

In addition, villagers often demonstrated a limited sense of agency—or ability to act of their own volition—which presents an important obstacle when trying to reduce sexual risk behaviors. In this regard economic and cultural factors reinforced each other. Poverty led villagers to talk about the conditions of their lives in fatalistic terms, frequently resigning themselves to God's will or attributing hardship to bad luck. Many villagers, particularly the poorest, least educated, and/or women, expressed such a fatalistic perspective on life. Their educational, cultural, and economic circumstances limited their aspirations and may have made it very challenging to navigate the links between their immediate needs and wider goals (Appadurai 2004). Recent research in rural Mwanza found that lack of agency was especially pronounced in relation to drought, theft, witchcraft, and health risks (Desmond 2009). However, we do not want to portray villagers as overwhelmingly resigned to events being inevitable. There were numerous counter examples, and talking in fatalistic terms may have sometimes been a conscious way for them to distance themselves from responsibility for making questionable choices (Desmond 2009).

Finally, in our study becoming infected with HIV was commonly referred to as being like an accident, as has also been found elsewhere in Tanzania (Setel 1999; Wijsen and Tanner 2002; Bastien 2009b). In neighboring Mara Region, where Dilger (2003, 30) had similar findings on young people's perspectives on sexuality and HIV, a youth encapsulated the apparent indifference towards possible HIV infection, saying, "AIDS has become normal—like an accident on the road. Some will die, others will take the next bus. However, nobody will give up traveling because of the accidents of others."

CONTEXTUAL FACILITATORS OF SEXUAL RISK REDUCTION

Our study also found various features of rural Tanzanian social life that might, potentially, facilitate sexual behavioral change and risk reduction.

Restrictive Norms

In rural Mwanza, young people's heterosexual activity—and particularly young women's—was constrained by the restrictive norms described in chapters 5 and 6, especially that school pupils should be abstinent, women should maintain their sexual respectability, couples should be faithful, and sex should only be discussed in particular social contexts. As in other regions of Tanzania (Dilger 2003), these norms were of far greater importance in restricting sexual behavior than the threat of HIV infection. However, the influence of these norms on sexual behavior was complex and mixed. Sometimes, for example, they contributed to greater secrecy among sexually active youth, which in turn could lead to higher risk sexual behavior. Campaigns for greater sexual fidelity in Uganda were found to have similar effects (Parikh 2007).

The norm of masculine sexual respectability was that men should be faithful to their wives and support them and their children financially, an ideal strongly endorsed by Christian and Muslim morality. This was in the interest of wives and their children, particularly as extramarital relationships were usually pursued at the cost of household income. Yet this restrictive norm was fundamentally incompatible with Sukuma custom, which historically gave husbands the right to have extramarital partners (Cory 1953). It also conflicted with the current esteem that men receive from their peers when they have multiple sexual partners, particularly amongst young men. Norms of masculine sexual respectability had far less influence on behavior than those of feminine sexual respectability, but the fact that these ideals were current in people's thoughts and were discussed—even if only when a man contravened them—suggests the potential for strengthening them.

Education and Religion

Two main social factors in rural Mwanza seemed to make some young people more averse to sexual risks. One was participation in formal education, and particularly an ambition to pursue further education. School boys typically had less sex than their out-of-school peers simply because they had less opportunities to earn money to exchange for sex. In addition, the small minority of youth with strong ambitions to go to secondary school were generally more averse to sexual risk. Similarly, studies elsewhere in sub-Saharan Africa have found that young people—especially young women—who complete secondary school are more likely to practice safer sex and less likely to be infected than those who did not attend secondary school (Bastien 2008; Hargreaves et al. 2008; Moyo et al. 2008; Hargreaves et al. 2010). This highlights the sexual health potential of generic interventions which increase young people's educational opportunities beyond primary school.

Furthermore, despite the great limitations of formal education in rural Mwanza that have already been discussed, the school system there as elsewhere in sub-Saharan Africa has a unique potential to reach a large number of youth with low cost health interventions. Given Mwanza's resource poor setting, the late age of most primary school leavers, and the low proportion that went on to secondary school in our study, primary schools were the only institution where an adolescent sexual health program could be implemented in rural Mwanza both on a large scale and at low cost at the start of the twenty-first century. A school-based intervention in that setting would have the added benefit of being potentially sustainable long-term, as primary school teachers are often some of the most literate and educated individuals in rural areas, and once trained, they would have the potential to deliver sexual health programs until they retired.

Devout religious experience was the other protective social factor that seemed to make some young people more averse to sexual risk. Specifically, young people who came from devout Christian or Muslim families were more likely to be abstinent or monogamous than other youth, especially if they shared their parents' strong religious beliefs. Even when they did not, religious disapproval and the threat of punishment could still be effective in reducing young people's sexual risk behaviors. However, parents' strong religious disapproval sometimes only seemed to prompt their children to be more secretive in their sexual behavior, contributing to greater risk. Furthermore, if a religious group prescribes abstinence or monogamy but specifically discourages condom use, youth might be even less likely than others to consider using condoms if they do have sex. A large Zambian study of 13–20-year-olds, for example, found that young women in conservative religious groups were more likely to report delayed sexual debut, but less likely to use condoms during first sex (Agha, Hutchinson, and Kusanthan 2006).

Parents' Concern for their Children's Health and Welfare

Parents in rural Mwanza were usually very concerned about the well-being and future prospects of their children, even though verbal or physical expression of affection between parents and their children was unusual. Parents' concern for their children was generally more evident in how they monitored their children's activities, taught them work skills, supported their educational goals, and provided them with day-to-day material support and long-term assets, such as land that they could farm themselves. Elsewhere in sub-Saharan Africa parents' close supervision of, and connection with, their children has been associated with children having healthier behaviors (Babalola, Tambashe, and Vondrasek 2005; Kumi-Kyereme et al. 2007; Amoran and Fawole 2008; Peltzer 2009; Biddlecom, Awusabo-Asare, and Bankole 2009).

Beyond parental love for their children, there was also a strong belief in the importance of continuing one's lineage, which remained a core part of villagers' identity. Furthermore with the government only providing the most basic social welfare, parents were almost entirely dependent on their children for care in old age. They therefore had multiple incentives to protect their children's health throughout their lives, which, if exploited, could make interventions much more meaningful and effective.

Village Conformity and Communal Activities

We found that village life was generally characterized by closely interknit social relationships, gender and generational hierarchies, widely shared beliefs, conventional practices, and enforced collective activities, although there were exceptions to this pattern, particularly in more heterogeneous fishing villages. Such communal conformity could result in conservatism that is a barrier to cultural change, but it could also provide an opportunity for preventive interventions, if the formal and informal opinion leaders within villages can be persuaded of the need for behavior change. To be effective, the values and beliefs that are confirmed and reproduced through social interaction must be health promoting rather than health jeopardizing. In addition, the widespread practice of communal village activities provides an opportunity to deliver interventions at a community level.

CONCLUSION

This innovative ethnography of young people's sexual relationships in rural Mwanza attempted to combine the validity of detailed qualitative research with the representativeness of a large scale study. The research setting is fairly representative of much of rural sub-Saharan Africa, where few adolescent sexual health programs existed even thirty years into the HIV epidemic.

We have described the typical patterns of sexual relationship formation in adolescent and early adult life in rural Mwanza, the variety of young people's relationships and practices, and the contradictory norms and expectations that lead their relationships to be concealed. We found that this concealment, combined with the common practice of material exchange for sex and poor understanding of HIV/AIDS, contributed to short sexual relationships, fast partner change, concurrent partnerships, and related sexual health risks. In this final chapter we have discussed the features of young people's social environment that perpetuate sexual risk behaviors, but we have also identified contextual factors which might facilitate sexual risk reduction.

A companion volume to this book will focus on adolescent sexual health intervention in sub-Saharan Africa (Plummer, forthcoming). That book will examine the process and impact of the multiple-component *MEMA kwa Vijana* adolescent sexual health program. It will also scrutinize the three internationally promoted "ABC" behavioral goals (abstinence, being faithful, and condom use), closely examining the motivations and experiences of the young people in our study who tried to practice such behaviors. Finally, this book's companion volume will describe and discuss ways that adolescent sexual health interventions in sub-Saharan Africa may be improved in the future.

Swahili and Sukuma Glossary

SWAHILI

Chama Cha Mapinduzi (CCM)	the Revolutionary Party of Tanzania, which has dominated national politics since independence in the 1960s
chapati	flat, unleavened bread
dagaa	small fish similar to whitebait
daladala	slang adopted from the English "dollar dollar" to refer to bicycle taxis, minibuses, or sexually promiscuous women
damu nzito	literally "heavy/thick blood," a condition believed to cause certain people (especially women) to be unattractive and to have difficulty attracting a sexual partner
geto	slang for a sleeping hut built by an unmarried man for his own use in his parents' compound; from the English "ghetto"
gongo	literally, "club" or "heavy stick," in this context homemade strong distilled alcohol
Halleluya	common holiday greeting that includes an expectation that, if a boy/man gives an unrelated girl/woman money, it will be reciprocated with sex later
hawara	lover or mistress, depending on context

hirizi	traditional protective amulet (e.g., contraceptive) made of animal hide and herbal medicine worn on a string around a woman's waist
kanga	rectangle(s) of colored patterned cotton cloth with a border and message, typically sold in pairs, one of which a woman wears wrapped around her waist like a skirt
kaswende	syphilis
katelelo	technique to arouse and lubricate a woman prior to intercourse reportedly practiced by the Haya, Zinza, and Longo ethnic groups
kisasa	modern
kisonono	gonorrhea
kitendo cha ndoa	literally "act of marriage," a euphemism for vaginal intercourse
kitongoji	(pl. *vitongoji*) a sub-village unit with its own leadership
kubaka	to rape
kubenchiana	when a male villager bids the highest amount to dance with the woman of his choice at a disco, effectively "benching" other bidders
kuchuna buzi	literally "to skin a goat," meaning a woman taking ample money from a man for sex
kufanya mapenzi	literally "making love," a euphemism for vaginal intercourse
kuhonga	literally "to bribe," in this context meaning material exchange for sex
kuliwa susa	multiple men having intercourse with one woman during one sexual encounter; women were rarely described as consenting in such incidents
kupenda	to like or to love
kusuluhisha	to conciliate, mediate, or make peace
kutongoza	to seduce
kutorosha	to elope
kuzalia nyumbani	literally "to give birth at home," meaning to have a child out-of-wedlock
magonjwa ya zinaa	literally "illnesses of fornication/adultery," meaning sexually transmitted infections
mahari	bridewealth, a payment of money or property given by or on behalf of a prospective husband to the bride's family
majini	evil spirits

malaya	prostitute(s)
mandazi	doughnuts
mboga	vegetable side dish that sometimes includes beans, fish, or (rarely) meat
mchango	(pl. *michango*) literally "intestinal worm" or "contribution," also a variety of illnesses believed to have supernatural causes and to be treated effectively with traditional medicine
mchumba	lover or fiancé/fiancée, depending on context
MEMA kwa Vijana	literally "Good Things for Youth," also the short form of *Mpango wa Elimu na Maadili kwa Vijana* (Health Education and Ethics Program for Youth), an adolescent sexual health intervention and trial
mhuni	(pl. *wahuni*) badly behaved person such as a thief, vagabond, or sexually promiscuous person
mkanda wa jeshi	literally "soldier's belt," a form of shingles (herpes zoster) associated with HIV infection that is characterized by a girdle-like outbreak on the torso
mkosi	jinx
moshi	literally "smoke," in this context homemade strong distilled alcohol
mpenzi	lover
mwarobaini	the neem tree (*Azadirechta indica*)
nakupenda	I like/love you
Nane nane	August 8th, the current Tanzanian Peasant's or Farmer's Day holiday
ngoma	traditional drumming/dancing events
Operesheni Vijiji	literally "Operation Villages," a national rural modernization campaign that required massive numbers of people who lived in remote areas to relocate to government-designated rural centers in 1973–1976
pombe	homemade beer
posta	literally "post office" or "mail," in this context an intermediary who facilitates sexual encounters
rafiki	friend
raha	pleasure, happiness
rika	literally, "peers of the same age," in this context a youth peer group that shares farming responsibilities and sometimes other activities such as *ngoma* competitions

Saba saba	July 7th, a Tanzanian national holiday; formerly Farmer's Day or Peasant's Day, currently International Trade Fair Day
Salama	literally "safety," also the main brand name for condoms in Tanzania
shamba	(pl. *mashamba*) a cultivated agricultural plot
Shikamoo	word used to greet someone of greater age or higher status with respect, particularly for children greeting adults
tamaa	desire, longing, greed, or lust
tangawizi	hot ginger drink or a ginger soda
uchafu	dirt or filth
uchawi	malevolent magic or witchcraft
udaga	pealed fermented cassava roots, used to make flour
ugali	stiff porridge staple made of maize, or maize and cassava mixed
uhuni	socially disapproved of behavior, such as theft, vagrancy, and sexual promiscuity
uji	maize- or millet-based porridge
UKIMWI	acronym for AIDS
Ukosefu wa Kinga ya Mwili	literally "lack of protection for the body," meaning Acquired Immunodeficiency Syndrome (AIDS)
virusi vya UKIMWI	literally "the AIDS virus," meaning Human Immunodeficiency Virus (HIV)
vitenge	large rectangles of colored patterned cotton cloth similar to *kanga* but less common and of higher quality
vitumbua	fried rice cakes
waganga wa kienyeji	traditional healers of different training and specialization, including diviners and herbalists
wazungu	white people or people of European heritage

SUKUMA

bafumu	traditional healers of different training and specialization, including diviners and herbalists
bagindu	men believed to break into a home at night, drug the inhabitants with a traditional medicine, and then have sex with one or more of the women before stealing trophies
budogo	dirt or filth

Bulabo	the Christian Eucharist holiday
bukwi	bridewealth, a payment of money or property given by or on behalf of a prospective husband to the bride's family
bukwilima	traditional Sukuma wedding
bulogi	malevolent magic or witchcraft
bunyolo	sexually transmitted infections
kabugume	when a pregnant woman is given traditional medicine without her knowledge to suspend fetal growth and delay childbirth
kasogone	gonorrhea
kikome	(pl. *shikome*) traditional fire in the center of a compound where men gather to eat meals and to socialize in the evening
kuchunyukila	tearing of the foreskin associated with first intercourse
kulehya	to elope
kupindya nda ku ngongo	literally "moving a pregnancy to the back," when a pregnant woman is given traditional medicine to suspend fetal growth and delay childbirth
kupondya	to rape
kutogwa	to like or to love
kwilala	vaginal intercourse
lupigi	traditional amulet made of wood, root and/or herbal medicine worn on a string around a woman's waist to prevent or promote pregnancy, or worn by a baby to prevent bewitchment and/or illness
lusumbo	bewitchment with a traditional illness that has symptoms similar to those of AIDS, believed to happen to people who have committed an offense such as theft
lwikilo	problematic, stalled childbirth believed to be caused by a woman's infidelity during pregnancy and to require traditional medicine
maji	sleeping hut built by an unmarried man for his own use in his parents' compound
masamva	ancestral spirits which are believed to have active influence on their descendants' lives
masinza	genital condition characterized by long-term growths; possibly genital warts
mbina	traditional drumming/dancing events
mhola	literally "cool," implying peace, purity, or wholeness
migilo	taboos common to all Sukumas or to specific clans and life circumstances

msela	(pl. ***basela***) female dancer hired by traveling disc jockey to dance with village men at discos for a fee
msimbe	(pl. ***wasimbe***) unmarried woman of reproductive age, such as a single mother, a divorced or widowed woman, and most never-married women who have been out of school for two or more years. Also referred to as ***shimbe*** or ***nshimbe*** (pl. ***bashimbe***).
mung'hya	girlfriend
nakutogagwa	I like/love you
nda	pregnancy, head, or lice
ngwekwe	fine paid from a man or his family to the parents of his wife after elopement
nsango	fine paid from a man or his family to the parents of a woman he made pregnant out-of-wedlock
nsebu	literally "hot," implying disruption, impurity or evil, such as witchcraft
nsumba	boyfriend
nyembe go ha nzila	literally "mango tree on a public path," suggesting fruit anyone can pick, a slang term for a promiscuous woman
nzoka	literally "snake," also a variety of illnesses believed to have supernatural causes and to be treated effectively with traditional medicine
sungusungu	village-level militia that works with village elders and government authorities to resolve cases of theft, property dispute, debt, witchcraft and adultery, often using intimidation and force to do so
Usukuma	area of northwestern Tanzania that historically consisted of many small, Sukuma chiefdoms; also known as Sukumaland

Bibliography

Abrahams, Ray G. 1967. *The peoples of Greater Unyamwezi, Tanzania (Nyamwezi, Sukuma Sumbwa, Kimbu, Konongo)*. London: International African Institute.

Abrahams, Ray G. 1978. Aspects of the distinction between the sexes in the Nyamwezi and some other African systems of kinship and marriage. In *Sex and age as principles of social differentiation, ASA Monograph 17*, ed. J. S. LaFontaine, 67–87. London: Academic Press.

Abrahams, Ray G. 1981. *The Nyamwezi today*. Cambridge: Cambridge University Press.

Abrahams, Ray G. 1987. Sungusungu: Village vigilante groups in Tanzania. *African Affairs* 86(343):179–96.

Abrahams, Ray G. 1989. Law and order and the state in the Nyamwezi and Sukuma area of Tanzania. *Africa* 59(3):356–70.

Adelore, O. O., M. G. Olujide, and R. A. Popoola. 2006. Impact of HIV/AIDS prevention promotion programs on behavioral patterns among rural dwellers in south western Nigeria. *Journal of Human Ecology* 20(1):53–58.

Adeokun, Lawrence A., and Rose M. Nalwadda. 1997. Serial marriages and AIDS in Masaka District. *Health Transition Review* 7(Supplement):49–66.

Agadjanian, Victor. 2005. Fraught with ambivalence: Reproductive intentions and contraceptive choices in a sub-Saharan fertility transition. *Population Research and Policy Review* 24:617–45.

Agha, Sohail, Paul Hutchinson, and Thankian Kusanthan. 2006. The effects of religious affiliation on sexual initiation and condom use in Zambia. *Journal of Adolescent Health* 38:550–55.

Agnew, Christopher R., and Timothy J. Loving. 1998. The role of social desirability in self-reported condom use attitudes and intentions. *AIDS and Behavior* 2(3):229–39.

Ahlberg, Beth Maina. 1994. Is there a distinct African sexuality? A critical response to Caldwell. *Africa* 64(2):220–42.

Akarro, Rocky R. J. 2009. Some factors associated with condom use among bar maids in Tanzania. *Journal of Biosocial Science* 41:125–37.

Allen, Caroline F., Nicola Desmond, Betty Chiduo, Lemmy Medard, Shelley S. Lees, Andrew Vallely, Suzanna C. Francis, David A. Ross, and Richard J. Hayes. 2010. Intravaginal and menstrual practices among women working in food and recreational facilities in Mwanza, Tanzania: Implications for microbicide trials. *AIDS Behavior* DOI 10.1007/s10461-010-9750-8.

Allen, Denise Roth. 2000. Learning the facts of life: Past and present experiences in a rural Tanzanian community. *Africa Today* 47(3/4):2–27.

Allen, Denise Roth. 2002. *Managing motherhood, managing risk: Fertility and danger in west central Tanzania.* Ann Arbor: University of Michigan.

Allen, Tim. 2007. Witchcraft, sexuality and HIV/AIDS among the Azande of Sudan *Journal of Eastern African Studies* 1(3):359–96.

Amoran, O. E., and O. Fawole. 2008. Parental influence on reproductive health behavior of youths in Ibadan, Nigeria. *African Journal of Medicine and Medical Sciences* 37(1):21–27.

Amuyunzu-Nyamongo, Mary, Ann E. Biddlecom, Christine Ouedraogo, and Vanessa Woog. 2005. *Qualitative evidence on adolescents' views on sexual and reproductive health in sub-Saharan Africa. Occasional Report No. 16.* New York: The Alan Guttmacher Institute.

Anand, A., R. W. Shiraishi, R. E. Bunnell, K. Jacobs, N. Solehdin, A. S. Abdul-Quader, L. H. Marum, J. N. Muttunga, K. Kamoto, J. M. Aberle-Grasse, and T. Diaz. 2009. Knowledge of HIV status, sexual risk behaviors and contraceptive need among people living with HIV in Kenya and Malawi. *AIDS* 23(12):1565–73.

Andersson, Neil, and Ari Ho-Foster. 2008. 13,915 reasons for equity in sexual offences legislation: A national school-based survey in South Africa. *International Journal for Equity in Health* 7:20 doi:10.1186/1475-9276-7-20.

Anglewicz, Philip A., Simona Bignami-Van Assche, Shelley Clark, and James Mkandawire. 2010. HIV risk among currently married couples in rural Malawi: What do spouses know about each other? *AIDS and Behavior* 14:103–12.

Ankrah, E. Maxine. 1989. AIDS: Methodological problems in studying its prevention and spread. *Social Science and Medicine* 29(3):265–76.

Anzala, O. A., N. J. D. Nagelkerke, J. J. Bwayo, D. Holton, S. Moses, E. N. Ngugi, J. O. Ndinya-Achola, and F. A. Plummer. 1995. Rapid progression to disease in African sex workers with human immunodeficiency virus type 1 infection. *Journal of Infectious Diseases* 171(3):686–89.

Appadurai, Arjun. 2004. The capacity to aspire: Culture and the terms of recognition. In *Culture and public action,* ed. V. Rao and M. Walton, 59–84. Palo Alto, California: Stanford University Press.

Aral, Sevgi O., and Betsy Foxman. 2003. Spatial mixing and bridging: Risk factors for what? *Sexually Transmitted Diseases* 30(10):750–51.

Aral, Sevgi O., and Mead Over, with Lisa Manhart and King K. Holmes. 2006. Sexually transmitted infections. In *Disease control priorities in developing countries, 2nd edition,* ed. Dean T. Jamison, Joel G. Breman, Anthony R. Measham, George Alleyne, Mariam Claeson, David B. Evans, Prabhat Jha, Anne Mills, and Philip Musgrove, 311–30. New York: The World Bank and Oxford University Press.

Arnfred, Signe. 2004. "African sexuality"/sexuality in Africa: Tales and silences. In *Re-thinking sexualities in Africa*, ed. Signe Arnfred, 59–78. Uppsala, Sweden: Nordiska Afrikainstitutet.

Arthur, Jo. 2001. Perspectives on educational language policy and its implementation in African classrooms: A comparative study of Botswana and Tanzania. *Compare* 31:347–62.

Ashforth, Adam. 2002. An epidemic of witchcraft? The implications of AIDS for the post-Apartheid state. *African Studies* 61:121–43.

Auvert, B., D. Taljaard, E. Lagarde, J. Sobngwi-Tambekou, R. Sitta, and A. Puren. 2005. Randomized, controlled intervention trial of male circumcision for reduction of HIV infection risk: The ANRS 1265 Trial. *PLoS Med*.2:e298.

Awusabo-Asare, K., and J. K. Anarfi. 1997. Health-seeking behavior of persons with HIV/AIDS in Ghana. *Health Transition Review* 7(Supplement):243–56.

Babalola, Stella, B. Oleko Tambashe, and Claudia Vondrasek. 2005. Parental factors and sexual risk-taking among young people in Côte d'Ivoire. *African Journal of Reproductive Health* 9(1):49–65.

Baddeley, Alan. 1979. The limitations of human memory: Implications for the design of retrospective surveys. In *The recall method of social surveys*, ed. Louis Moss and Harvey Goldstein, 13–27. London: University of London Institute of Education.

Bagenda, Danstan, Annette Nassali, Israel Kalyesubula, Becky Sherman, Dennis Drotar, Michael J. Boivin, and Karen Olness. 2006. Health, neurologic, and cognitive status of HIV infected, long-surviving, and antiretroviral naïve Ugandan children. *Pediatrics* 117:729–40.

Bagnol, Brigitte, and Esmerelda Mariano. 2008. Vaginal practices: Eroticism and implications for women's health and condom use in Mozambique. *Culture, Health and Sexuality* 10(6):573–85.

Bailey, Robert C., Stephen Moses, Corette B. Parker, Kawango Agot, Ian Maclean, John N. Krieger, Carolyn F. M. Williams, Richard T. Campbell, and Jeckoniah O. Ndinya-Achola. 2007. Male circumcision for HIV prevention in young men in Kisumu, Kenya: A randomized controlled trial. *Lancet* 369:643–56.

Balmer, D. H., E. Gikundi, M. C. Billingsley, F. G. Kihuho, M. Kimani, J. Wang'ondu, and H. Njoroge. 1997. Adolescent knowledge, values, and coping strategies: Implications for health in sub-Saharan Africa. *Journal of Adolescent Health* 21:33–38.

Bandura, A. 2004. Health promotion by social cognitive means. *Health Education and Behavior* 31:143–64.

Bankole, Akinrinola, Fatima H. Ahmed, Stella Neema, Christine Ouedraogo, and Sidon Konyani. 2007. Knowledge of correct condom use and consistency of use among adolescents in four countries in Sub-Saharan Africa. *African Journal of Reproductive Health* 11(3):197–220.

Bankole, Akinrinola, Susheela Singh, Rubina Hussain, and Gabrielle Oestreicher. 2009. Condom use for preventing STI/HIV and unintended pregnancy among young men in sub-Saharan Africa. *American Journal of Men's Health* 3(1):60–78.

Barnett, T., and A. Whiteside. 2002. *AIDS in the Twenty-First Century: Disease and globalization*. Basingstoke: Palgrave Macmillan.

Barreto, Thalia, Oona M. R. Campbell, J. Lynne Davies, Vincent Fauveau, Veronique G. A. Filippi, Wendy J. Graham, Masuma Mamdani, Cleone I. F. Rooney, and

Nahid F. Toubia. 1992. Investigating induced abortion in developing countries: Methods and problems. *Studies in Family Planning* 23(3):159–70.

Barrett, Angeline M. 2007. Beyond the polarization of pedagogy: Models of classroom practice in Tanzanian primary schools. *Comparative Education* 43(2):273–94.

Bastien, Sheri. 2008. Out-of-school and at risk? Socio-demographic characteristics, AIDS knowledge and risk perception among young people in northern Tanzania. *International Journal of Educational Development* 28:393–404.

Bastien, Sheri. 2009a. Access, agency and ambiguity: Communication about AIDS among young people in Northern Tanzania. *Culture, Health and Sexuality* 11(8):751–65.

Bastien, Sheri. 2009b. Reflecting and shaping the discourse: The role of music in AIDS communication in Tanzania. *Social Science and Medicine* 68(7):1357–60.

Baylies, Carolyn, and Janet Bujra. 2000. *AIDS, sexuality and gender in Africa*. London: Routledge.

Baylies, Carolyn, Janet Bujra, Tashisho Chabala, Naomi Kaihula, Beatrice Liatto-Katundu, Japhet Lutimba, Marjorie Mbilinyi, et al. 1999. Rebels at risk: Young women and the shadow of AIDS. In *Experiencing and understanding AIDS in Africa*, ed. Charles Becker, Jean-Pierre Dozon, Christine Obbo and Moriba Touré, 319–42. Dakar/Paris: Codesria/Editions Karthala/IRD.

Beguy, Donatien, Caroline W. Kabiru, Evangeline N. Nderu, and Moses W. Ngware. 2009. Inconsistencies in self-reporting of sexual activity among young people in Nairobi, Kenya. *Journal of Adolescent Health* 45:595–601.

Bell, David J., Yamika Kapitao, Rosemary Sikwese, Joep J. van Oosterhout, and David G. Lalloo. 2007. Adherence to antiretroviral therapy in patients receiving free treatment from a government hospital in Blantyre, Malawi. *Journal of Acquired Immune Deficiency Syndromes* 45(5):560–63.

Béné, Christophe, and Sonja Merten. 2008. Women and fish-for-sex: Transactional sex, HIV/AIDS and gender in African fisheries. *World Development* 36(5):875–99.

Benefo, Kofi D. 2008. Determinants of Zambian men's extra-marital sex: A multi-level analysis. *Archives of Sexual Behavior* 37:517–29.

Bennell, Paul, and Faustin Mukyanuzi. 2005. *Is there a teacher motivation crisis in Tanzania?* Brighton, UK: Knowledge and Skills for Development. Downloaded from www.eldis.org/vfile/upload/1/document/0709/Teacher_motivation_Tanzania .pdf on August 6, 2010.

Benson, Janie, Lori Ann Nicholson, Lynne Gaffikin, and Stephen N. Kinoti. 1996. Complications of unsafe abortion in sub-Saharan Africa: A review. *Health Policy and Planning* 11(2):117–31.

Benson, John. 2006. *"A complete education?" Observations about the state of primary education in Tanzania in 2005. HakiElimu Working paper no. 06.1.* Dar es Salaam: HakiElimu. Downloaded from www.hakielimu.org on August 6, 2010.

Berege, Zachariah, and Arnoud Klokke. 1997. Reducing HIV transmission via blood transfusion: A district strategy. In *HIV prevention and AIDS care in Africa: A district level approach,* ed. Japhet Ng'weshemi, Ties Boerma, John Bennett, and Dick Schapink, 292–304. Amsterdam: Royal Tropical Institute.

Bernard, H. Russell. 1995. *Research methods in anthropology: Qualitative and quantitative approaches.* Walnut Creek, California: AltaMira Press.

Bessire, Aimée, and Mark Bessire. 1997. *Sukuma.* New York: Rosen.

Bessire, Aimée. 2005. Sukuma figures, boundaries, and the arousal of spectacle. *African Arts* 38:36–49 and 93–94.

Biddlecom, Ann, Kofi Awusabo-Asare, and Akinrinola Bankole. 2009. Role of parents in adolescent sexual activity and contraceptive use in four African Countries. *International Perspectives on Sexual and Reproductive Health* 35(2):72–81.

Bingenheimer, Jeffrey B. 2010. Men's multiple sexual partnerships in 15 sub-Saharan African countries: Sociodemographic patterns and implications. *Studies in Family Planning* 41(1):1–17.

Binson, Diane, and Joseph A. Catania. 1998. Respondents' understanding of the words used in sexual behavior questions. *Public Opinion Quarterly* 62:190–208.

Birley, Martin H. 1982. Resource management in Sukumaland, Tanzania. *Africa* 52(2):1–28.

Birungi, H., F. Obare, J. F. Mugisha, H. Evelia, and J. Nyombi. 2009. Preventive service needs of young people perinatally infected with HIV in Uganda. *AIDS Care* 21(6):725–31.

Bisika, Thomas. 2009. Potential acceptability of microbicides in HIV prevention in stable marital relationships in Malawi. *Journal of Family Planning and Reproductive Health Care* 35(2):115–17.

Bledsoe, Caroline H., and Monica F. Goubaud. 1988. The reinterpretation and distribution of western pharmaceuticals: An example from the Mende of Sierra Leone. In *The context of medicines in developing countries*, ed. Sjaak van der Geest and Susan Reynolds Whyte, 253–76. Netherlands: Kluwer.

Bleek, Wolf. 1978. Induced abortion in a Ghanaian family. *African Studies Review* 21(1):103–20.

Bleek, Wolf. 1987. Lying informants: A fieldwork experience from Ghana. *Population and Development Review* 13(2):314–22.

Bloch, Maurice. 1989. The symbolism of money in Imerina. In *Money and the morality of exchange*, ed. M. Bloch and J. Perry, 165–90. Cambridge: Cambridge University Press.

Bloor, Michael, Jane Frankland, Michelle Thomas, and Kate Robson. 2001. *Focus groups in social research.* London: Sage.

Bodeker, G., D. Kabatesi, R. King, and J. Homsy. 2000. A regional task force on traditional medicine and AIDS. *Lancet* 355:1284.

Boerma, J. T., M. Urassa, S. Nnko, J. Ng'weshemi, R. Isingo, B. Zaba, and G. Mwaluko. 2002. Sociodemographic context of the AIDS epidemic in a rural area in Tanzania with a focus on people's mobility and marriage. *Sexually Transmitted Infections* 78(Supplement 1): 97–105.

Boerma, J. Ties, Simon Gregson, Constance Nyamukapa, and Mark Urassa. 2003. Understanding the uneven spread of HIV within Africa: Comparative study of biologic, behavioral, and contextual factors in rural populations in Tanzania and Zimbabwe. *Sexually Transmitted Diseases* 30(10):779–87.

Bogart, Laura M., and Sheryl Thorburn. 2005. Are HIV/AIDS conspiracy beliefs a barrier to HIV prevention among African Americans? *Journal of Acquired Immune Deficiency Syndromes* 38:213–18.

Boileau C., B. Vissandjee, V. K. Nguyen, S. Rashed, M. Sylla, and M. V. Zunzunegui. 2008. Gender dynamics and sexual norms among youth in Mali in the context of HIV/AIDS prevention. *African Journal of Reproductive Health* 12(3):173–84.

Bommier, Antoine, and Sylvie Lambert. 2001. Education demand and age at school enrollment in Tanzania. *Journal of Human Resources* 35:177–203.

Bond, Virginia, and Paul Dover. 1997. Men, women and the trouble with condoms: Problems associated with condom use by migrant workers in rural Zambia. *Health Transition Review* 7(Supplement):377–91.

Bongaarts, John, and Charles F. Westoff. 2000. The potential role of contraception in reducing abortion. *Studies in Family Planning* 31(3):193–202.

Bosmans, Marleen, Marie Noël Cikuru, Patricia Claeys, and Marleen Temmerman. 2006. Where have all the condoms gone in adolescent programs in the Democratic Republic of Congo. *Reproductive Health Matters* 14(28):80–88.

Bove, Riley, and Claudia Valeggia. 2009. Polygyny and women's health in sub-Saharan Africa. *Social Science and Medicine* 68:21–29.

Boyce, Carolyn, and Palena Neale. 2006. *Using mystery clients: A guide to using mystery clients for evaluation input. Pathfinder International Tool Series: Monitoring and Evaluation—3.* Downloaded on August 21, 2010 from www.pathfind.org/site/DocServer/m_e_tool_series_mystery_clients.pdf?docID=6303.

Brandström, P. 1999. Seeds and soil: The quest for life and the domestication of fertility in Sukuma-Nyamwezi thought and reality. In *The creative communion: African folk models of fertility and the regeneration of life*, ed. A. Jacobson-Widding and W. van Beek, 167–86. Stockholm, Sweden: Almqvist and Wiksell International.

Brewer, Devon D., Sharon B. Garrett, and Shalini Kulasingam. 1999. Forgetting as a cause of incomplete reporting of sexual and drug injection partners. *Sexually Transmitted Diseases* 26(3):166–76.

British Broadcasting Corporation. 2010a. Hundreds of Kenyan teachers sacked over sex abuse. Downloaded from www.bbc.co.uk/news/world-africa-11492499 on November 23, 2010.

British Broadcasting Corporation. 2010b. Nigerian senator Sani denies marrying girl of 13. Downloaded from http://news.bbc.co.uk/2/hi/africa/8651043.stm on May 15, 2010.

Brody, S., and J. J. Potterat. 2003. Assessing the role of anal intercourse in the epidemiology of AIDS in Africa. *International Journal of STD and AIDS* 14:431–36.

Brown, Judith E., and Richard C. Brown. 2000. Traditional intravaginal practices and the heterosexual transmission of disease: A review. *Sexually Transmitted Diseases* 27(4):183–87.

Bujra, Janet. 2000. Target practice: Gender and generational struggles in AIDS prevention work in Lushoto. In *AIDS, Sexuality and Gender in Africa*, ed. Carolyn Baylies and Janet Bujra, 113–31. London: Routledge.

Bulmer, Martin, and Donald P. Warwick. 2000. *Social research in developing countries: Surveys and censuses in the Third World.* London: University College London, London.

Buvé, A., E. Lagarde, M. Caraël, N. Rutenberg, B. Ferry, J. R. Glynn, M. Laourou, E. Akam, J. Chege, T. Sukwa, for the Study Group on Heterogeneity of HIV Epidemics in African Cities. 2001. Interpreting sexual behavior data: Validity issues in the multicentre study on factors determining the differential spread of HIV in four African cities. *AIDS* 15(Supplement 4):S117–26.

Buvé, Anne, Kizito Bishikwabo-Nsarhaza, and Gladys Mutangadura. 2002. The spread and effect of HIV-1 infection in sub-Saharan Africa. *Lancet* 359:2011–17.

Buvé, Anne. 2006. The HIV epidemics in sub-Saharan Africa: Why so severe? Why so heterogenous? An epidemiological perspective. In *The HIV/AIDS epidemic in sub-Saharan Africa in a historical perspective: Online edition*, ed. Philippe Denis and Charles Becker, 41–55. Downloaded on November 7, 2006 from www .refer.sn/rds/IMG/pdf/AIDSHISTORYALL.pdf.

Byakika-Tusiime, J., J. H. Oyugi, W. A. Tumwikirize, E. T. Katabira, P. N. Mugyenyi, and D. R. Bangsberg. 2005. Adherence to HIV antiretroviral therapy in HIV+ Ugandan patients purchasing therapy. *International Journal of STD and AIDS* 16(1):38–41.

Caldwell, John C. 1980. Mass education as a determinant of the timing of fertility decline. *Population and Development Review* 6(2):225–55.

Caldwell, John C., and Pat Caldwell. 1987. The cultural context of high fertility in sub-Saharan Africa. *Population and Development Review* 13(3):409–37.

Caldwell, John C., Pat Caldwell, and Pat Quiggin. 1989. The social context of AIDS in sub-Saharan Africa. *Population and Development Review* 15(2):185–234.

Caldwell, John C., Pat Caldwell, Bruce K. Caldwell, and Indrani Pieris. 1998. The construction of adolescence in a changing world: Implications for sexuality, reproduction, and marriage. *Studies in Family Planning* 29(2):137–53.

Camlin, Carol S., and Chiweni E. Chimbwete. 2003. Does knowing someone with AIDS affect condom use? An analysis from South Africa. *AIDS Education and Prevention* 15(3):231–44.

Camlin, Carol S., and Rachel C. Snow. 2008. Parental investment, club membership, and youth sexual risk behavior in Cape Town. *Health Education and Behavior* 35(4):522–40.

Campbell, C., and B. Williams. 1999. Beyond the biomedical and behavioral: Towards an integrated approach to HIV prevention in the South African mining industry. *Social Science and Medicine* 48:1625–39.

Campbell, Catherine. 2003. *"Letting them die": Why HIV/AIDS prevention programs fail*. Oxford, UK: James Currey.

Caraël, M., and K. Holmes. 2001. Dynamics of HIV epidemics in sub-Saharan Africa: Introduction. *AIDS* 215(Supplement 4):S1–4.

Caraël, Michel. 2006. Twenty years of intervention and controversy. In *The HIV/ AIDS epidemic in sub-Saharan Africa in a historical perspective: Online edition*, ed. Philippe Denis and Charles Becker, 29–40. Downloaded on November 7, 2006 from www.refer.sn/rds/IMG/pdf/AIDSHISTORYALL.pdf.

Carter, Marion W., Joan Marie Kraft, Todd Koppenhaver, Christine Galavotti, Thierry H. Roels, Peter H. Kilmarx, and Boga Fidzani. 2007. "A bull cannot be contained in a single kraal": Concurrent sexual partnerships in Botswana. *AIDS and Behavior* 11:822–30.

Castle, Mary Ann, Rosemary Likwa, and Maxine Whittaker. 1990. Observations on abortion in Zambia. *Studies in Family Planning* 21(4):231–35.

Castle, Sarah. 2003a. Factors influencing young Malians' reluctance to use hormonal contraceptives. *Studies in Family Planning* 34(3):186–99.

Castle, Sarah. 2003b. Doubting the existence of AIDS: A barrier to voluntary HIV testing and counseling in Mali. *Health Policy and Planning* 18:146–55.

Catania, Joseph A., David R. Gibson, Dale D. Chitwood, and Thomas J. Coates. 1990. Methodological problems in AIDS behavioral research: Influences on measurement error and participation bias in studies of sexual behavior. *Psychological Bulletin* 108(3):339–62.

Catania, Joseph A., Heather Turner, Robert C. Pierce, Eve Golden, Carol Stocking, Diane Binson, and Karen Mast. 1993. Response bias in surveys of AIDS related sexual behavior. In *Methodological issues in AIDS behavioral research*, ed. D. G. Ostrow and R. C. Kessler, 133–62. New York: Plenum Press.

Chen, Li, Prabhat Jha, Bridget Stirling, Sema K. Sgaier, Tina Daid, Rupert Kaul, Nico Nagelkerke, for the International Studies of HIV/AIDS Investigators. 2007. Sexual risk factors for HIV infection in early and advanced HIV epidemics in sub-Saharan Africa: Systematic overview of 68 epidemiological studies. *PLoS ONE* 10:e1001.

Chen, Susan, and David K. Guilkey. 2003. Determinants of contraceptive method choice in rural Tanzania between 1991 and 1999. *Studies in Family Planning* 34(4):263–76.

Chersich M. F., H. V. Rees, F. Scorgie, and G. Martin. 2009. Enhancing global control of alcohol to reduce unsafe sex and HIV in sub-Saharan Africa. *Globalization and Health* 5:16.

Chiao, Chi, and Vinod Mishra. 2009. Trends in primary and secondary abstinence among Kenyan youth. *AIDS Care* 21(7):881–92.

Chimwaza, A. F., and S. C. Watkins. 2004. Giving care to people with symptoms of AIDS in rural sub-Saharan Africa. *AIDS Care* 16:795–807.

Chirwa, B. U., and E. Sivile. 1989–1990. Enlisting the support of traditional healers in an AIDS education campaign in Zambia. *The International Quarterly of Community Health Education* 9:221–29.

Clark, Shelley, Judith Bruce, and Annie Dude. 2006. Protecting young women from HIV/AIDS: The case against child and adolescent marriage. *International Family Planning Perspectives* 32(2):79–88.

Clark, Shelley. 2010. Extra-marital sexual partnerships and male friendships in rural Malawi. *Demographic Research* 22(1):1–28.

Clift, S., A. Anemona, D. Watson-Jones, Z. Kanga, L. Ndeki, J. Changalucha, A. Gavyole, and D. A. Ross. 2003. Variations of HIV and STI prevalences within communities neighboring new gold mines in Tanzania: Importance for intervention design. *Sexually Transmitted Infections* 79:307–12.

Coast, Ernestina. 2007. Wasting semen: Context and condom use among the Maasai. *Culture, Health and Sexuality* 9(4):387–401.

Coffee, Megan P., Geoffrey P. Garnett, Makalima Mlilo, Hélène A. C. M. Voeten, Stephen Chandiwana, and Simon Gregson. Patterns of movement and risk of HIV infection in rural Zimbabwe. *Journal of Infectious Diseases* 191(Supplement 1):S159–67.

Cohen, Barney. 1998. The emerging fertility transition in sub-Saharan Africa. *World Development* 26(8):1431–61.

Colebunders, R., R. Ryder, H. Francis, W. Nekwei, Y. Bahwe, I. Lebughe, M. Ndilu, G. et al. 1991. Seroconversion rate, mortality, and clinical manifestations associated with the receipt of a human immunodeficiency virus-infected blood transfusion in Kinshasa, Zaire. *Journal of Infectious Diseases* 164(3):450–56.

Colvin, M., M. O. Bachmann, R. K. Homan, D. Nsibande, N. M. Nkwanyana, C. Connolly, and E. B. Reuben. 2006. Effectiveness and cost effectiveness of syndromic sexually transmitted infection packages in South African primary care: Cluster randomized trial. *Sexually Transmitted Infections* 82:290–94.

Cooksey, Brian, and Sibylle Riedmiller. Tanzanian education in the nineties: Beyond the diploma disease. *Assessment in Education* 4:121–35.

Cory, Hans. 1949. The ingredients of magic medicines. *Africa* 19(1):13–32.

Cory, Hans. 1953. *Sukuma law and custom*. London: Oxford University Press.

Cowan, Frances M., Lisa F. Langhaug, George P. Mashungupa, Tellington Nyamurera, John Hargrove, Shabbar Jaffar, Rosanna W. Peeling et al. 2002. School based HIV prevention in Zimbabwe: Feasibility and acceptability of evaluation trials using biological outcomes. *AIDS* 16:1673–78.

Cowan, Frances M., Lisa F. Langhaug, John W. Hargrove, Shabbar Jaffar, Lovemore Mhuriyengwe, Todd D. Swarthout, Rosanna Peeling et al. 2005. Is sexual contact with sex workers important in driving the HIV epidemic among men in rural Zimbabwe? *JAIDS: Journal of Acquired Immune Deficiency Syndromes* 40(3):371–76.

Crabbé, F., H. Carsauw, A. Buvé, M. Laga, J. P. Tchupo, and A. Trebucq. 1996. Why do men with urethritis in Cameroon prefer to seek care in the informal health sector? *Genitourinary Medicine* 72:220–22.

Davis, Karen R., and Susan C. Weller. 1999. The effectiveness of condoms in reducing heterosexual transmission of HIV. *Family Planning Perspectives* 31(6):272–79.

Day, Sophie. 1988. Prostitute women and AIDS: Anthropology (Editorial review). *AIDS* 2:421–28.

De Visser, R. O., and J. A. Smith. 2007. Alcohol consumption and masculine identity amongst young men. *Psychology and Health* 22:595–614.

De Zalduondo, B. J., and M. Bernard. 1995. Meanings and consequences of sexual-economic exchange. In *Conceiving sexuality: Approaches to sex research in a post-modern world*, ed. R. G. Parker and John H. Gagnon, 157–79. New York: Routledge.

Dehne, Karl L., and Gabriele Riedner. 2001. Adolescence: A dynamic concept. *Reproductive Health Matters* 9(17):11–15.

Desmond, Nicola, Caroline F. Allen, Simon Clift, Butolwa Justine, Joseph Mzugu, Mary L. Plummer, Deborah Watson-Jones, and David A. Ross. 2005. A typology of groups at risk of HIV/STI in a gold mining town in north-western Tanzania. *Social Science and Medicine* 60(8):1739–49.

Desmond, Nicola. 2009. *Ni kubahatisha tu!*—Its just a game of chance: Adaptation and resignation to socially constructed perceptions of risk in rural Tanzania. PhD thesis, Medical Research Council Social and Public Health Sciences Unit, University of Glasgow.

Devine, Owen J., and Sevgi O. Aral. 2004. The impact of inaccurate reporting of condom use and imperfect diagnosis of sexually transmitted disease infection in studies of condom effectiveness. *Sexually Transmitted Diseases* 31(10):588–95.

Dickinson, David. 2008. Traditional healers, HIV/AIDS and company programs in South Africa. *African Journal of AIDS Research* 7(3):281–91.

Dilger, H. 2003. Sexuality, AIDS, and the lures of modernity: Reflexivity and morality among young people in rural Tanzania. *Medical Anthropology* 22:23–52.

Dixon-Mueller, Ruth. 2009. Starting young: Sexual initiation and HIV prevention in early adolescence. *AIDS and Behavior* 13:100–9.

Doherty, Irene A., Stephen Shiboski, Jonathan M. Ellen, Adaora A. Adimora, and Nancy S. Padian. 2006. Sexual bridging socially and over time: A simulation model exploring the relative effects of mixing and concurrency on viral sexually transmitted infection transmission. *Sexually Transmitted Diseases* 33(6):368–73.

Doyle, Aoife M., David A. Ross, Kaballa Maganja, Kathy Baisley, Clemens Masesa, Aura Andreasen, Mary L. Plummer, et al. 2010. Long-term biological and behavioral impact of an adolescent sexual health intervention in Tanzania: Follow-up survey of the community-based MEMA kwa Vijana Trial. *PLoSMed* 7(6):e1000287.

Dunkle, K., R. Jewkes, H. Brown, G. Gray, J. Mcintyre, and S. Harlow. 2004. Transactional sex among women in Soweto, South Africa: Prevalence, risk factors and association with HIV. *Social Science and Medicine* 59:1581–92.

Dusenbury, Linda, Rosalind Brannigan, Mathea Falco, and William B. Hansen. 2005. Quality of implementation: Developing measures crucial to understanding the diffusion of preventive interventions. *Health Education Research* 20:308–13.

Dyer, Silke J. 2008a. Infertility in African countries: Challenges created by the HIV epidemic. *ESHRE Monographs* (1):48–53.

Dyer, Silke J. 2008b. Infertility-related reproductive health knowledge and help-seeking behavior in African countries. *ESHRE Monographs* (1):29–33.

Dyson, Tim. 2003. HIV/AIDS and urbanization. *Population and Development Review* 29(3):427–42.

Eaton, Liberty, Alan J. Flisher, and Leif E. Aarø. 2003. Unsafe sexual behavior in South African youth. *Social Science and Medicine* 56:149–65.

Erasmus, P. A. 1998. Perspectives on black masculinity: The abortion debate in South Africa. *South African Journal of Ethnology* 21(4):203–6.

Etkin, Nina L. 1992. "Side effects": Cultural constructions and reinterpretations of Western pharmaceuticals. *Medical Anthropology Quarterly* 6(2):99–113.

Ewing, Katherine. 1990. The illusion of wholeness: Culture, self and the experience of inconsistency. *Ethnos* 18:251–78.

Ezekiel, Mangi Job, Aud Talle, James M. Juma, and Knut-Inge Klepp. 2009. "When in the body, it makes you look fat and HIV negative": The constitution of antiretroviral therapy in local discourse among youth in Kahe, Tanzania. *Social Science and Medicine* 68:957–64.

Farmer, P. 1992. *AIDS and accusation: Haiti and the geography of blame.* Berkeley, CA: University of California Press.

Fawole, I. O., M. C. Asuzu, S. O. Oduntan, and W. R. Brieger. 1999. A school-based AIDS education program for secondary school students in Nigeria: A review of effectiveness. *Health Education Research* 14:675–83.

Fenton, K. A., A. M. Johnson, S. McManus, and B. Erens. 2001. Measuring sexual behavior: Methodological challenges in survey research. *Sexually Transmitted Infections* 77:84–92.

Ferguson, A. M. Pere, C. Morris, E. Ngugi, and S. Moses. 2004. Sexual patterning and condom use among a group of HIV vulnerable men in Thika, Kenya. *Sexually Transmitted Infections* 80:435–39.

Ferguson, Alan G., and Chester N. Morris. 2007. Mapping transactional sex on the Northern Corridor highway in Kenya. *Health and Place* 13(2):504–19.

Ferrand, R. A., E. L. Corbett, R. Wood, J. Hargrove, C. E. Ndhlovu, F. M. Cowan, E. Gouws, and B. G. Williams. 2009. AIDS among older children and adolescents in Southern Africa: Projecting the time course and magnitude of the epidemic. *AIDS* 23(15):2039–46.

Ferrand, R. A., R. Luethy, F. Bwakura, H. Mujuru, R. F. Miller, and E. L. Corbett. 2007. HIV infection presenting in older children and adolescents: A case series from Harare, Zimbabwe. *Clinical Infectious Diseases* 44:874–78.

Fihlani, Pumza. 2010. Is Zuma's sex life a private matter? BBC. Downloaded on February 3, 2010 from http://news.bbc.co.uk/2/hi/africa/8495446.stm.s.

Fishbein, Martin, and Willo Pequegnat. 2000. Evaluating AIDS prevention interventions using behavioral and biological outcome measures. *Sexually Transmitted Diseases* 27(2):101–10.

Fleming. D. T., and J. N. Wasserheit. 1999. From epidemiological synergy to public health policy and practice: The contribution of other sexually transmitted diseases to sexual transmission of HIV infection. *Sexually Transmitted Infections* 75(1):3–17.

Folkvord, Sigurd, Oystein Andreas Odegaard, and Johanne Sundby. 2005. Male infertility in Zimbabwe. *Patient Education and Counseling* 59:239–43.

Fortson, Jane G. 2008. The gradient in sub-Saharan Africa: Socioeconomic status and HIV/AIDS. *Demography* 45(2):303–22.

Foss, A. M., M. Hossain, P. T. Vickerman, and C. H. Watts. 2007. A systematic review of published evidence on intervention impact on condom use in sub-Saharan Africa and Asia. *Sexually Transmitted Infections* 83:510–16.

Fox, Matthew P., Kelly McCoy, Bruce A. Larson, Sydney Rosen, Margaret Bii, Carolyne Sigei, Douglas Shaffer, Fred Sawe, Monique Wasunna, and Jonathon L. Simon. 2010. Improvements in physical well being over the first two years on antiretroviral therapy in western Kenya. *AIDS Care* 22(2):137–45.

Francis, Dennis, and Crispin Hemson. 2009. Youth as research fieldworkers in a context of HIV/AIDS. *African Journal of AIDS Research* 8(2):223–30.

Freeman, Esther E., Helen A. Weiss, Judith R. Glynn, Pamela L. Cross, James A. Whitworth, and Richard J. Hayes. 2006. Herpes simplex virus 2 infection increases

HIV acquisition in men and women: Systematic review and meta-analysis of longitudinal studies. *AIDS* 20:73–83.

Gage-Brandon, Anastasia J., and Dominique Meekers. 1993. Sex, contraception and childbearing before marriage in sub-Saharan Africa. *International Family Planning Perspectives* 19:14–18.

Gagnon, John H., and William Simon. 1974. *Sexual conduct.* London: Hutchinson.

Gallant, M., and E. Maticka-Tyndale. 2004. School-based HIV prevention programs for African youth. *Social Science and Medicine* 58:1337–51.

Garcia-Calleja, J. M., E. Gouws, and P. D. Ghys. 2006. National population based HIV prevalence surveys in sub-Saharan Africa: Results and implications for HIV and AIDS estimates. *Sexually Transmitted Infections* 82(Supplement 3):iii64–70.

Gatell, Jose M. 2010. When and why to start antiretroviral therapy? *Journal of Antimicrobial Chemotherapy* 65:383–85.

Geissler, P. Wenzel, Lotte Meinert, Ruth Prince, Caherine Nokes, Jens Aagaard-Hansen, Jessica Jitta, and John H. Ouma. 2001. Self-treatment by Kenyan and Ugandan schoolchildren and the need for school-based education. *Health Policy and Planning* 16:362–71.

Gerbase, A. C., J. T. Rowley, D. H. L. Heymann, S. F. B. Berkley, and P. Piot. 1998. Global prevalence and incidence estimates of selected curable STDs. *Sexually Transmitted Infections* 74(Supplement 1):S12–16.

Gersovitz, M. 2007. HIV, ABC and DHS: Age at first sex in Uganda. *Sexually Transmitted Infections* 83:165–68.

Gersovitz, M., J. Jacoby, F. Dedy, and A. G. Tape. 1998. The balance of self-reported heterosexual activity in KAP surveys and the AIDS epidemic in Africa. *Journal of the American Statistical Association* 93(443):875–83.

Giddens, A. 1992. *The transformation of intimacy.* California: Stanford University Press.

Gleason, H. A. 1961. The role of tone in the structure of Sǫkúma [Book Review]. *Language* 37:294–308.

Goffman, E. 1959. *The presentation of self in everyday life.* USA: Anchor Books.

Goody, J. R. 1969. Inheritance, property and marriage in Africa and Eurasia. *Sociology* 3:55–76.

Gorbach, Pamina M., Bradley P. Stoner, Sevgi O. Aral, William L. H. Whittington, and King K. Holmes. 2002. "It takes a village: Understanding concurrent sexual partnerships in Seattle, Washington. *Sexually Transmitted Diseases* 29(8):453–62.

Gouws, E, P. J. White, J. Stover, and T. Brown. 2006. Short-term estimates of adult HIV incidence by mode of transmission: Kenya and Thailand as examples. *Sexually Transmitted Infections* 82(Supplement 3):iii51–55.

Grady, Denise. 2009. The deadly toll of abortion by amateurs. *New York Times*, downloaded on June 1, 2009 from www.nytimes.com/2009/06/02/health/02abort.html.

Gray, Ronald H., Godfrey Kigozi, David Serwadda, Frederick Makumbi, Stephen Watya, Fred Nalugoda, Noah Kiwanuka, et al. 2007. Male circumcision for HIV prevention in men in Rakai, Uganda: A randomized controlled trial. *Lancet* 369:657–66.

Green, Edward C. 1988. Can collaborative programs between biomedical and African indigenous health practitioners succeed? *Social Science and Medicine* 27:1125–30.

Green, Edward C. 1992a. Sexually transmitted disease, ethnomedicine and health policy in Africa. *Social Science and Medicine* 35:121–30.

Green, Edward C. 1992b. The anthropology of sexually transmitted disease in Liberia. *Social Science and Medicine* 35:1457–68.

Green, Edward C. 1997. The participation of African healers in AIDS/ TD prevention programmes. *Tropical Doctor* 27(Supplement 1):56–59.

Green, Edward C., Annemarie Jurg, and Armando Djedje. 1993. Sexually transmitted diseases, AIDS and traditional healers in Mozambique. *Medical Anthropology* 15:261–81.

Gregson, Simon, Constance A. Nyamukapa, Geoffrey P. Garnett, Peter R. Mason, Tom Zhuwau, Michel Caraël, Stephen K. Chandiwana, and Roy M. Anderson. 2002. Sexual mixing patterns and sex-differentials in teenage exposure to HIV infection in rural Zimbabwe. *Lancet* 359:1896–1903.

Gregson, Simon, Tom Zhuwau, Roy M. Anderson, and Stephen K. Chandiwana. 1998. Is there evidence for behavior change in response to AIDS in rural Zimbabwe? *Social Science and Medicine* 46(3):321–30.

Grimes, David A., Janie Benson, Susheela Singh, Mariana Romero, Bela Ganatra, Friday E. Okonofua, and Iqbal H. Shah. 2006. Unsafe abortion: The preventable pandemic. *Lancet* 368:1908–19.

Grosskurth, Heiner, Frank Mosha, James Todd, Ezra Mwijarubi, Arnoud Klokke, Kesheni Senkoro, Phillipe Mayaud et al. 1995. Impact of improved treatment of sexually transmitted diseases on HIV infection in rural Tanzania: Randomized controlled trial. *Lancet* 346:530–36.

Gueye, Mouhamadou, Sarah Castle, and Mamadou Kani Konate. 2001. Timing of first intercourse among Malian adolescents: Implications for contraceptive use. *International Family Planning Perspectives* 27(2):56–62 and 70.

Gumodoka, Balthazar, Isabelle Favot, and Wil Domans. 1997. Medical care-related transmission. In *HIV prevention and AIDS care in Africa: A district level approach,* ed. Japhet Ng'weshemi, Ties Boerma, John Bennett, and Dick Schapink, 280–91. Amsterdam: Royal Tropical Institute.

Gunderson, Frank. 2001. From 'dancing with porcupines' to 'twirling a hoe': Musical labor transformed in Sukumaland, Tanzania. *Africa Today* 48(4):3–25.

Hageman, Kathy M., Hazel M. B. Dube, Owen Mugurungi, Loretta E. Gavin, Shannon L. Hader, and Michael E. St. Louis. 2010. Beyond monogamy: Opportunities to further reduce risk for HIV infection among married Zimbabwean women with only one lifetime partner. *AIDS and Behavior* 14:113–24.

Hallett, Timothy B., John Stover, Vinod Mishra, Peter D. Ghys, Simon Gregson, and Ties Boerma. 2010. Estimates of HIV incidence from household-based prevalence surveys. *AIDS* 24(1):147–52.

Halperin, Daniel T., and Helen Epstein. 2004. Concurrent sexual partnerships help to explain Africa's high HIV prevalence: Implications for prevention. *Lancet* 364:4–6.

Haram, L. 2004. 'Prostitutes' or modern women? Negotiating respectability in northern Tanzania. In *Re-thinking sexualities in Africa*, ed. S. Arnfred, 211–29. Uppsala, Sweden: Nordiska Afrikainstitutet.

Haram, Liv. 1995. Negotiating sexuality in times of economic want: The young and modern Meru women. In *Young people at risk: Fighting AIDS in northen Tanzania*, ed. K. I. Klepp, P. M. Biswalo, and A. Talle, 31–48. Oslo: Scandinavian University Press.

Hardon, Anita, Sheila Davey, Trudie Gerrits, Catherine Hodgkin, Henry Irunde, Joyce Kgatlwane, John Kinsman, Alice Nakiyemba, and Richard Laing. 2006. *From access to adherence: The challenges of antiretroviral treatment: Studies from Botswana, Tanzania, and Uganda.* Geneva: World Health Organization.

Hargreaves J. R., and L. D. Howe. 2010. Changes in HIV prevalence among differently educated groups in Tanzania between 2003 and 2007. *AIDS* 24(5):755–61.

Hargreaves J. R., C. P. Bonell, T. Boler, D. Boccia, I. Birdthistle, A. Fletcher, P. M. Pronyk, and J. R. Glynn. 2008. Systematic review exploring time trends in the association between education attainment and risk of HIV infection in sub-Saharan Africa. *AIDS* 22:403–14.

Harrison, Abigail, and Lucia F. O'Sullivan. 2010. In the absence of marriage: Long-term concurrent partnerships, pregnancy, and HIV risk dynamics among South African young adults. *AIDS and Behavior* DOI 10.1007/s10461-010-9687-y.

Harrison, Abigail, Lucia F. O'Sullivan, Susie Hoffman, Curtis Dolezal, and Robert Morrell. 2006. Gender role and relationship norms among young adults in South Africa: Measuring the context of masculinity and HIV risk. *Journal of Urban Health* 83(4):709–22.

Hart, G. J., R. Pool, G. Green, S. Harrison, S. Nyanzi, and J. A. G. Whitworth. 1999. Women's attitudes to condoms and female-controlled means of protection against HIV and STDs in southwestern Uganda. *AIDS Care* 11(6):687–98.

Harwood-Lejeune, Audrey. 2000. Rising age at marriage and fertility in southern and eastern Africa. *European Journal of Population* 17:261–80.

Hatchett, L. A., C. P. N. Kaponda, C. N. Chihana, E. Chilemba, M. Nyando, A. Simwaka, and J. Levy. 2004. Health-seeking patterns for AIDS in Malawi. *AIDS Care* 16:827–33.

Hattori, Megan Klein, and F. Nii-Amoo Dodoo. 2007. Cohabitation, marriage, and "sexual monogamy" in Nairobi's slums. *Social Science and Medicine* 64:1067–78.

Hayes, Richard J., John Changalucha, David A. Ross, Awene Gavyole, Jim Todd, Angela I. N. Obasi, Mary L. Plummer, Daniel Wight, David C. Mabey, and Heiner Grosskurth. 2005. The MEMA kwa Vijana Project: Design of a community-randomized trial of an innovative adolescent sexual health intervention in rural Tanzania. *Contemporary Clinical Trials* 26:430–42.

Hayes, Richard, Maria Wawer, Ron Gray, James Whitworth, Heiner Grosskurth, and David Mabey. 1997. Randomized trials of STD treatment for HIV prevention: Report of an international workshop. *Genitourinary Medicine* 73:432–43.

Heald, Suzette. 1995. The power of sex: Some reflections on the Caldwells "African sexuality" thesis. *Africa* 65(4):489–505.

Heimer, Carol A. 2007. Old inequalities, new disease: HIV/AIDS in Sub-Saharan Africa. *Annual Review of Sociology* 33:551–77.

Helleringer, Stéphane, and Hans-Peter Kohler. 2007. Sexual network structure and the spread of HIV in Africa: Evidence from Likoma Island, Malawi. *AIDS* 21(17):2323–32.

Helle-Valle, Jo. 1999. Sexual mores, promiscuity and 'prostitution' in Botswana. *Ethnos* 64(3):372–96.

Helle-Valle, Jo. 2004. Understanding sexuality in Africa: Diversity and contextualized dividuality. In *Re-thinking sexualities in Africa*, ed. Signe Arnfred, 195–210. Uppsala, Sweden: Nordiska Afrikainstitutet.

Hess, Rosanna F. 2007. Women's stories of abortion in southern Gabon, Africa. *Journal of Transcultural Nursing* 18(1):41–48.

Hilber, Adriane Martin, Terence H. Hull, Eleanor Preston-Whyte, Brigitte Bagnol, Jenni Smit, Chintana Wacharasin, Ninuk Widyantoro, for the WHO GSVP Study Group. 2010. A cross cultural study of vaginal practices and sexuality: Implications for sexual health. *Social Science and Medicine* 70(3):392–400.

Hinde, Andrew, and Akim J. Mturi. 2000. Recent trends in Tanzanian fertility. *Population Studies* 54(2):177–91.

Hingson, Ralph, and Lee Strunin. 1993. Validity, reliability, and generalizability in studies of AIDS knowledge, attitudes, and behavioral risks based on subject self-report (Commentary). *American Journal of Preventive Medicine* 9(1):62–64.

Hirsch, Jennifer S., Holly Wardlow, Daniel Jordan Smith, Harriet M. Phinney, Shanti Parikh, and Constance A. Nathanson. 2009. *The secret: Love, marriage, and HIV*. Nashville: Vanderbilt University Press.

Homsy, Jaco, Rachel King, Dorothy Balaba, and Donna Kabatesi. 2004. Traditional health practitioners are key to scaling up comprehensive care for HIV/AIDS in sub-Saharan Africa. *AIDS* 18:1723–25.

Hrdy, D. 1987. Cultural practices contributing to the transmission of human immunodeficiency virus in Africa. *Review of Infectious Diseases* 9(6):1109–19.

Hudson, M. 1999. *Our grandmothers' drums*. London: Vintage.

Hunter, M. 2002. The materiality of everyday sex: Thinking beyond 'prostitution'. *African Studies*, 61(1):99–120.

Hunter, Mark. 2009. Providing love: Sex and exchange in twentieth-century South Africa. In *Love in Africa*, ed. Jennifer Cole and Lynn M. Thomas, 135–56. Chicago: University of Chicago Press.

Huygens, Pierre, Ellen Kajura, Janet Seeley, and Tom Barton. 1996. Rethinking methods for the study of sexual behavior. *Social Science and Medicine* 42(2):221–31.

IFAD (International Fund for Agricultural Development). 2001. *Rural poverty report 2001: The challenge of ending rural poverty*. Oxford: Oxford University Press.

Illife, John. 1979. *A modern history of Tanganyika*. Cambridge: Cambridge University Press.

Ingstad, Benedicte. 1990. The cultural construction of AIDS and its consequences for prevention in Botswana. *Medical Anthropology Quarterly* 4:28–40.

Isingo, Raphael, Basia Zaba, Milly Marston, Milalu Ndege, Julius Mngara, Wambura Mwita, Alison Wringe, David Beckles, John Changalucha, and Mark Urassa. 2007. Survival after HIV infection in the pre-antiretroviral therapy era in a rural Tanzanian cohort. *AIDS* 21(Supplement 6):S5–13.

Izugbara, Chimaraoke O. 2007. Representations of sexual abstinence among rural Nigerian adolescent males. *Sexuality Research and Social Policy* 4(2):74–87.

Izugbara, Chimaraoke Otutubikey, and Felicia Nwabuawele Modo. 2007. Risks and benefits of multiple sexual partnerships: Beliefs of rural Nigerian adolescent males. *American Journal of Men's Health* 1(3):197–207.

Jana, M., M. Nkambule, and D. Tumbo. 2008. *Onelove: Multiple and concurrent sexual partnerships. A ten country research report.* Soul City Institute Regional Program, Adelie Publishing.

Jankowiak, William R., and Edward F. Fischer. 1992. A cross-cultural perspective on romantic love. *Ethnology* 31(2):149–55.

Jewkes, Rachel, Helen Rees, Kim Dickson, Heather Brown, and Jonathan Levin. 2005. The impact of age on the epidemiology of incomplete abortions in South Africa after legislative change. *BJOG: An International Journal of Obstetrics and Gynaecology* 112(3):355–59.

Jewkes, Rachel, Jonathan Levin, Nolwazi Mbananga, and Debbie Bradshaw. 2002. Rape of girls in South Africa. *Lancet* 359:319–20.

Joel, M., A. Chukwuemeka, B. Amusa, and K. Klindera. 2004. Youth-friendly HIV voluntary counseling and testing services—from a youth perspective. 15th International AIDS Conference. Bangkok, Thailand. 11–16 July 2004. Abstract no. TuPeD5111.

Johnson, David. 2008. *The changing landscape of education in Africa: Quality, equality and democracy.* Oxford: Symposium Books.

Johnson-Hanks, Jennifer. 2005. When the future decides: Uncertainty and intentional action in contemporary Cameroon. *Current Anthropology* 46(3):363–85.

Juma, Waziri. 1960. The Sukuma societies for young men and women. *Tanganyika Notes and Records* 54:27–29.

Kaaya, Sylvia F., Alan J. Flisher, Jessie K. Mbwambo, Herman Schaalma, Leif Edvard Aarø, and Knut-Inge Klepp. 2002. A review of studies of sexual behavior of school students in sub-Saharan Africa. *Scandinavian Journal of Public Health* 30:148–60.

Kaijage, F. J. 1993. AIDS control and the burden of history in northwestern Tanzania. *Population and Environment* 14(3):279–300.

Kajubi, P., M. R. Kamya, H. F. Raymond, S. Chen, G. W. Rutherford, J. S. Mandel, and W. McFarland. 2008. Gay and bisexual men in Kampala, Uganda. *AIDS and Behavior* 12(3):492–504.

Kale, Rajendra. 1995. Traditional healers in South Africa: A parallel health care system. *British Medical Journal* 310:1182–85.

Kaler, Amy. 2001. "Many divorces and many spinsters": Marriage as an invented tradition in southern Malawi, 1946–1999. *Journal of Family History* 26(4):529–56.

Kaler, Amy. 2004a. AIDS-talk in everyday life: The presence of HIV/AIDS in men's informal conversation in Southern Malawi. *Social Science and Medicine* 59:285–97.

Kaler, Amy. 2004b. The moral lens of population control: Condoms and controversies in southern Malawi. *Studies in Family Planning* 35(2):105–15.

Kalichman, S. C., and L. Simbayi. 2004. Traditional beliefs about the cause of AIDS and AIDS-related stigma in South Africa. *AIDS Care* 16:572–80.

Kamali, Anatoli, John Kinsman, Norah Nalweyiso, Kirsten Mitchell, Edward Kanye-sigye, Jane F. Kengeya-Kayondo, Lucy M. Carpenter, Andrew Nunn, and James A. G. Whitworth. 2002. A community randomized controlled trial to investigate impact of improved STD management and behavioral interventions on HIV incidence in rural Masaka, Uganda: Trial design, methods and baseline findings. *Tropical Medicine and International Health* 7:1053–63.

Kapiga, S. H., and J. L. P. Lugalla. 2002. Sexual behavior patterns and condom use in Tanzania: Results from the 1996 Demographic and Health Survey. *AIDS Care* 14(4):455–69.

Karim, S. S. Abdool, Q. Abdool Karim, E. Preston-Whyte, and N. Sankar. 1992. Reasons for lack of condom use among high school students. *South African Medical Journal* 82(2):107–10.

Katapa, R. S. 2004. Caretakers of AIDS patients in rural Tanzania. *International Journal of STDs and AIDS* 15:673–78.

Katz, Itamar. 2006. Explaining the increase in condom use among South African young females. *Journal of Health Communication* 11:737–53.

Kaufman, C. E., and S. E. Stavrou. 2004. "Bus fare, please": The economics of sex and gifts among young people in urban South Africa. *Culture, Health and Sexuality* 6(5):377–91.

Kazaura, Method R., and Melkiory C. Masatu. 2009. Sexual practices among unmarried adolescents in Tanzania. *BMC Public Health* 9:373.

Kenyatta, J. 1938. *Facing Mount Kenya: The tribal life of the Gikuyu.* London: Heinemann.

Kessler, Ilana. 2006. *What went right in Tanzania: How nation building and political culture have produced forty-four years of peace.* Thesis submitted in partial fulfillment of the requirements for the award of Honors in International Politics and the African Studies Certificate in the Edmund A. Walsh School of Foreign Service of Georgetown University. Downloaded on September 10, 2010 from http://aladinrc.wrlc.org/bitstream/1961/3688/1/Kessler_Ilana_Thesis.pdf.

Kiapi-Iwa, L., and G. J. Hart. 2004. The sexual and reproductive health of young people in Adjumani district, Uganda: Qualitative study of the role of formal, informal and traditional health providers. *AIDS Care* 16:339–47.

Kim, Julia C., and Charlotte Watts. 2005. Gaining a foothold: Tackling poverty, gender equality, and HIV in Africa. *British Medical Journal* 331:769–72.

Kimuna, S., and Y. Djamba. 2005. Wealth and extramarital sex among men in Zambia. *International Family Planning Perspectives* 31(2):83–89.

Kinsman, J., J. Nakiyingi, A. Kamali, and J. Whitworth. 2001. Condom awareness and intended use: Gender and religious contrasts among school pupils in rural Masaka. *AIDS Care* 13(2):215–20.

Kinsman, J., S. Harrison, J. Kengeya-Kayondo, E. Kanyesigye, S. Musoke, and J. Whitworth. 1999. Implementation of a comprehensive AIDS education program for schools in Masaka district, Uganda. *AIDS Care* 11:591–601.

Kirk, Dudley, and Bernard Pillet. 1998. Fertility levels, trends, and differentials in sub-Saharan Africa in the 1980s and 1990s. *Studies in Family Planning* 29(1):1–22.

Kleiner-Bossaller, Anke. 1993. Kwantacce, the "sleeping pregnancy," a Hausa concept. In *Focus on women in Africa*, ed. Gudrun Ludwar-Ene and Mechthild Reh, 17–30. Bayreuth. Germany: African Studies Series, No. 26.

Konings, E., G. Bantebya, M. Caraël, D. Bagenda, and T. Mertens. 1995. Validating population surveys for the measurement of HIV/STD prevention indicators. *AIDS* 9:375–82.

Kraut-Becher, Julie R., and Sevgi O. Aral. 2003. Gap length: An important factor in sexually transmitted disease transmission. *Sexually Transmitted Diseases* 30(3):221–25.

Kretzschmar, Mirjam, Richard G. White, and Michel Caraël. 2010. Concurrency is more complex than it seems. *AIDS* 24:313–15.

Kuhn, L., M. Steinberg, and C. Mathews. 1994. Participation of the school community in AIDS education: An evaluation of a high school programme in South Africa. *AIDS Care* 6:161–71.

Kumi-Kyereme, Akwasi, Kofi Awusabo-Asare, Ann Biddlecom, and Augustine Tanle. 2007. Influence of social connectedness, communication and monitoring on adolescent sexual activity in Ghana. *African Journal of Reproductive Health* 11(3):133–47.

Kusimba, J., H. A. C. M. Voeten, H. B. O'hara, J. M. Otido, J. D. F. Habbema, J. O. Ndinya-Achola, and J. J. Bwayo. 2003. Traditional healers and the management of sexually transmitted diseases in Nairobi, Kenya. *International Journal of STD and AIDS* 14:197–201.

Laga, Marie, Bernhard Schwärtlander, Elisabeth Pisani, Papa Salif Sow, and Michel Caraël. 2001. To stem HIV in Africa, prevent transmission to young women. *AIDS* 15(7):931–34.

Lagarde, E., M. Schim van der Loeff, C. Enel, B. Holmgren, R. Dray-Spira, G. Pison, J. P. Piau et al. 2003. Mobility and the spread of human immunodeficiency virus into rural areas of West Africa. *International Journal of Epidemiology* 32:744–52.

Lagarde, Emmanuel, Bertran Auvert, Michel Caraël, Martin Laourou, Benoît Ferry, Evina Akam, Tom Sukwa et al. 2001. Concurrent sexual partnerships and HIV prevalence in five urban communities of sub-Saharan Africa. *AIDS* 15:877–84.

Lamptey, Peter, and Gail A. W. Goodridge. 1991. Condom issues in AIDS prevention in Africa. *AIDS* 5(Supplement 1):S183–91.

Landman, Keren Z., Grace D. Kinabo, Werner Schimana, Wil M. Dolmans, Mark E. Swai, John F. Shao, and John A. Crump. 2006. Capacity of health-care facilities to deliver HIV treatment and care services, northern Tanzania, 2004 *International Journal of STD and AIDS* 17:459–62.

Larke, Natasha, Bernadette Cleophas-Mazige, Mary L. Plummer, Angela I. N. Obasi, Merdard Rwakatare, Jim Todd, John Changalucha, Helen A. Weiss, Richard J. Hayes, and David A. Ross. 2010. Impact of the *MEMA kwa Vijana* adolescent sexual and reproductive health interventions on use of health services by young people in rural Mwanza, Tanzania: Results of a cluster randomized trial. *Journal of Adolescent Health* 47(5):512–22.

Larsen, Ulla, and Marida Hollos. 2003. Women's empowerment and fertility decline among the Pare of Kilimanjaro region, Northern Tanzania. *Social Science and Medicine* 57:1099–115.

Larsen, Ulla. 2000. Primary and secondary fertility in sub-Saharan Africa. *International Journal of Epidemiology* 29:285–91.

Larsen, Ulla. 2003. Primary and secondary infertility in Tanzania. *Journal of Health and Population in Developing Countries* 5:1–15.

Laumann, E. O., J. H. Gagnon, R. T. Michael, and S. Michaels. 1994. *The social organization of sexuality: Sexual practices in the United States.* Chicago: Chicago University Press.

Lawi, Yusufu Qwaray. 2007. Tanzania's Operation *Vijiji* and local ecological consciousness: The case of eastern Iraqwland, 1974–1976. *Journal of African History* 48:69–93.

Le Blanc, Marie-Nathalie, Deidre Meintel, and Victor Piche. 1991. The African sexual system: Comment on Caldwell et al. *Population and Development Review* 17(3):497–505.

Leclerc-Madlala, S. 2003. Transactional sex and the pursuit of modernity. *Social Dynamics* 29(2):213–33.

Leclerc-Madlala, Suzanne. 2008. Age-disparate and intergenerational sex in southern Africa: The dynamics of hypervulnerability. *AIDS* 22(Supplement 4):S17–25.

Leclerc-Madlala, Suzanne. 2009. Cultural scripts for multiple and concurrent partnerships in southern Africa: Why HIV prevention needs anthropology. *Sexual Health* 6(2):103–10.

Lees, Shelley, Nicola Desmond, Caroline Allen, Gilbert Bugeke, Andrew Vallely, and David Ross. 2009. Sexual risk behavior for women working in recreational venues in Mwanza, Tanzania: Considerations for the acceptability and use of vaginal microbicide gels. *Culture, Health and Sexuality* 11(6):581–95.

Leiva, Anya, Matthew Shaw, Katie Paine, Kebba Manneh, Keith McAdam, and Philippe Mayaud. 2001. Management of sexually transmitted diseases in urban pharmacies in the Gambia. *International Journal of STD and AIDS* 12:444–52.

Levinson, David. 1998. *Ethnic groups worldwide: A ready reference handbook.* Phoenix, AZ: Oryx Press.

Lewis, I. M. 1976. *Social anthropology in perspective.* Harmondsworth: Penguin.

Lillie, Tiffany, Julie Pulerwitz, and Barbara Curbow. 2009. Kenyan in-school youths' level of understanding of abstinence, being faithful, and consistent condom use terms: Implications for HIV prevention programs. *Journal of Health Communication* 14(3):276–92.

Lindan, Christina, Susan Allen, Michel Caraël, F. Nsengumuremyi, P. Van de Perre, A. Serufilina, J. Tice, D. Black, T. Oates, and S. Hulley. 1991. Knowledge, attitudes, and perceived risk of AIDS among urban Rwandan women: Relationship to HIV infection and behavior change. *AIDS* 5(8):993–1002.

Lindenbaum, S. 1991. Anthropology rediscovers sex: Introduction. *Social Science and Medicine* 33(8):865–66.

Little, Kenneth. 1973. *African women in towns: An aspect of African's social revolution.* New York: Cambridge University Press.

Lloyd, Cynthia B., and Paul Hewett. 2009. Educational inequalities in the midst of persistent poverty: Diversity across Africa in educational outcomes. *Journal of International Development* 21:1137–51.

Longfield, K., A. Glick, M. Waithaka, and J. Berman. 2004. Relationships between older men and younger women: Implications for STIs/HIV in Kenya. *Studies in Family Planning* 35(2):125–34.

Lowe-McConnell, R. 1994. The changing ecosystem of Lake Victoria, East Africa. *Freshwater Forum* 4(2):76–89.

Luke, Nancy. 2003. Age and economic asymmetries in the sexual relationships of adolescent girls in sub-Saharan Africa. *Studies in Family Planning* 34(2):67–86.

Lurie, Mark N., and Samantha Rosenthal. 2010. Concurrent partnerships as a driver of the HIV epidemic in Sub-Saharan Africa? The evidence is limited. *AIDS and Behavior* 14(1):17–24.

Lurie, Mark N., Brian G. Williams, Khangelani Zuma, David Mkaya-Mwamburi, Geoff P. Garnett, Michael D. Sweat, Joel Gittelsohn, and Salim S. Abdool Karim. 2003. Who infects whom? HIV-1 concordance and discordance among migrant and nonmigrant couples in South Africa. *AIDS* 17:2245–52.

Lutz, Brian. 2005. Marital status, sexual behavior and sexually transmitted infection in rural Tanzanian villages. Thesis for Master of Science in Epidemiology, London School of Hygiene and Tropical Medicine, UK.

Macintyre, K., N. Rutenberg, L. Brown, and A. Karim. 2004. Understanding perceptions of HIV risk among adolescents in KwaZulu-Natal. *AIDS and Behavior* 8(3):237–50.

Macintyre, Kate, Lisanne Brown, and Stephen Sosler. 2001. Its not what you know, but who you knew: Examining the relationship between behavior change and AIDS mortality in Africa. *AIDS Education and Prevention* 13(2):160–74.

Mack, Natasha, Cynthia Woodsong, Kathleen M. Macqueen, Greg Guest, and Emily Namey. 2005. *Qualitative research methods: A data collector's field guide*. Research Triangle Park, NC: Family Health International.

MacPhail, Catherine, and Catherine Campbell. 2001. 'I think condoms are good, but, aai, I hate those things': Condom use among adolescents and young people in a Southern African township. *Social Science and Medicine* 52(11):1613–27.

MacPhail, Catherine, Audrey Pettifor, Sophie Pascoe, and Helen Rees. 2007. Predictors of dual method use for pregnancy and HIV prevention among adolescent South African women. *Contraception* 75:383–89.

Madriz, Esther. 2000. Focus groups in feminist research. In *Handbook of qualitative research*, ed. Norman K. Denzin and Yvonna S. Lincoln, 835–50. Thousand Oaks, CA: Sage.

Madulu, Ndalahwa F. 1998. *Changing lifestyles in farming societies of Sukumaland: Kwimba District, Tanzania. De-Agrarianisation and Rural Employment Network Working Paper Vol. 27*. Leiden, the Netherlands: Afrika-Studiecentrum.

Mafeje, Archie. 1991. *Kingdoms of the Great Lakes Region: Ethnography of African social formations*. Kampala, Uganda: Fountain Publishers.

Maganja, R., S. Maman, A. Groves, and J. Mbwambo. 2007. Skinning the goat and pulling the load: Transactional sex among youth in Dar es Salaam, Tanzania. *AIDS Care* 19(8):974–81.

Maharaj, Pranitha. 2006. Reasons for condom use among young people in KwaZulu-Natal: Prevention of HIV, pregnancy or both? *International Family Planning Perspectives* 32(1):28–34.

Mapunjo, S., and D. P. Urassa. 2007. Quality standards in provision of facility based HIV care and treatment: A case study from Dar es Salaam Region, Tanzania. *East African Journal of Public Health* 4(1):12–18.

Marandu, Edward E., and Mbaki A. Chamme. 2004. Attitudes towards condom use for prevention of HIV infection in Botswana. *Social Behavior and Personality* 32(5):491–510.

Marchant, T., A. K. Mushi, R. Nathan, O. Mukasa, S. Abdulla, C. Lengeler, and J. R. M. Armstrong Schellenberg. 2004. Planning a family: Priorities and concerns in rural Tanzania. *African Journal of Reproductive Health* 8(2):111–23.

Marck, J. 1997. Aspects of male circumcision in sub-equatorial African culture history. *Health Transit Review* 7(Supplement):337–60.

Marston, Milly, Basia Zaba, Joshua A. Salomon, Heena Brahmbatt, and Danstan Bagenda. 2005. Estimating the net effects of HIV on child mortality in African populations affected by generalized HIV epidemics. *Journal of Acquired Immune Deficiency Syndromes* 38:219–27.

Matasha, E., T. Ntembelea, P. Mayaud, W. Saidi, J. Todd, B. Mujaya, and L. Tendo-Wambua. 1998. Sexual and reproductive health among primary and secondary school pupils in Mwanza, Tanzania: Need for intervention. *AIDS Care* 10(5):571–82.

Maticka-Tyndale, Eleanor, Richmond Tiemoko, and Paulina Makinwa-Adebusoye (eds). 2007. *Human sexuality in Africa: Beyond reproduction.* Auckland Park, South Africa: Fanele.

Mauss, Marcel. 2002. *The gift: The form and reason for exchange in archaic societies.* London: Routledge.

Mavhu, Webster, Lisa Langhaug, Bothwell Manyongo, Robert Power and Frances Cowan. 2008. What is "sex" exactly? Using cognitive interviewing to improve the validity of sexual behavior reporting among young people in rural Zimbabwe. *Culture, Health and Sexuality* 10(6):563–72.

Mbonile L., and E. J. Kayombo. 2008. Assessing acceptability of parents/guardians of adolescents towards introduction of sex and reproductive health education in schools at Kinondoni Municipal in Dar es Salaam city. *East African Journal of Public Health* 5(1):26–31.

Meekers, Dominique, and Anne-Emmanuele Calvès. 1997. "Main" girlfriends, girlfriends, marriage, and money: The social context of HIV risk behavior in sub-Saharan Africa. *Health Transition Review* 7(Supplement):361–75.

Meekers, Dominique. 1992. The process of marriage in African societies: A multiple indicator approach. *Population and Development Review* 18(1):61–78.

Mehryar, Amir. 1995. Condoms: Awareness, attitudes and use. In *Sexual behavior and AIDS in the developing* world, ed. John Cleland and Benoît Ferry, 124–56. London: Taylor and Francis.

Mensch, B., D. Bagah, W. H. Clark, and F. Binka. 1999. The changing nature of adolescence in the Kassena-Nankana District of Northern Ghana. *Studies in Family Planning* 30(2):95–111.

Mensch, Barbara S., Paul C. Hewett, and Annabel S. Erulkar. 2003. The reporting of sensitive behavior by adolescents: A methodological experiment in Kenya. *Demography* 40(2):247–68.

Mesaki, S. 1994. Witch-killing in Sukumaland. In *Witchcraft in contemporary Tanzania*, ed. R. Abrahams, 47–60. Cambridge: African Studies Centre, University of Cambridge.

Messersmith, Lisa J., Thomas T. Kane, Adetanwa I. Odebiyi, and Alfred A. Adewuyi. 2000. Who's at risk? Men's STD experience and condom use in southwest Nigeria. *Studies in Family Planning* 31(3):203–16.

Mgalla, Zaida, and J. Ties Boerma. 2001. The discourse of infertility in Tanzania. In *Women and infertility in sub-Saharan Africa: A multi-disciplinary perspective*, ed. J. Ties Boerma and Zaida Mgalla, 189–200. Amsterdam, Netherlands: Royal Tropical Institute, KIT Publishers.

Miguel, Edward. 2005. Poverty and witch killing. *Review of Economic Studies* 72:1153–72.

Miller, N., and R. Rockwell. 1988. *AIDS in Africa: The social and policy impact*. Lewiston/Queenston: Edwin Mellen.

Mills, Edward J., Jean B. Nachega, David R. Bangsberg, Sonal Singh, Beth Rachlis, Ping Wu, Kumanan Wilson, Iain Buchan, Christopher J. Gill, and Curtis Cooper. 2006. Adherence to HAART: A systematic review of developed and developing nation patient-reported barriers and facilitators. *PLoS Medicine* 3(11):2039–64.

Mills, Edward J., Jean B. Nachega, Iain Buchan, Jame Orbinski, Amir Attaran, Sonal Singh, S., Beth Rachlis et al. 2006. Adherence to antiretroviral therapy in sub-Saharan Africa and North America: A meta-analysis. *Journal of the American Medical Association* 296(6):679–90.

Minnis, A. M., M. J. Steiner, M. F. Gallo, L. Warner, M. M. Hobbs, A. van der Straten, T. Chipato, M. Macaluso, and N. S. Padian. 2009. Biomarker validation of reports of recent sexual activity: Results of a randomized controlled study in Zimbabwe. *American Journal of Epidemiology* 170(7):918–24.

Mirambo, Immaculate. 2004. Oral literature of the Sukuma. *Folklore* 26:113–22.

Mishra, V. and S. Bignami-Van Assche. 2009. Concurrent sexual partnerships and HIV infection: Evidence from national population-based surveys. *DHS Working Papers*, 62.

Mitsunaga, Tisha M., Antonia M. Powell, Nathan J. Heard, and Ulla M. Larsen. 2005. Extramarital sex among Nigerian men: Polygyny and other risk factors. *JAIDS: Journal of Acquired Immune Deficiency Syndromes* 39(4):478–88.

Mlangwa, Susan. 2009. *The social construction of gender in response to HIV/AIDS: The case of Tanzanian professional couples*. PhD thesis. University of Minnesota, Minneapolis, USA.

Mlemya, B., V. Justine, and Z. Mgalla. 1997. Country watch: Tanzania. *AIDS/STD Health Promotion Exchange* 1:5–6.

Mmbaga, Elia J., Germana H. Leyna, Kagoma S. Mnyika, Akhtar Hussain, and Knut-Inge Klepp. 2009. Prevalence and predictors of failure to return for HIV-1 posttest counseling in the era of antiretroviral therapy in rural Kilimanjaro, Tanzania: Challenges and opportunities. *AIDS Care* 21(2):160–67.

Mnyika, K. S., G. Kvåle, and K. I. Klepp. 1995. Perceived function of and barriers to condom use in Arusha and Kilimanjaro regions of Tanzania. *AIDS Care* 7(3):295–305.

Mogensen, Hanne Overgaard. 1997. The narrative of AIDS among the Tonga of Zambia. *Social Science and Medicine* 44:431–39.

Montgomery, C. M., M. Gafos, S. Lees, N. S. Morar, O. Mweemba, A. Ssali, J. Stadler, and R. Pool. 2010. Reframing microbicide acceptability: Findings from the MDP301 trial. *Culture, Health and Sexuality* 12(6):649–62.

Montgomery, C. M., S. Lees, J. Stadler, N. S. Morar, A. Ssali, B. Mwanza, M. Mntambo, J. Phillip, C. Watts and R. Pool. 2008. The role of partnership dynamics in determining the acceptability of condoms and microbicides. *AIDS Care* 20(6):733–40.

Morgan, Dilys, Cedric Mahe, Billy Mayanja, J. Martin Okongo, Rosemary Lubega, and James A. G Whitworth. 2002. HIV-1 infection in rural Africa: Is there a difference in median time to AIDS and survival compared with that in industrialized countries? *AIDS* 16:597–603.

Moyo, Witness, Brooke A. Levandowski, Catherine MacPhail, Helen Rees, and Audrey Pettifor. 2008. Consistent condom use in South African youth's most recent sexual relationships. *AIDS and Behavior* 12:431–40.

Mpangile, Gottlieb S., M. T. Leshabari, and David J. Kihwele. 1993. Factors associated with induced abortion in public hospitals in Dar es Salaam, Tanzania. *Reproductive Health Matters* 1(2):21–31.

Mshana, Gerry Hillary, Joyce Wamoyi, Joanna Busza, Basia Zaba, John Changalucha, Samuel Kaluvya, and Mark Urassa. 2006. Barriers to accessing antiretroviral therapy in Kisesa, Tanzania: A qualitative study of early rural referrals to the national program. *AIDS Patient Care and STDs* 20(9):649–57.

Mshana, Gerry, Mary L. Plummer, Joyce Wamoyi, Zachayo S. Shigongo, David A. Ross, and Daniel Wight. 2006. "She was bewitched and caught an illness similar to AIDS": AIDS and sexually transmitted infection causation beliefs in rural northern Tanzania. *Culture, Health and Sexuality* 8(1):45–58.

Msisha, Wezi M., Saidi H. Kapiga, Felton Earls, and S. V. Subramanian. 2008. Socioeconomic status and HIV seroprevalence in Tanzania: A counterintuitive relationship. *International Journal of Epidemiology* 37(6):1297–303.

Msiska, R., E. Nangawe, D. Mulenga, M. Sichone, J. Kamanga, and P. Kwapa. 1997. Understanding lay perspectives: Care options for STD treatment in Lusaka, Zambia. *Health Policy and Planning* 12:248–52.

Muela, Susanna Hausmann, Adiel K. Mushi, and Joan Muela Ribera. 2000. The paradox of the cost and affordability of traditional and government health services in Tanzania. *Health Policy and Planning* 15:296–302.

Mukoma, Wanjiru, Alan J. Flisher, Nazeema Ahmed, Shahieda Jansen, Catherine Mathews, Knut-Inge Klepp, and Herman Schaalma. 2009. Process evaluation of a school-based HIV/AIDS intervention in South Africa. *Scandinavian Journal of Public Health* 37(Supplement 2):37–47.

Mundigo, Axel I. 1999. Research methodology: Lessons learnt. In *Abortion in the developing world*, ed. Axel I. Mundigo and Cynthia Indriso, 465–76. New York: Zed Books.

Mundigo, Axel I. 2003. The challenge of induced abortion research: Transdisciplinary perspectives. In *The sociocultural and political aspects of abortion: Global perspectives*, ed. Alaka Malwade Basu, 49–63. Westport, CT: Praeger.

Murcott, A. 1980. The social construction of teenage pregnancy: A problem in the ideologies of childhood and reproduction. *Sociology of Health and Illness* 2(1):1–23.

Myer, Landon, Louise Kuhn, Zena A. Stein, Thomas C. Wright, and Lynette Denny. 2005. Intravaginal practices, bacterial vaginosis, and women's susceptibility to HIV infection: Epidemiological evidence and biological mechanisms. *Lancet Infectious Diseases* 5:786–94.

Nachega, J. B., D. M. Stein, D. A. Lehman, D. Hlatshwayo, R. Mothopeng, R. E. Chaisson, and A. S. Karstaedt. 2004. Adherence to antiretroviral therapy in HIV-infected adults in Soweto, South Africa. *AIDS Research and Human Retroviruses* 20(10):1053–56.

Nachtigall, Robert D. 2006. International disparities in access to infertility services. *Fertility and Sterility* 85(4):871–75.

Namisi, F. S., A. J. Flisher, S. Overland, S. Bastien, H. Onya, S. Kaaya, and L. E. Aarø. 2009. Sociodemographic variations in communication on sexuality and HIV/AIDS with parents, family members and teachers among in-school adolescents: A multisite study in Tanzania and South Africa. *Scandinavian Journal of Public Health* 37(Supplement 2):65–74.

National Bureau of Statistics and ICF Macro. 2010. *Tanzania Demographic and Health Survey 2010: Preliminary report.* Dar es Salaam, Tanzania: National Bureau of Statistics and ICF Macro.

National Bureau of Statistics and Macro International Inc. 2000. *Tanzania Reproductive and Child Health Survey 1999.* Calverton, Maryland: National Bureau of Statistics and Macro International Inc.

National Bureau of Statistics and ORC Macro. 2004. *2002 Population and Housing Census: The Regional and District Census Data in Brief (Volume IV).* Dar es Salaam, Tanzania: National Bureau of Statistics and ORC Macro.

National Bureau of Statistics and ORC Macro. 2005. *Tanzania Demographic and Health Survey 2004–05.* Dar es Salaam, Tanzania: National Bureau of Statistics and ORC Macro.

National Research Council. 2002. *Geographic information for sustainable development in Africa.* Washington DC: National Academies Press.

Ndinda, Catherine, Chiweni Chimbwete, Nuala McGrath, and Robert Pool. 2008. Perceptions of anal intercourse in rural South Africa. *Culture, Health and Sexuality* 10(2):205–12.

Ndulo, Jane, Elisabeth Faxelid, Carol Tishelman, and Ingela Krantz. 2000. "Shopping" for sexually transmitted disease treatment: Focus group discussions among lay persons in rural and urban Zambia. *Sexually Transmitted Diseases* 27:496–503.

Neighbors, Clayton, Amanda J. Dillard, Melissa A. Lewis, Rochelle L. Bergstrom, and Teryl A. Neil. 2006. Normative misperceptions and temporal precedence of perceived norms and drinking. *Journal of Studies on Alcohol* 67(2):290–99.

Nelson, Sara J., Lisa E. Manhart, Pamina M. Gorbach, David H. Martin, Bradley P. Stoner, Sevgi O. Aral, and King K. Holmes. 2007. Measuring sex partner concurrency: It's what's missing that counts. *Sexually Transmitted Diseases* 34(10):801–7.

Neumann, A. K., and P. Lauro. 1982. Ethnomedicine and biomedicine linking. *Social Science and Medicine* 16:1817–24.

Ngalula, J., M. Urassa, G. Mwaluko, R. Isingo, and J. T. Boerma. 2002. Health service use and household expenditure during terminal illness due to AIDS in rural Tanzania. *Tropical Medicine and International Health* 7:873–77.

Nilsson, Paula. 2003. *Education for all: Teacher demand and supply in Africa. Education International Working Papers no. 12.* Brussels: Education International.

Nnko, Soori, and Robert Pool. 1997. Sexual discourse in the context of AIDS: Dominant themes on adolescent sexuality among primary school pupils in Magu district, Tanzania. *Health Transition Review* 7(Supplement 3):85–90.

Nnko, Soori, Boerma J. Ties, Mark Urassa, Gabriel Mwaluko, and Basia Zaba. 2004. Secretive females or swaggering males? An assessment of the quality of sexual partnership reporting in rural Tanzania. *Social Science and Medicine* 59:299–310.

Nnko, Soori, Robert Washija, Mark Urassa, and J. Ties Boerma. 2001. Dynamics of male circumcision practices in northwest Tanzania. *Sexually Transmitted Diseases* 28(4):214–18.

Nyanzi, S., J. Kinsman, and R. Pool. 2004. Mobility, sexual networks and exchange among bodabodamen in southwest Uganda. *Culture, Health and Sexuality* 6(3):239–254.

Nyanzi, S., R. Pool, and J. Kinsman. 2001. The negotiation of sexual relationships among school pupils in south western Uganda. *AIDS Care* 13(1):83–98.

Nzioka, C. 2001. Perspectives of adolescent boys on the risks of unwanted pregnancy and sexually transmitted infections: Kenya. *Reproductive Health Matters* 9(17):108–17.

Nzioka, Charles. 2004. Unwanted pregnancy and sexually transmitted infection among young women in rural Kenya. *Culture, Health and Sexuality* 6(1):31–44.

O'Farrell, Nigel. 1999. Increasing prevalence of genital herpes in developing countries: Implications for heterosexual HIV transmission and STI control programs. *Sexually Transmitted Infections* 75(6):377–84.

O'Hara, H. B., H. A. C. M. Voeten, A. G. Kuperus, J. M. Otido, J. Kusimba, J. D. F. Habbema, J. J. Bwayo, and J. O. Ndinya-Achola. 2001. Quality of health education during STD case management in Nairobi, Kenya. *International Journal of STD and AIDS* 12:315–22.

Obasi, A. I., B. Cleophas, D. A. Ross, K. L. Chima, G. Mmassy, A. Gavyole, M. L. Plummer, M. Makokha, B. Mujaya, J. Todd, D. Wight, H. Grosskurth, D. C. Mabey, and R. J. Hayes. 2006. Rationale and design of the *MEMA kwa Vijana* adolescent sexual and reproductive health intervention in Mwanza Region, Tanzania. *AIDS Care* 18(4):311–22.

Okonofua, Friday E., James I. Ogonor, Franscisca I. Omorodion, Miriam T. Temin, Paul A. Coplan, Joan A. Kaufman, and H. Kristian Heggenhougen. 1999. Assessment of health services for treatment of sexually transmitted infections among Nigerian adolescents. *Sexually Transmitted Diseases* 26:184–90.

Omari, C. K. 1987. Ethnicity, politics and development in Tanzania. *African Study Monographs* 7:65–80.

Omorodion, Francisca Isi. 1993. Sexual networking among market women in Benin City, Bendel State, Nigeria. *Health Transition Review* 3(Supplement):1–11.

Oraby, Doaa, Cherif Soliman, Sherif Elkamhawi, and Rawya Hassan. 2008. *Assessment of youth friendly clinics in teaching hospitals in Egypt. Family Health International Assessment Report.* Downloaded on August 21, 2010 from www.fhi .org/NR/rdonlyres/esvin7blgv2r3bq6dqhpiwbyzthu3wvu7oa7gzqaunnsctfnohdiad wcy4bjqep66xubgutujbhykm/Assessmentreportmay28final2.pdf.

O-saki, Kalafunja Mlang'a, and Augustine Obeleagu Agu. 2002. A study of classroom interaction in primary schools in the United Republic of Tanzania. *Prospects* 32:103–16.

Oyugi, Jessica H., Jayne Byakika-Tusiime, Kathleen Ragland, Oliver Laeyendecker, Roy Mugerwa, Cissy Kityo, Peter Mugyenyi, Thomas C. Quinn, and David R. Bangsberg. 2007. Treatment interruptions predict resistance in HIV-positive individuals purchasing fixed-dose combination antiretroviral therapy in Kampala, Uganda. *AIDS* 21(8):965–71.

Paciotti, Brian, and Craig Hadley. 2003. The ultimatum game in southwestern Tanzania: Ethnic variation and institutional scope. *Current Anthropology* 44(3): 427–32.

Paciotti, Brian, and Monique Borgerhoff Mulder. 2004. Sungusungu: The role of pre-existing and evolving social institutions among Tanzanian vigilante organizations. *Human Organization* 63(1):112–24.

Paciotti, Brian, Craig Hadley, Christopher Mulder, and Monique Borgerhoff. 2005. Grass-roots justice in Tanzania. *American Scientist* 93(1):58–65.

Page, Randy M., and Cougar P. Hall. 2009. Psychosocial distress and alcohol use as factors in adolescent sexual behavior among sub-Saharan African adolescents. *Journal of School Health* 79(8):369–79.

Painter, Thomas M., Kassamba L. Diaby, Danielle M. Matia, Lillian S. Lin, Toussaint S Sibailly, Moïse K. Kouassi, Ehounou R. Ekpini, Thierry H Roels, and Stefan Z. Wiktor. 2007. Faithfulness to partners: A means to prevent HIV infection, a source of HIV infection risks, or both? A qualitative study of women's experiences in Abidjan, Côte d'Ivoire. *African Journal of AIDS Research* 6(1):25–31.

Palmer, Robert, Ruth Wedgwood and Rachel Hayman, with Kenneth King and Neil Thin. 2007. *Educating out of poverty? A synthesis report on Ghana, India, Kenya, Rwanda, Tanzania and South Africa. Department for International Development: Educational Paper no. 70.* Edinburgh, UK: Centre of African Studies, University of Edinburgh.

Panos Institute. 2003. *Beyond victims and villains: Addressing sexual violence in the education sector. PANOS Report No. 47.* London: Panos.

Parikh, Shanti A. 2007. The political economy of marriage and HIV: The ABC approach, safe infidelity, and managing moral risk in Uganda. *American Journal of Public Health* 97(7):1198–208.

Parker, R. G., G. Herdt, and M. Carballo. 1991. Sexual culture, HIV transmission, and AIDS research. *The Journal of Sex Research* 28(1):77–98.

Parker, Richard G., Delia Easton, and Charles H. Klein. 2000. Structural factors and facilitators in HIV prevention: A review of international research. *AIDS* 14(Supplement 1):S22–32.

Parkes, Alison, Daniel Wight, Marion Henderson, and Graham Hart. 2007. Explaining associations between adolescent substance use and condom use. *Journal of Adolescent Health* 40:180e1–18.

Partnership for Child Development. 1998. Implications for school-based health programs of age and gender patterns in the Tanzanian primary school. *Tropical Medicine and International Health* 3:850–53.

Pellati, Donatella, Ioannis Mylonakis, Giulio Bertoloni, Cristina Fiore, Alessandra Andrisani, Guido Ambrosini, and Decio Armanini. 2008. Genital tract infections and infertility. *European Journal of Obstetrics and Gynecology and Reproductive Biology* 140:3–11.

Peltzer, K. 2009. Health behavior and protective factors among school children in four African countries. *International Journal of Behavioral Medicine* 16(2):172–80.

Pettifor, Audrey E., Ariane van der Straten, Megan S. Dunbar, Stephen C. Shiboski, and Nancy S. Padian. 2004. Early age of first sex: A risk factor for HIV infection among women in Zimbabwe. *AIDS* 18:1435–42.

Phetla, G., J. Busza, J. R. Hargreaves, P. M. Pronyk, J. C. Kim, L. A. Morison, C. Watts, and J. D. H. Porter. 2008. They have opened our mouths: Increasing women's skills and motivation for sexual communication with young people in rural South Africa. *AIDS Education and Prevention* 20(6):504–18.

Pickering, H., M. Okongo, K. Bwanika, B. Nnalusiba, and J. Whitworth. 1997. Sexual behavior in a fishing community on Lake Victoria, Uganda. *Health Transition Review* 7:13–20.

Pickering, Helen, Jim Todd, J. Dunn, J. Pepin, and A. Wilkins. 1992. Prostitutes and their clients: A Gambian survey. *Social Science and Medicine* 34(1):75–88.

Pilcher, Christopher D., Hsiao Chuan Tien, Joseph J. Eron Jr., Pietro L. Vernazza, Szu-Yun Leu, Paul W. Stewart, Li-Ean Goh, and Myron S. Cohen, for the Quest Study and the Duke-UNC-Emory Acute HIV Consortium. 2004. Brief but efficient: Acute HIV infection and the sexual transmission of HIV. *Journal of Infectious Diseases* 189:1785–92.

Pinkerton, S. D., P. M. Layde, W. DiFranceisco, H. W. Chesson, and the NIMH Multisite Prevention Trial Group. 2003. All STDs are not created equal: An analysis of the differential effects of sexual behavior changes on different STDs. *International Journal of STD and AIDS* 14:320–28.

Plummer, M. L. Promoting abstinence, being faithful and condom use with young rural Africans: Findings from a large qualitative study within an intervention trial in Tanzania. Lanham, MD: Lexington Books, forthcoming.

Plummer, M. L., D. A. Ross, D. Wight, J. Changalucha, G. Mshana, J. Wamoyi, J. Todd et al. 2004. 'A bit more truthful': The validity of adolescent sexual behavior data collected in rural northern Tanzania using five methods. *Sexually Transmitted Infections* 80(Supplement 2):ii49–56.

Plummer, Mary L., D. Wight, J. Wamoyi, K. Nyalali, T. Ingall, G. Mshana, Z. S. Shigongo, A. I. N. Obasi, and D. A. Ross. 2007. Are schools a good setting for adolescent sexual health promotion in rural Africa? A qualitative assessment from Tanzania. *Health Education Research* 22(4):483–99.

Plummer, Mary L., Daniel Wight, David A. Ross, Rebecca Balira, Alessandra Anemona, Jim Todd, Zachayo Salamba et al. 2004. Asking semiliterate adolescents about sexual behavior: The validity of assisted self-completion questionnaire (ASCQ) data in rural Tanzania. *Tropical Medicine and International Health* 9:737–54.

Plummer, Mary L., Daniel Wight, Joyce Wamoyi, Gerry Mshana, Richard J. Hayes and David A. Ross. 2006. Farming with your hoe in a sack: Condom attitudes, access, and use in rural Tanzania. *Studies in Family Planning* 37(1):29–40.

Plummer, Mary L., Gerry Mshana, Joyce Wamoyi, Zachayo S. Shigongo, Richard J. Hayes, David A. Ross, and Daniel Wight. 2006. "The man who believed he had AIDS was cured": AIDS and sexually transmitted infection treatment-seeking behavior in rural Mwanza, Tanzania. *AIDS Care* 18(5):460–66.

Plummer, Mary L., Joyce Wamoyi, Kija Nyalali, Gerry Mshana, Zachayo S. Shigongo, David A. Ross, and Daniel Wight. 2008. Aborting and suspending pregnancy in rural Tanzania: An ethnography of young people's beliefs and practices. *Studies in Family Planning* 39(4):281–92.

Plummer, Mary L., Joyce Wamoyi, Zachayo S. Shigongo, Gerry Mshana, Angela I. N. Obasi, David A. Ross, and Daniel Wight. 2010. "Seek any means, and keep it your secret": Young women's attempts to control their reproduction through contraceptive and fertility practices in rural Tanzania. *Tanzania Journal of Health Research* (12)3:178–93.

Pool, R. 1997. Anthropological research on AIDS. In *HIV prevention and AIDS care in Africa: A district level approach*, ed. J. Ng'weshemi, J. T. Boerma, J. Bennett, and D. Schapink, 69–83. Amsterdam: Royal Tropical Institute.

Pool, R., A. Kamali, and J. A. G. Whitworth. 2006. Understanding sexual behavior change in rural southwest Uganda: A multi-method study. *AIDS Care* 18(5): 479–88.

Pool, R., and W. Geissler. 2005. *Medical anthropology*. Berkshire, England: Open University Press.

Pool, Robert, and Ndatulu Robert Washija. 2001. Traditional healers, STDs and infertility in northwest Tanzania. In *Women and infertility in sub-Saharan Africa*, ed. J. T. Boerma and Z. Mgalla, 241–55. Amsterdam: KIT.

Povinelli, Elizabeth A. 2006. *The empire of love: Toward a theory of intimacy, genealogy, and carnality*. Durham, USA: Duke University.

Price, Neil, and Kirstan Hawkins. 2002. Researching sexual and reproductive behavior: A peer ethnographic approach. *Social Science and Medicine* 55(8):1325–36.

Radcliffe-Brown, Alfred Reginald. 1950. Introduction. In *African systems of kinship and marriage*, ed. Alfred Reginald Radcliffe-Brown and Cyril Daryll Forde, 1–85. Oxford: Oxford University Press.

Rajani, Rakesh, and Mustafa Kudrati. 1996. The varieties of sexual experience of the street children of Mwanza. In *Learning about sexuality: A practical beginning*, ed. S. Zeidenstein and K. Moore, 301–23. New York: The Population Council.

Ramjee, Gita, and E. Gouws. 2002. The prevalence of HIV among truck drivers visiting sex workers in KwaZulu-Natal, South Africa. *Sexually Transmitted Diseases* 29:44–49.

Rasch, Vibeke, and Mathias A. Lyaruu. 2005. Unsafe abortion in Tanzania and the need for involving men in postabortion contraceptive counseling. *Studies in Family Planning* 36(4):301–10.

Rasch, Vibeke, Hamed Muhammad, Ernest Urassa, and Staffan Bergström. 2000. Self-reports of induced abortion: An empathetic setting can improve the quality of data. *American Journal of Public Health* 90(7):1141–44.

Rasch, Vibeke, Siriel Massawe, Fortunata Yambesi, and Staffan Bergstrom. 2004. Acceptance of contraceptives among women who had an unsafe abortion in Dar es Salaam. *Tropical Medicine and International Health* 9(3):399–405.

Reniers, Georges, and Rania Tfaily. 2008. Polygyny and HIV in Malawi. *Demographic Research* 19:1781–1800.

Reniers, Georges, and Susan Watkins. 2010. Polygyny and the spread of HIV in sub-Saharan Africa: A case of benign concurrency. *AIDS* 24:299–307.

Reniers, Georges. 2008. Marital strategies for regulating exposure to HIV. *Demography* 45(2):417–38.

Renju, J., and K. Nyalali. 2008. *Scaling up adolescent sexual health education in rural primary schools in Tanzania: Evaluation of teacher training 2005–2006.* Research report from the Tanzanian National Institute for Medical Research and the Liverpool School of Tropical Medicine. Downloaded on March 7, 2010 from www.memakwavijana.org.

Renne, Elisha P. 1997. *Changing patterns of child-spacing and abortion in a northern Nigerian town. Princeton University Office of Population Research Working Paper No. 97-1.* Downloaded on June 5, 2007 from http://opr.princeton.edu/papers/opr9701.pdf.

Research to Prevention. 2009. *Concurrent partnerships and HIV/AIDS in Tanzania: Evidence from the literature, June 2009.* Baltimore, Maryland: John Hopkins University Center for Communication Programs.

Robins, S. 2009. Foot soldiers of global health: Teaching and preaching AIDS science and modern medicine on the frontline. *Medical Anthropology* 28(1):81–107.

Rosenwein, Barbara H. 2002. Worrying about emotions in history. *The American Historical Review* 107(3):821–45.

Ross, David A., John Changalucha, Angela I. Obasi, Jim Todd, Mary L. Plummer, Bernadette Cleophas-Mazige, Alessandra Anemona et al. 2007. Biological and behavioral impact of an adolescent sexual health intervention in Tanzania: A community-randomized trial. *AIDS* 21(14):1943–55.

Roura, Maria, Joanna Busza, Alison Wringe, Doris Mbata, Mark Urassa, and Basia Zaba. 2009. Barriers to sustaining antiretroviral treatment in Kisesa, Tanzania: A follow-up study to understand attrition from the antiretroviral program. *AIDS Patient Care and STDs* 23(3):203–10.

Rushton, J. P., and A. Bogaert. 1989. Population differences in susceptibility to AIDS: An evolutionary analysis. *Social Science and Medicine* 28:1211–20.

Rutenberg, Naomi, and Susan Cotts Watkins. 1997. The buzz outside of clinics: Conversations and contraception in Nyanza Province, Kenya. *Studies in Family Planning* 28(4):290–307.

Rutherford, George W. 2008. Condoms in concentrated and generalized HIV epidemics. *Lancet* 372:275–76.

Rwebangira, M., and R. Liljestrom (eds). 1998. *Haraka haraka . . . Look before you leap: Youth at the crossroad of custom and modernity.* Uppsala: Nordic African Institute.

Rwebangire, Magdalena Kamugisha. 1994. What has the law got to do with it? In *Chelewa, chelewa: The dilemma of teenage girls*, ed. Zubeida Tumbo-Masabo and Rita Liljeström, 187–210. Sweden: Scandinavian Institute of African Studies.

Rweyemamu, Datius, and Minou Fuglesang. 2008. *Multiple and concurrent sexual relationships among youth in Tanzania; A research study commissioned by Femina HIP in preparation for a regional youth MCP campaign.* Dar es Salaam: Femina HIP.

Sambisa, William, and C. Shannon Stokes. 2006. Rural/urban residence, migration, HIV/AIDS, and safe sex practices among men in Zimbabwe. *Rural Sociology* 71(2):183–211.

Samuelsen, Helle. 2006. Love, lifestyles and the risk of AIDS: The moral worlds of young people in Bobo-Dioulasso, Burkina Faso. *Culture, Health and Sexuality* 8(3):211–24.

Sanders, Stephanie A., Brandon J. Hill, William L. Yarber, Cynthia A. Graham, Richard A. Crosby, and Robin R. Milhausen. 2010. Misclassification bias: Diversity in conceptualizations about having "had sex". *Sexual Health* 7(1):31–34.

Sayles, Jennifer N., Audrey Pettifor, Mitchell D. Wong, Catherine MacPhail, Sung-Jae Lee, Ellen Hendriksen, Helen V. Rees, and Thomas Coates. 2006. Factors associated with self-efficacy for condom use and sexual negotiation among South African youth. *Journal of Acquired Immune Deficiency Syndromes* 43:226–33.

Schapink, Dick, Japhet Ng'weshemi, Gabriel Mwaluko, and Venanmce Nyonyo. 2001. *The Bwana Kiko story: An interactive health education method to promote safe sexual behavior for controlling the spread of STD/HIV.* Amsterdam: KIT Publishers.

Schoepf, B. 1991. Sex, gender and society in Zaire. In *Sexual behavior and networking: Anthropological and socio-cultural studies on the transmission of HIV*, ed. T. Dyson, 353–75. Liege, Belgium: International Union for the Scientific Study of Population.

Schoepf, B. G. 1992a. Women at risk: Case studies from Zaire. In *The time of AIDS: Social analysis, theory and method*, ed. G. Herdt and S. Lindenbaum, 259–86. Newbury Park, CA: Sage.

Schoepf, B. G. 1992b. AIDS, sex and condoms: African healers and the reinvention of tradition in Zaire. *Medical Anthropology* 14:225–42.

Schomogyi, Mark, Anna Wald, and Lawrence Corey. 1998. Herpes Simplex Virus-2: An emerging disease? *Infectious Disease Clinics of North America* 12(1):47–61.

Schwandt, M., C. Morris, A. Ferguson, E. Ngugi, and S. Moses. 2006. Anal and dry sex in commercial sex work, and relation to risk for sexually transmitted infections and HIV in Meru, Kenya. *Sexually Transmitted Infections* 82:392–96.

Scorgie, Fiona, Busisiwe Kunene, Jennifer Smit, Ntsiki Manzini, Matthew Chersich, and Eleanor Preston-Whyte. 2009. In search of sexual pleasure and fidelity: Vaginal practices in kwaZulu-Natal, South Africa. *Culture, Health and Sexuality* 11(3)67–83.

Sedere, Upali M., Helima Mengele, and Teferi Kajela. 2008. *Evaluation of the Education Quality Improvement Through Pedagogy (EQUIP) Project in Shinyanga, Tanzania. Full report, Oxfam GB Programme Evaluation December 2008.* Downloaded from www.oxfam.org.uk/resources/evaluations/downloads/1208_p00048 _tanzania_pedagogy_education_exec.pdf on August 6, 2010.

Seeley, J., S. Malamba, A. Nunn, D. Mulder, J. Kengeya-Kayonde, and T. Barton. 1994. Socioeconomic status, gender, and risk of HIV-1 infection in a rural community in southwest Uganda. *Medical Anthropology Quarterly* 8(1):78–89.

Seeley, Janet, Stefan Dercon, and Tony Barnett. 2010. The effects of HIV/AIDS on rural communities in East Africa: A 20-year perspective. *Tropical Medicine and International Health* 15(3):329–35.

Selikow, Terry-Ann, Nazeema Ahmed, Alan J. Flisher, Catherine Mathews, and Wanjiru Mukoma. 2009. I am not "umqwayito": A qualitative study of peer pressure and sexual risk behavior among young adolescents in Cape Town, South Africa. *Scandinavian Journal of Public Health* 37(Supplement 2):107–12.

Setel, Philip W. 1999a. Comparative histories of sexually transmitted diseases and HIV/AIDS in Africa: An introduction. In *Histories of sexually transmitted diseases and HIV/AIDS in sub-Saharan Africa*, ed. Philip W. Setel, Milton Lewis, and Maryinez Lyons, 1–15. Westport, CT: Greenwood Press.

Setel, Philip W. 1999b. *A plague of paradoxes: AIDS, culture and demography in northern Tanzania.* Chicago: University of Chicago Press.

Sharma S. K., M. SaiRam, G. Ilavazhagan, K. Devendra, S. S. Shivaji, and W. Selvamurthy. 1996. Mechanism of action of NIM-76: A novel vaginal contraceptive from neem oil. *Contraception* 54:373–78.

Shelton, James D. 2007. Ten myths and one truth about generalized HIV epidemics. *Lancet* 370:1809–11.

Shuey, Dean A., Bernadette B. Babishangire, Samuel Omiat, and Henry Bagarukayo. 1999. Increased sexual abstinence among in-school adolescents as a result of school health education in Soroti district, Uganda. *Health Education Research* 14: 411–19.

Silberschmidt, Margrethe, and Vibeke Rasch. 2001. Adolescent girls, illegal abortions and "sugar daddies" in Dar es Salaam: Vulnerable victims and active social agents. *Social Science and Medicine* 52:1815–26.

Singh, Susheela, Deirdre Wulf, Renee Samara, and Yvette P. Cuca. 2000. Gender differences in the timing of first intercourse: Data from 14 countries. *International Family Planning Perspectives* 26(1):21–28 and 43.

Singh, Susheela. 2006. Hospital admissions resulting from unsafe abortion: Estimates from 13 developing countries. *Lancet* 368:1887–92.

Smith, Daniel Jordan. 2009. Managing men, marriage, and modern love: Women's perspectives on intimacy and male infidelity in southeastern Nigeria. In *Love in Africa*, ed. Jennifer Cole and Lynn M. Thomas, 157–80. Chicago: University of Chicago Press.

Smith, Jennifer S., Stephen Moses, Michael G. Hudgens, Corette B. Parker, Kawango
    Agot, Ian Maclean, Jeckoniah O. Ndinya-Achola, Peter J. F. Snijders, Chris J. L.
    M. Meijer, and Robert C. Bailey. 2010. Increased risk of HIV acquisition among
    Kenyan men with Human Papillomavirus infection. *Journal of Infectious Diseases*
    201(11):1677–85.
Smith, Peter G., and Richard H. Morrow. 1996. *Field trials of health interventions:*
    A Toolbox. Oxford: Macmillan.
Sobngwi-Tambekou, Joelle, Dirk Taljaard, Pascale Lissouba, Kevin Zarca, Adrian
    Puren, Emmanuel Lagarde, and Bertran Auvert. 2009. Effect of HSV-2 serostatus
    on acquisition of HIV by young men: Results of a longitudinal study in Orange
    Farm, South Africa. *Journal of Infectious Diseases* 199(7):958–64.
Somi, G., M. Matee, C. L. Makene, J. Van Den Hombergh, B. Kilama, K. I. Ya-
    hyamalima, P. Masako et al. 2009. Three years of HIV/AIDS care and treatment
    services in Tanzania: Achievements and challenges. *Tanzania Journal of Health*
    Research 11(3):136–43.
Sommer, Marni. 2009. Ideologies of sexuality, menstruation and risk: Girls' experi-
    ences of puberty and schooling in northern Tanzania. *Culture Health and Sexuality*
    11(4):383–98.
Stadler, Jonathan. 2003. Rumor, gossip and blame: Implications for HIV/AIDS
    prevention in the South African lowveld. *AIDS Education and Prevention* 15(4):
    357–68.
Stambach, Amy. 2003. *Kutoa mimba*: Debates about school girl abortion in Ma-
    chame, Tanzania. In *The sociocultural and political aspects of abortion: Global*
    perspectives, ed. Alaka Malwade Basu, 79–102. Western, CT: Praeger.
Steinberg, Jonny. 2009. *Three letter plague. A young man's journey through a great*
    epidemic. London: Vintage.
Stroeken, Koen. 2001. Defying the gaze: *Exodelics* for the bewitched in Sukumaland
    and beyond. *Dialectical Anthropology* 26:285–309.
Stroeken, Koen. 2006. 'Stalking the stalker': A Chwezi initiation into spirit pos-
    session and experiential structure. *Journal of the Royal Anthropological Institute*
    (N.S.) 12:785–802.
Stycos, J. Mayone. 2000. Sample surveys for social science in underdeveloped areas.
    In *Social research in developing countries: Surveys and censuses in the Third*
    World, ed. Martin Bulmer and Donald P. Warwick, 53–64. London: University
    College London.
Sundby, Johanne, Reuben Mboge, and Sheriff Sonko. 1998. Infertility in the Gambia:
    Frequency and health care seeking. *Social Science and Medicine* 46(7):891–99.
Swidler, A., and S. Watkins. 2007. Ties of dependence: AIDS and transactional sex
    in rural Malawi. *Studies in Family Planning* 38(3):147–62.
Talwar, G. P., S. Shah, S. Mukherjee, and R. Chabra. 1997. Induced termination of
    pregnancy by purified extracts of *Azadirachta indica* (Neem): Mechanisms in-
    volved. *American Journal of Reproductive Immunology* 37(6):485–91.
Tamale, Sylvia. 2006. Eroticism, sensuality, and 'women's secrets' among the
    Baganda. *IDS Bulletin* 37(5):89–97.
Tanner, R. E. S. 1955a. Maturity and marriage among the northern Basukuma of
    Tanganyika. *African Studies* 14(3):123–33.

Tanner, R. E. S. 1955b. The sexual mores of the Basukuma, Tanganyika. *International Journal of Sexology* 8(4):238–41.

Tanner, R. E. S. 1956a. An introduction to the northern Basukuma's idea of the Supreme Being. *Anthropological Quarterly* 29(2):45–56.

Tanner, R. E. S. 1956b. The sorcerer in northern Sukumaland, Tanganyika. *Southwestern Journal of Anthropology* 12(4):437–43.

Tanner, R. E. S. 1957. The magician in northern Sukumaland, Tanganyika. *Southwestern Journal of Anthropology* 13(4):344–51.

Tanner, R. E. S. 1959. The spirits of the dead: An introduction to the ancestor worship of the Sukuma of Tanganyika. *Anthropological Quarterly* 32(2):108–24.

Tanzania Commission for AIDS (TACAIDS), National Bureau of Statistics (NBS), and ORC Macro. 2005. *Tanzania HIV/AIDS Indicator Survey 2003–04.* Calverton, MD: TACAIDS, NBS, and ORC Macro.

Tanzania Commission for AIDS (TACAIDS), Zanzibar AIDS Commission (ZAC), National Bureau of Statistics (NBS), Office of Chief Government Statistician (OCGS), and Macro International Inc. 2008. *HIV/AIDS and Malaria Indicator Survey 2007–08.* Dar es Salaam, Tanzania: TACAIDS, ZAC, NBS, OCGS, and Macro International Inc.

Tassiopoulos, Katherine K., George R. Seage, Noel E. Sam, Trong T. H. Ao, Elisante J. Masenga, Michael D. Hughes, and Saidi H. Kapiga. 2006. Sexual behavior, psychosocial and knowledge differences between consistent, inconsistent and nonusers of condoms: A study of female bar and hotel workers in Moshi, Tanzania. *AIDS and Behavior* 10:405–13.

Tawfik, L., and S. C. Watkins. 2007. Sex in Geneva, sex in Lilongwe, and sex in Balaka. *Social Science and Medicine*, 64:1090–101.

Taylor, Christopher C. 1990. Condoms and cosmology: The 'fractal' person and sexual risk in Rwanda. *Social Science and Medicine* 31(9):1023–28.

Terceira, Nicola, Simon Gregson, Basia Zaba, and Peter R. Mason. 2003. The contribution of HIV to fertility decline in rural Zimbabwe, 1985–2000. *Population Studies* 57(2):149–64.

Thomas, Lynn M., and Jennifer Cole. 2009. Thinking through love in Africa. In *Love in Africa*, ed. Jennifer Cole and Lynn M. Thomas, 1–30. Chicago: University of Chicago Press.

Thomsen, S., M. Stalker, and C. Toroitich-Ruto. 2004. Fifty ways to leave your rubber: How men in Mombasa rationalize unsafe sex. *Sexually Transmitted Infections* 80(6):430–34.

Tobian, Aaron A. R., David Serwadda, Thomas C. Quinn, Godfrey Kigozi, Patti E. Gravitt, Oliver Laeyendecker, Blake Charvat, et al. 2009. Male circumcision for the prevention of HSV-2 and HPV infections and syphilis. *New England Journal of Medicine* 360(13):1298–309.

Todd, J., J. Changalucha, D. A. Ross, F. Mosha, A. I. N. Obasi, M. Plummer, R. Balira, H. Grosskurth, D. C. W. Mabey, and R. Hayes. 2004. The sexual health of pupils in years 4 to 6 of primary schools in rural Tanzania. *Sexually Transmitted Infections* 80:35–42.

Todd, Jim, and Longin Barongo. 1997. Epidemiological methods. In *HIV prevention and AIDS care in Africa: A district level approach,* ed. Japhet Ng'weshemi, Ties

Boerma, John Bennett, and Dick Schapink, 51–69. Amsterdam: Royal Tropical Institute.

Topan, Farouk. 2008. Tanzania: The development of Swahili as a national and official language. In *Language and national identity in Africa*, ed. Andrew Simpson, 252–66. New York: Oxford University Press.

Townsend, P. 1979. *Poverty in the United Kingdom*. Suffolk: Allen Lane.

Towse, Peter, David Kent, Funja Osaki, and Noah Kirua. 2002. Nongraduate teacher recruitment and retention: Some factors affecting teacher effectiveness in Tanzania. *Teaching and Teacher Education* 18:637–52.

Tschann, J. M., N. E. Adler, S. G. Millstein, J. E. Gurvey, and J. M Ellen. 2002. Relative power between sexual partners and condom use among adolescents. *Journal of Adolescent Health* 31(1):17–25.

Turner, Abigail Norris, Alana E. De Kock, Amy Meehan-Ritter, Kelly Blanchard, Mohlatlego H. Sebola, Anwar A. Hoosen, Nicol Coetzee, and Charlotte Ellertson. 2009. Many vaginal microbicide trial participants acknowledged they had misreported sensitive sexual behavior in face-to-face interviews. *Journal of Clinical Epidemiology* 62(7):759–65.

Twa-Twa, Jeremiahs, Immaculate Nakanaabi, and Deogratius Sekimpi. 1997. Underlying factors in female sexual partner instability in Kampala. *Health Transition Review* 7(Supplement):83–88.

Uiso, F. C., E. J. Kayombo, Z. H. Mbwambo, Y. Mgonda, R. L. A. Mahunnah, and M. J. Moshi. 2006. Traditional healer's knowledge and implications to the management and control of HIV/AIDS in Arusha, Tanzania. *Tanzania Health Research Bulletin* 8(2):95–100.

UNAIDS and WHO. 2006. *2006 report on the global AIDS epidemic: A UNAIDS 10th anniversary special edition*. Geneva: UNAIDS and WHO.

UNAIDS and WHO. 2009. *AIDS epidemic update December 2009*. Geneva: UNAIDS and WHO.

UNAIDS. 2000. *Collaboration with traditional healers in HIV/AIDS prevention and care in sub-Saharan Africa*. Geneva: UNAIDS.

UNAIDS. 2002. AIDS care and prevention: An integrated model in the United Republic of Tanzania. In *Ancient remedies, new disease: Involving traditional healers in increasing access to AIDS care and prevention in East Africa*. Geneva: UNAIDS.

UNAIDS. 2008. *2008 Report on the global AIDS epidemic*. Geneva: UNAIDS.

UNAIDS. 2010. *Young people are leading the HIV prevention revolution*. Geneva: UNAIDS.

Undie, Chi-Chi, and Kabwe Benaya. 2006. The state of knowledge on sexuality in sub-Saharan Africa: A synthesis of literature. *Jenda: A Journal of Culture and African Women Studies* (8):1–33.

Undie, Chi-Chi, Joanna Crichton, and Eliya Zulu. 2007. Metaphors we love by: Conceptualizations of sex among young people in Malawi. *African Journal of Reproductive Health* 11(3):221–35.

UNICEF. 1998. *The state of the world's children*. New York: Oxford University Press.

United Nations. 2002. *Abortion policies: A global review.* New York: United Nations.

United Nations. 2004. *World population to 2300 [Publication no. ST/ESA/SER.A/236].* New York: United Nations.

United Nations. 2007. *World urbanization prospects: The 2006 revision: Executive Summary [Publication no. ST/ESA/SER.A/261/ES].* New York: United Nations.

United Republic of Tanzania. 1997. *Mwanza Region socioeconomic profile: Joint publication of the Planning Commission and the Regional Commissioner's Office.* Dar es Salaam: United Republic of Tanzania.

United Republic of Tanzania. 1999. *Education for all: The 2000 assessment. National report, second draft.* Dar es Salaam: United Republic of Tanzania.

United Republic of Tanzania. 2002. *Guidelines for implementing HIV/AIDS/STDs and life skills education in schools and teachers' colleges: January 2002, Version 2.0.* Dar es Salaam: United Republic of Tanzania.

United Republic of Tanzania. 2003. *Basic statistics in education 2003: Regional data.* Dar es Salaam: United Republic of Tanzania.

Van den Borne, Francine. 2007. Using mystery clients to assess condom negotiation in Malawi: Some ethical concerns. *Studies in Family Planning* 38(4):322–30.

van der Geest, S. 1987. Self-care and the informal sale of drugs in South Cameroon. *Social Science and Medicine* 25:293–305.

Van Dyk, Alta C. 2008. Perspectives of South African school children on HIV/AIDS, and the implications for education programs *African Journal of AIDS Research* 7(1):79–93.

Van Eeuwijk, B. Obrist, and S. Mlangwa S. 1997. Competing ideologies: Adolescence, knowledge and silence in Dar es Salaam. In *Power, reproduction and gender: The inter-generational transfer of knowledge,* ed. Wendy Harcourt, 35–57. London: Zed Books.

Van Reeuwijk, Miranda. 2010. *Because of temptations: Children, sex and HIV/AIDS in Tanzania.* Diemen: AMB Publishers.

Vance, Carol. 1991. Anthropology rediscovers sexuality: A theoretical comment. *Social Science and Medicine* 33(8):875–84.

Vanwesenbeeck, I., G. van Zessen, R. Ingham, E. Jaramazovic, and D. Stevens. 1999. Factors and processes in heterosexual competence and risk: An integrated review of the evidence. *Psychology and Health* 14(1):25–50.

Varkevisser, Corlien M. 1973. *Socialization in a changing society: Sukuma childhood in rural and urban Mwanza, Tanzania.* The Hague: Centre for the Study of Education in Changing Societies.

Vaughan, Meghan. 2009. *The history of romantic love in sub-Saharan Africa.* Presented as part of the Raleigh Lecture on History series at the British Academy, 26 February 2009. Podcast downloaded on February 5, 2010 from www.britac.ac.uk/events/archive/raleigh-podcast.cfm.

Vissers, Debby C. J., Helene A. C. M. Voeten, Mark Urassa, Raphael Isingo, Milalu Ndege, Yusufu Kumogola, Gabriel Mwaluko, Basia Zaba, Sake J. De Vlas, and J. Dik F. Habbema. 2008. Separation of spouses due to travel and living apart raises HIV risk in Tanzanian couples. *Sexually Transmitted Diseases* 35(8):714–20.

Voétèn, Helene A. C. M., Omar B. Egesah, and J. Dik F. Habbema. 2004. Sexual behavior is more risky in rural than in urban areas among young women in Nyanza Province, Kenya. *Sexually Transmitted Diseases* 31(8):481–87.

Vos, T. 1994. Attitudes to sex and sexual behavior in rural Matabeleland, Zimbabwe. *AIDS Care* 6(2):193–203.

Waako, Paul J., Richard Odoi-adome, Celestino Obua, Erisa Owino, Winnie Tumwikirize, Jasper Ogwal-okeng, Willy W. Anokbonggo, Lloyd Matowe, and Onesky Aupont. 2009. Existing capacity to manage pharmaceuticals and related commodities in East Africa: An assessment with specific reference to antiretroviral therapy. *Human Resources for Health* 7:21.

Wald, A., and K. Link. 2002. Risk of human immunodeficiency virus infection in herpes simplex virus type 2-seropositive persons: A meta-analysis. *Journal of Infectious Diseases* 185:45–52.

Walker, A. Sarah, Veronica Mulenga, Frederick Sinyinza, Kennedy Lishimpi, Andrew Nunn, Chifumbe Chintu, Diana M. Gibb, and the CHAP Trial Team. 2006. Determinants of survival without antiretroviral therapy after infancy in HIV-1-infected Zambian children in the CHAP trial. *Journal of Acquired Immune Deficiency Syndromes* 42:637–45.

Wamoyi, Joyce M., Danny Wight, Mary Plummer, Gerry Hillary Mshana, and David Ross. 2010. Transactional sex amongst young people in rural northern Tanzania: An ethnography of young women's motivations and negotiation. *Reproductive Health* 7:2.

Wamoyi, Joyce, Angela Fenwick, Mark Urassa, Basia Zaba, and William Stones. 2010. "Women's bodies are shops": Beliefs about transactional sex and implications for understanding gender power and HIV prevention in Tanzania. *Archives of Sexual Behavior* DOI 10.1007/s10508-010-9646-8.

Warenius, Linnea, Karen Pettersson, Eva Nissen, Bengt Hojer, Petronella Chishimba and Elisabeth Faxelid. 2007. Vulnerability and sexual and reproductive health among Zambian secondary school students. *Culture, Health and Sexuality* 9(5):533–44.

Watkins, Susan Cotts, and Anne Swidler. 2006. *Hearsay ethnography: Capturing culture in action. California Center for Population Research On-Line Working Paper Series (University of California, Los Angeles), Paper CCPR-007-06.* Downloaded on December 5, 2007 from http://repositories.cdlib.org/ccpr/olwp/CCPR-007-06.

Wawer, Maria J., Ronald H. Gray, Nelson K. Sewankambo, David Serwadda, Xian bin Li, Oliver Laeyendecker, Noah Kiwanuka et al. 2005. Rates of HIV-1 transmission per coital act, by stage of HIV-1 infection, in Rakai, Uganda. *Journal of Infectious Diseases* 191:1403–9.

Weinreb, Alexander A. 2006. The limitations of stranger-interviewers in rural Kenya. *American Sociological Review* 71:1014–39.

Weiser, Sheri, William Wolfe, David Bangsberg, Ibou Thior, Peter Gilbert, Joseph Makhema, Poloko Kebaabetswe et al. 2003. Barriers to antiretroviral adherence for patients living with HIV infection and AIDS in Botswana. *Journal of Acquired Immune Deficiency Syndromes* 34(3):281–88.

Weiss, Eric A. 1998. *A comprehensive guide to wilderness and travel medicine, 2nd edition.* USA: Adventure Medical Kits.

Weiss, H. A., S. L. Thomas, S. K. Munabi, and R. J. Hayes. 2006. Male circumcision and risk of syphilis, chancroid, and genital herpes: A systematic review and meta-analysis. *Sexually Transmitted Infections* 82(2):101–9.

Weiss, Helen A., Mary L. Plummer, John Changalucha, Gerry Mshana, Zachayo S. Shigongo, Jim Todd, Daniel Wight, Richard J. Hayes, and David A. Ross. 2008. Circumcision among adolescent boys in rural northwestern Tanzania. *Tropical Medicine and International Health* 13(8):1054–61.

Werner, David, Carol Thuman, and Jane Maxwell. 1992. *Where there is no doctor*. Berkeley, CA: Hesperian.

Westercamp, N., and R. C. Bailey. 2006. Acceptability of male circumcision for prevention of HIV/AIDS in sub-Saharan Africa: A review. *AIDS and Behavior* 11:341–55.

Westhoff, Carolyn. 2003. Depot-medroxyprogesterone acetate injection (Depo-Provera): A highly effective contraceptive option with proven long-term safety. *Contraception* 68:75–87.

WHO and UNAIDS. 2007. *New data on male circumcision and HIV prevention: Policy and programme implications: Conclusions and recommendations*. Geneva: UNAIDS.

WHO. 1997. *Promoting health through schools: Report of a WHO Expert Committee on Comprehensive School Health Education and Promotion*. Geneva: WHO.

WHO. 2001. *Global prevalence and incidence of selected curable sexually transmitted infections: Overview and estimates. WHO/CDS/CSR/EDC/2001.10*. Geneva: WHO.

WHO. 2003. *Skills for health: Skills-based health education including life skills: An important component of a child-friendly/health-promoting school. Information Series on School Health, Document 9*. Geneva: WHO.

WHO. 2004. *Unsafe abortion: Global and regional estimates of incidence of unsafe abortion and associated mortality in 2000*. Geneva: WHO.

WHO. 2007. *Helping parents in developing countries improve adolescents' health*. Geneva: WHO.

Wight, Daniel, and Marion Henderson. 2004. The diversity of young people's sexual behavior. In *Young people and sexual health: Social, political and individual contexts*, ed. Mary Duffy and Elizabeth Burtney, 15–33. London: Palgrave.

Wight, Daniel, Mary L. Plummer, Gerry Mshana, Joyce Wamoyi, Zachayo S. Shigongo, and David A. Ross. 2006. Contradictory sexual norms and expectations for young people in rural northern Tanzania. *Social Science and Medicine* 62:987–97.

Wijsen, Frans, and Ralph Tanner. 2002. *"I am just a Sukuma": Globalization and identity construction in northwest Tanzania*. Amsterdam: Rodopi.

Williamson, Lisa M., Alison Parkes, Daniel Wight, Mark Petticrew, and Graham J. Hart. 2009. Limits to modern contraceptive use among women in developing countries: A systematic review of qualitative research. *Reproductive Health* 6:3.

Witte, Frans, Tijs Goldscmidt, Jan Wanink, Martien van Oijen, Kees Goudswaard, Els Witte-Maas and Niels Bouton. 1992. The destruction of an endemic species flock: Quantitative data on the decline of the haplochromine cichlids of Lake Victoria. *Environmental Biology of Fishes* 34:1–28.

Wood, Kate, and Rachel Jewkes. 2006. Blood blockages and scolding nurses: Barriers to adolescent contraceptive use in South Africa. *Reproductive Health Matters* 14(27):109–18.

Woodsong, Cynthia, and Patty Alleman. 2008. Sexual pleasure, gender power and microbicide acceptability in Zimbabwe and Malawi. *AIDS Education and Prevention* 20(2):171–87.

World Bank. 2004. *User fees in primary education.* Washington DC: The World Bank.

World Bank. 2005. *World development report 2006: Equity and development.* Washington DC: World Bank.

World Bank. 2006. *World development report 2007: Development and the next generation.* Washington DC: World Bank.

Yamba, C. B. 1997. Cosmologies in turmoil: Witchfinding and AIDS in Chiawa, Zambia. *Africa* 67:200–23.

Żaba, B., R. Isingo, A. Wringe, M. Marston, E. Slaymaker, and M. Urassa. 2009. Influence of timing of sexual debut and first marriage on sexual behavior in later life: Findings from four survey rounds in the Kisesa cohort in northern Tanzania. *Sexually Transmitted Infections* 85(Supplement 1):i20–26.

Zablotska I. B., R. H. Gray, D. Serwadda, F. Nalugoda, G. Kigozi, N. Sewankambo, T. Lutalo, F. W. Mangen, and M. Wawer. 2006. Alcohol use before sex and HIV acquisition: A longitudinal study in Rakai, Uganda. *AIDS* 20(8):1191–96.

Zachariah, R., W. Nkhoma, A. D. Harries, V. Arendt, A. Chantulo, M. P. Spielmann, M. P. Mbereko, and L. Buhendwa. 2002. Health seeking and sexual behavior in patients with sexually transmitted infections: The importance of traditional healers in Thyolo, Malawi. *Sexually Transmitted Infections* 78:127–29.

Index

About the Authors

Mary Louisa Plummer is a consultant to the UK Medical Research Council's Social and Public Health Sciences Unit. Her academic background is in social sciences, biology, and languages (Swahili, Mandarin Chinese, and German). She has worked in HIV education, curriculum development, and program evaluation since 1988. Her HIV-related work in Tanzania began with the development and testing of a secondary school curriculum in urban Mwanza in 1994. This was followed by process evaluations of two rural Mwanza primary school programs in 1997–1998. From 1999–2009, Mary was employed by the London School of Hygiene and Tropical Medicine, UK, first as a research fellow and then as a lecturer. From 1999–2002, she was also the Social Science Coordinator for the *MEMA kwa Vijana* adolescent sexual health trial in Mwanza. In that capacity she was responsible for co-designing and managing quantitative and qualitative social science research, including the HALIRA Project that is the basis for this book. Mary has a PhD in comparative social and natural science methods (2004) and she is a British Academy postdoctoral fellow (2005–2008). She lives in Dar es Salaam, Tanzania with her husband and three children.

Daniel Wight heads the Sexual Health and Families Program at the UK Medical Research Council's Social and Public Health Sciences Unit in Glasgow, Scotland. He trained as a social anthropologist, conducting a participant observation community study in Scotland. Subsequently he conducted qualitative research on young men's sexual behavior in Glasgow and went on to lead the development of a theoretically based, teacher-delivered sex education program (SHARE), and its process and impact evaluation in twenty-five schools. His involvement in African research began in Uganda in 1992. He started collaborating with the London School of Hygiene and Tropical Medicine and the Tanzanian National Institute for Medical Research in Mwanza in 1997, and led the design and supervision of the HALIRA Project to accompany the *MEMA kwa Vijana* trial. He is currently involved in the development of a community-based sexual health program in Tanzania. Daniel's research interests include young people's lifestyles, parent-child relationships, perceptions of risk, the influence of the media, developing research capacity in Africa and the development and evaluation of behavioral interventions, both in Britain and sub-Saharan Africa.